PHARMATECTURE™

Minimizing Medications To Maximize Results

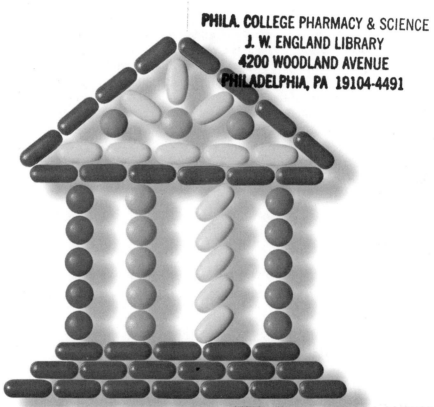

by

GIDEON BOSKER, MD FACEP

Pharmatecture™: Minimizing Medications To Maximize Results

Copyright 1996 by Facts and Comparisons, A Wolters Kluwer Company.

Trademarks by Gideon Bosker, MD

All rights reserved. No part of this publication may be reproduced or transmitted in any form or by any means, electronic or mechanical, including photocopy, recording, stored in a data base or any information storage or retrieval system or put into a computer, without prior permission in writing from Facts and Comparisons, the publisher.

ISBN 0-932686-64-8

Printed in the United States of America

The information contained in this publication is intended to supplement the knowledge of health care professionals regarding drug information. This information is advisory only and is not intended to replace sound clinical judgment or individualized patient care in the delivery of health care services. The views expressed in this text are the author's and do not necessarily represent those of Facts and Comparisons. Facts and Comparisons disclaims all warranties, whether expressed or implied, including any warranty as to the quality, accuracy or suitability of this information for any particular purpose.

Published by
Facts and Comparisons
111 West Port Plaza, Suite 300
St. Louis, Missouri 63146-3098
314/878-2515
Toll free customer service 800/223-0554

Acknowledgements

This book has been many years in the making and its completion has required the talents, insights, recommendations, and counsel of many distinguished professionals who have made a major impact in the area of drug therapy and clinical pharmacology. I would first like to thank Sue Sewester, President of Facts & Comparisons, who had the vision to recognize the need for publishing a hands-on, therapeutics-oriented resource that would synthesize clinical, pharmacoeconomic, and patient considerations into a practical, drug prescribing system. Her pivotal role in launching the project and marshalling the appropriate resources is to be commended.

No project of this kind comes to completion without a trusted and proven retinue of pharmacological consultants and advisors. In this regard, I would like to gratefully acknowledge the invaluable insights, meticulous review, and strategic guidance of Bernie R. Olin, PharmD, Editor-in-Chief of Facts and Comparisons. In his quiet and perspicacious manner, Dr. Olin was kind enough to apply his lifelong experience in the field of clinical pharmacology to every phase of this project. I sincerely appreciate his mid-course manuscript corrections, which not only assured the accuracy of drug-related information, but substantially enhanced the book's usefulness in the clinical and pharmacy setting.

I am especially gratified to note that Dr. Olin's recommendations were complimented by the careful, insightful reviews of the distinguished clinical pharmacists Michael T. Reed, PharmD and David Tatro, PharmD. Drs. Reed's and Tatro's extensive experience in the fields of psychopharmacology, cardiovascular drug therapy, drug information, and drug interactions generated a significant body of pharmacotherapeutic pearls, strategies, and suggestions that were incorporated into the final manuscript. Their intelligent, experienced commentaries regarding drug therapy dramatically improved the final product, and are gratefully acknowledged.

The developmental editor for a project of this scope is faced with the impossible task of mixing, monitoring, and matching manuscript materials, marketing strategies, and graphic designers with personalities and deadlines in order to achieve a seamless and elegant end-result. Accomplishing this Herculean task requires a unique, highly committed individual with the intelligence and vision to make the whole equal to something that is much greater than the sum of its parts. With this in mind, it is with great respect and admiration that I acknowledge the invaluable assistance of JoAnn Amore, my developmental editor, who, from the inception of this project had all the right stuff. Her unique resources in the subjective arenas of author encouragement, cajoling, and personality management were perfectly balanced by her state-of-the-art skills in the area of book design, manuscript production, and project development. Her collaboration, insights, and recommendations are sincerely appreciated and it has been a pleasure and honor to have her as the project manager. My thanks also go to Ingrid Reaves, who admirably assisted Ms. Amore in maintaining manuscript flow and communication.

The marketing and sales department at Facts & Comparisons provided invaluable information as to how this book might best reach a wide audience of physicians, pharmacists, and other prescribers. For their wise counsel in this area, I would like to thank Barb Wright, Director of Marketing, and Brad Strothkamp, Marketing Specialist, both of whom provided useful suggestions that helped me to focus on strategies that would help this book reach those prescribers who might benefit most from this material.

There is a critical point in time when a book manuscript takes the fragile leap from a "work in progress" to a full-fledged, etched-in-stone manuscript worthy of publication. This hands-on process of weaving together diverse visual and graphic elements, text inserts, reviewers' commentaries, and author-generated changes to create a confluent manuscript requires intelligence, diligence, and a commitment to excellence. These are the qualities that best describe Cathy Reilly, the book's production editor. I would like to thank Ms. Reilly for her superior editorial skills, which not only played a pivotal role in providing quality assurance, but were instrumental in giving the manuscript its final layer of polish.

Gideon Bosker, MD FACEP

Table of Contents

Preface

In the world of clinical medicine, experience is frequently the best guide. After more than 15 years of evaluating and treating patients who were suffering from the consequences of excessive, inappropriate, or suboptimal drug prescribing, I felt there was a need for a source of practical information that would present a systematic approach for constructing safe and cost-effective drug regimens for the outpatient setting. Against the backdrop of mounting cost-containment pressures that required prescribers to accomplish more with less, this approach would have to address real world issues that balanced institutional needs with those of individual patients and their families. As this drug prescribing system evolved, it became clear to me that its primary objective was to direct physicians and pharmacists toward prescribing approaches that would minimize medications in order to maximize clinical results.

With these issues in clear focus, this book is intended as a guide for all prescribers—physicians, pharmacists, nurse practitioners, physician assistants—who are faced with the daily challenge of selecting drugs that will meet therapeutic objectives without adversely affecting quality of life. In particular, the strategies in this book are consistent with a new mission statement for choosing medications that encompass *all* of the factors that enter into the equation for drug selection. These considerations include: cost, side effects, compliance, quality assurance, and risk management issues such as drug-drug and drug-disease interactions, smartness and productivity levels of medications, regimen durability, dose stability, duration of therapy, and the relative noise levels of drugs vs the noise levels of the disease against which they are directed.

If, based on the prescribing principles contained in this book, prescribers can improve therapeutic outcomes while maintaining quality-of-life for their patients, Pharmatecture™ will have achieved its purpose.

Gideon Bosker, MD FACEP

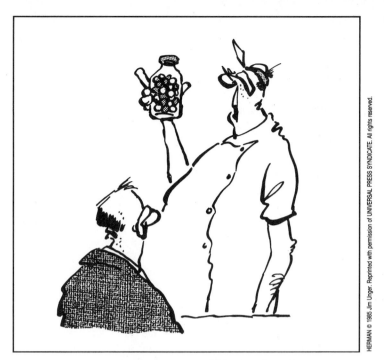

"I'm not sure what these are, but take them for a couple of weeks and let me know how you feel."

Introduction

Better living through pharmacology has become a way of life. When appropriately used and wisely combined, drugs are fundamental to optimizing clinical outcome and maintaining good health. Appropriately prescribed medications keep people alive. They sometimes cure fatal diseases. They make it possible for people to lead more productive, active, pain-free lives.

Stated simply, drugs are some of the most ingenious biomolecular solutions ever devised. That is the good news. The bad news is that a wide array of pharmacological options are available for human use, complicating choices for physicians, and therefore, increasing the risk of polypharmacy and drug interactions.

In light of the importance of drug therapy in clinical disease, constructing safe, cost-effective drug regimens, especially for chronic conditions managed in the outpatient setting, is one of the most important clinical challenges facing health care providers. [1,2,3,4] It should be emphasized that attitudes toward outpatient drug therapy have changed dramatically over the past decade.[5,6,7,8] The mounting pressures of cost containment in health care, the emergence of public policy mandates encouraging out-of-hospital management of both acute and chronic diseases, the financial and clinical hazards associated with polypharmacy, and the introduction of increasingly potent oral agents are just some of the factors inducing physicians and formulary managers to develop innovative pharmaco-therapeutic strategies.[7,9,10,11]

In this regard, it should be stressed that the whole issue of drug prescribing is more than just a day-to-day, patient-to-patient clinical activity. It is a public policy issue. There will be increasing pressure during the next decade and beyond to use drugs in the most cost effective manner possible. To achieve these public policy goals—most are clearly aimed at containment of health care expenditures—a new discipline, pharmacoeconomics, has evolved to focus attention on and evaluate total outcome costs associated with different pharmacotherapeutic interventions. In an age characterized by vigilant cost management in health care, the day may come when pharmacists and physicians are restricted in the number of different prescription ingredients permitted for patients. Healthcare maintenance organizations (HMOs), in an attempt to curb drug costs, are likely to introduce capitated pharmacological maintenance programs in which predetermined dollar amounts will be allotted for patients with various medical disorders. For example, depending on the clinical disorder, insurance companies, managed care networks, and HMOs will allocate, let's say, $280 per year for drug treatment of a patient with hypertension, $440 per year to manage the patient with coronary artery disease, $440 to manage the individual with major depression, $580 to manage diabetes mellitus, and so on.

Operating under these stringent fiscal group rules, pharmacists and physicians will be free to choose whatever drugs they please, but the annual drug expenditures will have to conform to the capitated limits established by third-party, government-funded, or HMO payor organizations. This new world order in clinical pharmacotherapeutics has made "necessity the mother of invention" when it comes to drug prescribing and, in turn, is fueling the development of new approaches, such as Pharmatecture™, to guide long-term drug regimen construction.[12,13,14]

Good News, Bad News

Perceptions also are changing about the relative risks and benefits of drug therapy.[15,16,17,18,19] Although clinicians may think of coronary angiograms and surgical interventions as invasive procedures, the fact is, prescribing a drug has the potential for being one of the most invasive acts in which a physician or consulting pharmacists can participate. When used in a systematic, rational manner, drugs have the capacity to reduce morbidity, improve or relieve symptoms, enhance the quality of life, and prolong survival. But there also are other, more problematic aspects to long-term pharmacologic intervention—side effects, financial hardship, and the potential for quality-of-life impairment.

Clinical studies demonstrate that the majority of drugs used in the outpatient environment have the potential for producing adverse effects, including subtle impairments in cognitive, sexual, sleep, and emotional function.[1,12,20] I am reminded of the patient who, during an office visit with his physician, explained, "I feel a lot better since I ran out of those pills you gave me." If a patient takes regular medication for a chronic condition, but endures negative side effects, then something is wrong. Consequently, in the case of many chronic diseases managed in the ambulatory environment, committing a patient to a medication for 5, 10, or 15 years can be characterized as an invasive act, carrying with it all the attendant responsibilities of risk-to-benefit analyses, clinical vigilance, the need for meticulous follow-up, and continuous reevaluation of the need for medication.

Increasingly, how patients *feel* while taking their medications, to what extent a drug preserves quality-of-life, and its negative side effects have become just as important as whether or not a particular medication gets the job done. Put another way, "pill-wise, patient-foolish" approaches to drug therapy no longer are acceptable. More and more, the selection of a drug depends as much on its efficacy as on its ability to maintain the patient's functional status with minimal side effects.

To be sure, the growing number of pharmacotherapeutic choices allows physicians to treat patients more safely, rapidly, and effectively than ever before. Progress, however, also has pitfalls. With increased drug use comes the potential for drug interactions. For example, many drugs that function well in *isolation* of other agents can induce drug interactions when *combined* with other medications. With the dramatic expansion of drug classes and a growing menu of potentially useful pharmacologic interventions, physicians are not only given new opportunities for drug-based management, but also face the increased risk of producing drug-induced side effects, quality-of-life impairment, and interactions.

The Pharmacological Imperative

The pharmacological imperative is upon us: Drugs are playing an increasingly pivotal role in the management of clinical disorders. In turn, as drug therapy succeeds in prolonging life, new conditions emerge that require additional pharmacological palliation. As a result, the number of prescription ingredients in an average drug regimen seems to have swelled dangerously out of control. Considering the recent explosion in the number of useful chemical agents, it is not surprising that polypharmacy is common in the treatment of elderly patients with chronic disease. In searching for an antidote to these trends, drug therapy consultants and physicians have forged new, comprehensive approaches to treatment. Prescribing methods are being developed that take into account all the factors influencing safety, value, efficacy, and cost-effectiveness of long-term drug regimens. Objectives include identifying drugs associated with good medication compliance, galvanizing strategies for optimizing drug selection within drug classes, using drugs in appropriate combinations, improving techniques for detecting drug toxicity and adverse drug reactions, and improving quality of life.

Achieving these goals will not be easy, but one thing is clear: The pharmacological imperative forces physicians to re-examine traditional approaches to drug regimen construction. In the United States, approximately two thirds of all physician visits result in a drug prescription.[1] It has been estimated that a patient visiting a U.S. physician for a specific complaint receives approximately four times more medication than a person with similar complaints in Scotland. Other studies show that up to 60% of physicians prescribe antibiotics to treat the common cold.[1]

The sheer number of pharmacological options creates the need for a simple, clinically applicable, and systematic approach to drug regimen design. There are presently 13,000 prescription drugs available in the United States, and the annual expenditure on prescription drugs is estimated to be in excess of $28 billion. In 1994, physicians generated 2.8 billion prescriptions, or about eight prescriptions for every man, woman, and child in the country. The increase in prescription drug use was accompanied by a corresponding increase in adverse reactions to drugs. It was estimated that between 10% and 15% of all hospitalized patients experience an adverse reaction to a drug at some point during their hospital stay.[6,7,21,22] Other studies show that 25% of all hospital admissions of patients over 65 years of age are associated with, or precipitated by, a drug-related incident.[16,23,24] Although many adverse drug reactions are relatively minor and have predictable occurrences, estimates of adverse reactions serious enough to cause hospitalization range from 0.5% to as high as 8%.[1,25,26,27]

The Information Gap

Not surprisingly, the staggering explosion in our pharmacopoeia has created a profound information and education gap that, to some extent, threatens the safety and quality of pharmacy-based medicine as it is practiced in the contemporary medical environment. For example, by the time a physician completes a three-year residency program, five years have elapsed since his or her course in clinical pharmacology. During this interval, approximately 100 new drugs will become available,[1] and the majority of drugs prescribed will be for agents about which the physicians received no formal education. Against the backdrop of rapidly expanding pharmacologic options, the Health and Public Policy Committee of the American College of Physicians points out that, "After completion of formal medical school and house officer training, there is no exposure to intelligent, informative, and unbiased assessments of drug therapy." This white paper goes on to comment that "the entire [educational] process can be characterized as largely random, incomplete and subject to distortion."[1]

Because drug therapy is the primary defense against common illnesses, more and more the art of clinical pharmacology—as well as the art of medicine, for that matter—has become synonymous with how well and how wisely a drug regimen is constructed. With so many new therapeutic agents tumbling into the pharmacist's and physician's arsenal, however, designing safe, cost-effective, quality-of-life enhancing drug regimens is increasingly problematic. In developing a rational, systematic, hands-on approach to drug regimen construction, several things appear necessary. For one, prescribing drugs *reflexively* must give way to prescribing drugs *selectively*. Moreover, opportunities for reducing overall *pharmacologic* burden—i.e. the number, frequency, and dosage level of medications—must be considered by physicians at every point in the therapeutic decision-making process. State-of-the-art drug prescribing in the contemporary medical environment, as well as in the future, should not only emphasize introducing drugs to normalize test results and objective parameters (i.e., blood pressure control, blood sugar and cholesterol levels, pulmonary function tests, etc.), but should consider quality of life, side effects, compliance, cost, drug-drug interactions, drug-disease interactions, and the "smartness" of prescription ingredients, i.e., the number of target organs and clinical endpoints that can be serviced within the context of a *single* prescription ingredient.

In previous decades, physicians were preoccupied simply with "getting the numbers (abnormal laboratory values, physiological parameters, etc.) square" on a piece of paper. In recent years, however, their pharmacotherapeutic mandate has expanded to include maintaining quality-of-life as an essential criterion against which the success of a drug regimen is measured.

Stated simply, we are in the midst of an epidemic of excessive, inappropriate, and suboptional drug prescribing in middle-aged and older Americans.[1,21,23,28] Developing viable solutions to this problem requires us to understand the full scope of the problem. In 1994, North Americans spent $14 billion hospitalizing 265,000 patients for drug-related problems.[1] During this same interval,[9,16,17] it is estimated that $10.5 billion was spent servicing noncompliance-induced disease deterioration. In other words, the health-care sector spent almost $11 billion on drugs, clinical services, and hospitalizations for individuals whose clinical conditions became worse or who developed complications simply because of poor medication compliance. Noncompliance with medications is an issue of special concern, because physicians are able to exert little control over factors influencing noncompliance. Clearly, innovative approaches relying on some combination of patient education reassurance, cost-savings, and reduction of daily dose frequency are required for noncompliant patients.

Pharmatecture ™

With these issues in clear focus, the purpose of this book is to provide pharmacists and physicians a hands-on approach to drug regimen construction in the outpatient environment. This new approach called Pharmatecture, is a drug prescribing system that weds pharmacology with architectural concepts to provide a practical, clinically useful strategy for the construction of outpatient drug regimens. Since pharmatecture represents a systematic drug selection system that employs an architectural metaphor to help guide the construction of optimal drug regimens, it can be applied to new regimens as well as to the remodeling, deconstruction, and reconstruction of preexisting polypharmacy combinations. The strategies that underpin the pharmatecture-based approach to drug selection are not only designed to increase patient compliance and reduce side effects, but also to ensure therapeutic efficacy, cost-effective drug selection, and to increase safety of drug prescribing.[27]

---

[1]American College of Physicians. Improving medical education in therapeutics. Ann Intern Med 1988; 108:145-47.

[2]Colley CA, Lucas LM. Polypharmacy: the cure becomes the disease. (Review) J Gen Intern Med 1993 May; 8(5):278-83.

[3]De Santis G, Harvey KJ, Howard D, Mashford ML, Moulds RF. Improving the quality of antibiotic prescription patterns in general practice. The role of intervention. Med J Aust 1994 April 18; 160(8):502-5.

[4]Kahl A, Blandford DH, Krueger K, Zwick DI. Geriatric education centers address medication issues affecting older adults. Public Health Reports-Hyattsville 1992 Jan-Feb; 107(1):37-47.

[5]Peck CC, Temple R, Collins JM. Understanding consequences of concurrent therapies. JAMA1993 March 24; 269(12):1550-52.

[6]Poulsen RL. Some current factors influencing the prescribing and use of psychiatric drugs. Public Health Reports-Hyattsville 1992 Jan-Feb; 107(1):47-53.

[7]Safavi KT, Hayward RA. Choosing between apples and apples: physicians' choices of prescription drugs that have similar side effects and efficacies. J Gen Intern Med 1992 Jan-Feb; 7(1):32-7.

[8]Wetle T. Age as a risk factor for inadequate treatment. (Editorial) JAMA 1987; 258:516.

[9]Lamy PP. Compliance in long-term care. Geriatrika 1985; 1(8)32.

[10]Peck CC, Temple RJ, Collins JM. Drug interactions: The death pen. (Letter) JAMA 1993 Sept 15; 270(11):1317.

[11]Valentine C. Use computers to detect inappropriate prescriptions. (Letter, Comment) BMJ 1993 July 3; 307(6895):61.

[12]Hux JE, Levinton CM, Naylor CD. Prescribing propensity; influence of life-expectancy gains and drug cost. J Gen Intern Med 1994 April; 9(4);195-201.

[13]Inman W, Pearce G. Prescriber profile and post-marketing surveillance. Lancet 1993 Sept 11; 342(8872):658-61.

[14]Jones JK. Assessing potential risk of drugs: The elusive target. Ann Intern Med 1992 Oct 15; 117(8):691-92.

[15]Belitsos NJ. Overprescribing of benzodiazepine hypnotic drugs in the elderly. (Letter, comment). Am J Med 1991 Sept; 91(3):321.

[16]Bloom JA, Frank JW, Shafir MS, Martiquet P. Potentially undesirable prescribing and drug use among the elderly. Measurable and remediable. Canadian Family Physician 1993 Nov; 39:2337-45.

[17]Burns LR, Denton M, Goldfein S. Warrick L. Morenz B, Sales B. The use of continuous quality improvement methods in the development and dissemination of medical practice guidelines. QRB 1992 Dec; 18(12):434-9.

[18]Grob PR. Antibiotic prescribing practices and patient compliance in the community. (Review) Scand J Infect Dis Suppl 1992; 83:7-14.

[19]Hamilton IJ, Reay LM, Sullivan FM. A survey of general practitioners' attitudes to benzodiazepine overprescribing. Health Bulletin 1990 Nov; 48(6):299-03.

[20]Chinburapa V, Larson LN. The importance of side effects and outcomes in differentiating between prescription drug products. J Clin Pharm Ther 1992 Dec; 17(6):333-42.

[21]Ashburn PE. Polypharmacy in skilled-nursing facilities. (Letter, Comment) Ann Intern Med 1993 April 15; 118(8):649-51.

[22]Swanson PO. Drug treatment of Parkinson's disease: is "polypharmacy" best? (Review) J Neurol Neurosurg Psychiatry 1994 April; 57(4):401-3.

[23]Beers MH, Ouslander JG, Fingold SF, Morgenstern H, Ruben DB, Rogers W, Zeffren MJ, Beck JC. Inappropriate medication prescribing in skilled-nursing facilities. Ann Intern Med 1992 Oct 15; 117(8):684-9.

[24]Bliss MR. Prescribing for the elderly. BMJ 1981; 282:203-6.

[25]Huszonek JJ, Dewan MJ, Koss M, Hadoby WJ, Ispahani A. Antidepressant side effects and physician prescribing patterns. Ann Clin Psychiatry 1993 March; 5(1):7-11.

[26]Jordan LK, Jordan LO. Prudent prescribing. Prescribing suggestions for physicians. North Carolina Medical Journal 1992 Nov; 53(11):585-8.

[27]Lamy PP. Adverse drug effects. Clin Geriatr Med 1990; 6:293-305.

[28]Beers MH, Fingold SF, Ouslander JG, Ruben DB, Morgenstern H, Beck JC. Characteristics and quality of prescribing by doctors practicing in nursing homes. J Am Geriatr Soc 1993 Aug; 41(8):802-7.

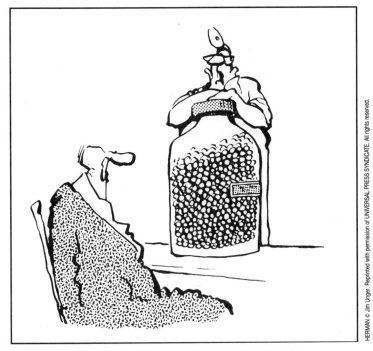

"I hope you're not one of those people who have trouble swallowing pills."

Pharmatecture™
A Systematic Approach to Pharmacologic Assessment and Drug Prescribing

Pharmatecture™ is a new drug prescribing system that melds time-honored architectural principles and concepts used for the construction of three-dimensional structures, with the objectives, strategies, and clinical approaches that comprise the foundations of clinical pharmacology. Put simply, pharmatecture is the science of designing drug regimens for the 1990s and beyond. Why pharmatecture? Because in much the same way architects design three-dimensional houses and skyscrapers out of glass, steel, and stone, clinicians are in the business of designing "drug houses" for their patients. Not only are the analogies between designing structures for the built landscape and fabricating a chemical environment using prescription ingredients quite striking, but they provide the underpinnings for an approach that can shape, simplify, and streamline drug prescribing in day-to-day clinical practice.

When it comes to constructing drug regimens, pharmacists and physicians mix, match, layer, and combine medications much like architects stitch together diverse building materials to form an integrated composition.[1,2,3] While architects work with granite, wood, glass, stone, and steel, clinicians usually draw on pharmacologic building blocks—i.e., selective serotonin reuptake inhibitors (SSRIs), calcium channel antagonists, prostaglandin inhibitors, and beta agonists—for their therapeutic constructions. Consequently, for the purpose of analogy, one can think of pharmacists and physicians, who engage primarily in pharmacotherapeutic interventions as "pharmatects". They are builders of pharmacologic environments or, pharmatecturally speaking, "drug houses," for their patients. By the term "drug house," of course, is meant a pharmacologic environment consisting of one or more prescription medications.

One can think of these drug houses as chemical environments that are both *built* and *maintained* by pharmacists and physicians. For example, when a physician prescribes a beta-blocker for angina, an aspirin a day for secondary prevention of myocardial infarction, a calcium blocker for hypertension, an angiotensin converting enzyme (ACE) inhibitor for congestive heart failure, and a nonsteroidal anti-inflammatory drug (NSAID) for arthritis, he or she has constructed a pharmacologic environment in which a patient may have to live for many years.[4,5] The final architecture of this drug house—its building blocks, its framework, its safety considerations, its foundation—are the primary determinants of its durability, cost-effectiveness, and patient-friendliness.

Pharmacologic Framework

From a pharmatectural perspective, how safe this drug house is over time, how effectively it meets functional objectives, how much it costs, and how good the patient feels living inside that house, are the most important criteria against which the success and durability of a drug regimen can be measured. Clearly, drug houses designed by physicians are not three-dimensional environments as are skyscrapers, museums, and private residences, but they are quantifiable environments, nevertheless, with the capacity to produce distinct side effect profiles and outcomes.[1,6,7] A drug house can be thought of as a pharmacologically determined milieu, consisting of many different prescription ingredients with active biochemical properties. These building blocks sometimes interact to produce positive results, and sometimes they create negative effects for the patient living within its pharmacologic framework.[8,9] Over time, pharmacologic building blocks may even become obsolete or unsafe. The introduction of better materials may necessitate remodeling a drug house, that is, deconstructing and reconstructing it according to the best materials (i.e., drugs) currently available. In the final analysis, like a work of architecture, a drug house must satisfy specific functional, and quality-of-life objectives.

Interestingly, many of the same criteria against which the success, quality, and suitability of a work of architecture is measured, also apply to pharmacologic environments constructed by practitioners trying to achieve optimal therapeutic outcomes. The manner in which building materials are chosen in the architectural world is similar to the way pharmacologic building blocks are selected in the therapeutic sphere. For example, architectural works are fabricated from a wide variety of building materials, including glass, steel, wood, stone, plastic, aluminum, granite, marble, stucco, and terra cotta. Within budgetary constraints, an architect has the freedom to choose among these options. Extensive catalogues consisting of thousands and thousands of building materials—many of them very similar except for slight differences in color, texture, or weight—are consulted to evaluate the desirability of one product over another.

A similar process guides the selection of medications. Physicians consult many different types of references—formulary lists, drug catalogues, clinical monographs, such established resources as *Drug Facts and Comparisons,* as well as software programs—to guide their selection of pharmacologic building blocks. This is a necessary process because all the options within a given drug class are not created equal. There are, in fact, better drugs and worse drugs, with some drugs making better building blocks and some drugs making inferior building blocks.[10,11,12,13,14] For example, some nonsteroidal anti-inflammatory drugs (ibuprofen, Motrin®) are more likely to cause renal deterioration than others (sulindac, Clinoril®), while some H_2 blockers (cimeditine, Tagamet®) have a greater propensity for causing drug interactions through inhibition of P450 cytochrome oxidase system than other H_2 blockers (famotidine, Pepcid).[7,15] Moreover, advantages and disadvantages of drugs vary according to the drug class. In some cases, pharmacologic inferiority and superiority may be determined by the risk of drug interactions, in others by compliance patterns, and in other classes, by side effect profiles. For example, some potentially very effective antibiotics (e.g., erythromycin) have a high incidence of side effects and, therefore, are associated with higher discontinuation rates, making them therapeutically less effective. To maximize pharmatectural effectiveness, physicians must select among various options in order to determine which pharmacotherapeutic choices (building blocks for drug regimens) offer unique advantages in some patients but might pose a risk in others and, therefore, should be avoided.

Safe Construction

Architecture has been called "the beautiful necessity," a description that underscores the fact that the building arts do not exist for beauty's sake alone. At the very minimum, a work of architecture has to satisfy certain functional criteria. First and foremost among these are safety considerations: No matter what other goals are accomplished, a house must meet certain building codes pertaining to electrical, heating, plumbing, and waste disposal systems. To be sure, once these rudimentary criteria are met, the best works of architecture also function on a spiritual level. Ideally, they please the eye with a well-chosen color, elevate the mood by the way light is apportioned in a space, or excite the imagination with a properly chosen ornament.

Similarly, much like an architectural work, drug houses designed by pharmacists or physicians should address both *safety* and *life quality* issues. First, the risk of producing mild or serious side effects should be minimized. All organ systems—renal, pulmonary, cardiovascular, neurological, dermatological—should be protected. In addition, drugs used to build a pharmacologic environment should not adversely affect underlying diseases or interact with other medications in ways that might produce clinically significant side effects.[16] Moreover, the safety of a drug should be confirmed in the patient population in whom its use is being contemplated. "Safety first" is a mandate that applies equally to both architecture and pharmatecture. Finally, drug houses also must meet functional objectives.[17,18,19,20,21]

But safety is only the beginning. Once the basic pharmacologic building codes are met, with all organ systems operative, and side effect safety checks completed, the *livability* of a drug house becomes an extremely important pharmatectural issue. If architecture is the beautiful necessity, then pharmatecture can be characterized as the *endurable* necessity. In other words, if patients cannot endure living in their drug houses, the fragile walls of their chemical abode eventually will come tumbling down. Noncompliance will undermine therapeutic results, and new problems will surface that may require patching with still more drugs.[22,23] In the world of pharmatecture, then, livability, affordability, and endurability are of paramount importance. Like great works of architecture, the best-designed drug houses also make their inhabitants feel better, more optimistic about life, and healthier for living within their pharmacological walls.[24,25] These subjective aspects of long-term drug therapy are increasingly important features that should be incorporated into the final therapeutic equation.

Less Is More

There also are important *quantitative* parameters that govern the construction of contemporary drug houses. Like modern architecture, pharmatecture subscribes to the guiding principle that, "Less is more." In other words, the more a physician can achieve in the way of desired clinical effects using the *fewest* number of prescription ingredients, at the *lowest* dosage, for the *shortest* duration permissible, and at *lowest* daily dose frequency, the better off the patient will be. In this regard, studies demonstrate that the risk of scheduling errors, drug toxicity, and drug-related adverse side effects are most closely correlated with the total number of prescription ingredients a patient is taking and to the total pill count in the daily drug regimen.[4,8,9,11,24,26,27,28,29,30,31]

Moreover, studies of drug use consistently show a negative relationship between medication compliance and the number of drugs taken by the patient.[1,28,29,31,32,33] Specifically, taking three or more drugs increases the likelihood that the patient will be either deliberately or unknowingly noncompliant. Compliance also tends to decrease with time. For example, patients are more likely to take antibiotics in the first stages of treatment than the later stages, with one study showing that only 8% of patients prescribed a 10-day course of antibiotics were actually taking the medication on the tenth day of therapy.[28,29] With respect to long-term therapy, the percentage of patients who adhere faithfully to treatment plans for hypertension and other chronic diseases rapidly declines after the initial diagnosis and early months of treatment. With respect to daily dose frequency, compliance studies show a decrease in medication compliance with increasing daily dose frequency.[31] Many pitfalls, both financial and clinical, associated with polypharmacy can be minimized by subscribing to the "less is more" approach for drug regimen design.

Foundation Drugs

While architects work within a certain structural framework to ensure sound physical construction, physicians operate within a conceptual framework governed by such issues as comfort, cost, and quality-of-life issues associated with drug therapy. Architects emphasize that a house is only as good as its foundation. And so it is with drug regimens. It is important to identify so-called *foundation drugs,* that is, those agents that will stand the test of time in terms of drug and disease interactions, and that can be used as *monotherapy* for long durations. In other words, to avoid excessive costs and other problems associated with altering drug regimens over time, physicians should prescribe agents that safely allow addition of other drugs, without incurring the risk of drug-drug or drug-disease interactions.[34,35]

These are the broad brush strokes of a drug prescribing system that is designed to promote cost-effective pharmacologic intervention in the outpatient setting. The following sections discuss specific parameters of this system in detail and their implementation in clinical practice.

PHARMATECTURE™: THE SYSTEM IN PRACTICE

For all practical purposes, pharmatecture can be seen as the science of *building* drug regimens. Science, in this case, means generating a logical, systematic approach for drug regimen design in the outpatient setting. This is an approach that stresses optimizing drug selection, enhancing patient medication compliance, and streamlining drug regimens, always with an eye toward drug reduction, elimination, simplification, and consolidation (DRESC™). (See Chapter 5)

WINDOWS

Architects pay special attention to windows in their building designs. Physicians also must consider windows—windows of *opportunity* and *vulnerability* as they relate to the selection of individual drugs, and the design of long-term, outpatient drug regimens.

Windows of Vulnerability

By window of vulnerability is meant that noncompliance with medications is recognized as a public health problem. Noncompliance is associated with staggering clinical and economic consequences.[29,36,37,38] For example, Americans now spend almost $11 billion annually servicing poor therapeutic outcomes associated with medication noncompliance.[33,39] Noncompliance-induced disease deterioration has been observed in such chronic conditions as hypertension, seizures, and diabetes mellitis, as well as in acute diseases such as sexually transmitted disorders, especially chlamydial infections. Most studies demonstrate that noncompliance with medications is exacerbated by increasing daily dose frequency, lack of patient education, and cost of the drug.[40,41,42] Attention to these factors promotes improved medication compliance, and as a result, better therapeutic outcomes. Not surprisingly, the pharmatectural approach to drug prescribing highlights pharmacology-, physician-, and patient-oriented strategies designed to enhance drug compliance.[29,30,31,43]

Inappropriate drug use takes many forms and can produce a wide range of undesirable consequences. Consider the following patient scenarios as glimpses into the window of vulnerability associated with poor medication compliance:

A 62-year-old gentleman with high blood pressure discontinues his medication because its side effects make him feel worse than he does when he is not on medication. His hypertension is no longer in control and he eventually has a stroke leading to prolonged hospitalization, subsequent rehabilitation, and permanent disability.

Analysis: In this example, the side effects of the antihypertensive drug are more uncomfortable than the disease (silent hypertension). As expected, the patient opts for the "silence" of the disease rather than the excessive "noise level" of the medication. The end result is noncompliance-mediated therapeutic failure, increased morbidity, and poor outcome.

A 35-year old woman suffering from depression stops taking her antidepressant drug because she sees no improvement in her condition after 1 week of drug therapy. She grows more and more depressed and, eventually, has her employment terminated because she is unable to perform her job duties. When asked why she stopped taking her medicine, she indicates she was not aware that the benefits of some antidepressants become apparent only after the drug has been taken for several weeks.

Analysis: This patient received inadequate education from her physician or pharmacist regarding the relationship between duration of antidepressant therapy and onset of therapeutic benefits. The result is premature discontinuation of drug therapy and exacerbation of symptoms associated with her depression.

A 55-year-old patient taking diuretics and digoxin for congestive heart failure stops taking his potassium supplement because he finds it unpalatable. Eventually, his serum potassium level drops. The potassium deficiency, in combination with the digoxin therapy, produces a potentially life-threatening heart rhythm disturbance necessitating an emergency department visit and subsequent hospitalization.[36]

Analysis: In this patient, discontinuation of one drug (potassium) potentiates the side effects of another drug (digoxin). This case also illustrates the risk of medication noncompliance and clinical consequences associated with construction of complex (i.e., three or more different prescription ingredients) drug regimens. Lack of patient education might also have played a role. The importance of maintaining potassium levels should have been stressed. Finally, simplification of the drug regimen might have prevented this patient's deterioration caused by a heart rhythm disturbance. In this regard, a combination drug that combines a diuretic with a potassium-sparing drug (e.g., aldactone with hydrochlorothiazide, Aldactazide®; triamterene with hydrochlorothiazide, Maxzide®) would have simplified drug intake, enhanced compliance, and minimized the risk of hypokalemia-induced potentiation of digoxin toxicity.

An 82-year-old woman on a fixed income stops taking her anti-anginal medication because she feels she can no longer afford it. Within one week of discontinuing her drug, she experiences increasing frequency of angina and severity of chest discomfort. These symptoms precipitate an emergency department visit and subsequent short-term hospitalization. She is discharged on a less expensive anti-anginal agent. The cost of her hospitalization is $6,543.45.

Analysis: This case illustrates the potentially devastating consequences of *cost-mediated* medication noncompliance. The irony is that the discontinuation of the drug because of cost considerations resulted in an expensive hospitalization. Although the cost of medications is frequently justified, especially for once-daily drugs with few side effects, for many individuals cost is the bottom line affecting long-term adherence to a therapeutic program. When managing individuals who are extremely sensitive to drug cost, less expensive agents might produce better overall clinical outcomes, even if these drugs have other features (complicated dosing schedule, side effects, etc.) usually associated with poor compliance.[36,38,39,44]

Compliance Problems

Noncompliance is widespread among ambulatory patients, especially the elderly. The extent of noncompliance generally is estimated at about 40%, although some studies place the estimate as a high as 75%.[22,36,45,46] Omission or underuse of medications is the most common form of noncompliance, with some studies reporting that among older persons on long-term therapy, 59% of patients made one or more errors and that 26% made potentially serious errors.[36,39,44] Nearly 66% of the patients who made errors omitted prescribed medications. Interestingly, not only was underuse the most prevalent type of noncompliance, but researchers found that many elderly patients who omit drugs do so *deliberately,* primarily because they think they do not need the medication in the dosage prescribed.[47,48] In general, the major reason medications are underused is a dissatisfaction with some part of the drug regimen, i.e., with the type, amount, dosage schedule, or side effects. Because of these concerns, patients make adjustments in their drug therapy, often omitting medications to suit their perceived needs.

Patient education plays an important role in promoting medication compliance. Despite laws mandating pharmacists to instruct patients about safe and effective use of new prescriptions, in a recent Seattle, Washington study, only 44% of those regularly using prescription drugs could recall pharmacists instructing them on use, whereas 80% recalled that their physician had done so.[28,49] Only 52% reported their physician had instructed them about possible side effects, and only 30% reported receiving this information from their pharmacist. The fact is, a large percentage of patients, especially the elderly, lack basic information about their drugs.[33,50,148] They are uninformed about the name and purpose of their prescription drugs, the dosage schedules, as well as the duration of therapy, possible side effects, and adverse consequences. Fortunately, these problems have solutions. While mastery of this basic information does not guarantee compliance, there are numerous studies suggesting it is at least a necessary condition for ensuring compliance.[28,30,44,51,52] It is well-established, for example, that when patients are provided with specific and detailed instructions about their particular drug regimen, compliance improves. Moreover, individualized instruction is effective when the mode of communication is either oral or written.[48,51,53,54,55]

Economic Barriers. Another barrier to compliance is economic: patients' inability to afford prescription medications in the quantity called for by prescription directions. In one study of 290 chronically ill patients discharged from a general hospital in Canada, it was found that the financial burden imposed by drug costs was the primary reason given by patients for noncompliance with drug treatment.[53] Examining the relationship between drug expenditures and the rate of noncompliance, the study revealed that the average monthly cost of drugs prescribed for noncompliant patients was almost three times higher than the cost of drugs for those who did comply.[49,55] These studies argue for the importance of taking cost factors into consideration when building drug regimens.[44,47,55,56]

Intelligent Noncompliance. Usually, patient omission of drugs undermines therapeutic efficacy. However, there are situations when omission of drugs or self-administration of lower than prescribed dosages of drugs may actually be beneficial. It may be appropriate for patients with side effects from taking too many drugs, an excessive dose of a single drug, to cut back on their medication intake.[52] This type of behavior is called, "intelligent noncompliance," and is best able to serve the patient's interest when undertaken in *collaboration* with the physician or pharmacist.[52] Intelligent noncompliance requires that open doors of communication are maintained between patient and physician or pharmacist, so that alterations perceived as necessary by the patient are managed within the context of the overall drug regimen.

Noncompliance and Polypharmacy. Pharmatecturally speaking, the journey from the prescription pad to an optimal clinical outcome is oftentimes derailed by poor medication compliance. Selecting the appropriate drug for the appropriate patient is simply not enough to guarantee desirable outcomes. For example, one may prescribe the indicated drug for a condition, but the therapeutic result may be compromised by less-than-optimal medication intake. Of special concern is the observation that *being noncompliant with a medication actually increases the patient's risk of receiving additional, unnecessary drugs.*[36,38,39,48,53]

In other words, noncompliance with medications can be dangerous. As ironic as it may seem, patients who fail to take their medications as prescribed actually *increase* the likelihood that they will become victims of unnecessary polypharmacy. Why? Because when a patient is noncompliant with medication, poor therapeutic results are observed. As a rule, poor therapeutic results are expressed in patients as abnormal test results. Almost without exception, the way physicians respond to abnormal disease parameters is by: (1) initiating pharmacologic therapy; (2) continuing existing drug therapy but at a higher dose; (3) adding a new drug to the regimen, or; (4) eliminating the drug that is perceived as ineffective and substituting an agent from a different therapeutic class.

Herein lies the pharmacological rub. In so many cases, when poor medication intake produces unsatisfactory results, patients are given additional, unnecessary drugs that are prescribed by physicians to correct the problem. Although less is *usually* more when it comes to drug therapy, the opposite is generally true when *patients* decide on their own that they can get by with fewer medications than prescribed.

Drugs are prescribed for many different reasons, but abnormal laboratory values or measurable physiological parameters are the primary inducements to initiating therapy with prescription drugs. In most situations, unless noncompliance is recognized by the clinician, to normalize these abnormal end points, the physician either increases the dose of the medication the patient already has failed to take appropriately, or even worse, the clinician will add another medication to the drug regimen. This is the beginning of a cycle in which noncompliance-mediated disease deterioration induces excessive drug prescribing. Thus, noncompliance not only has the potential for fueling polypharmacy, but it is often-times associated with cost-ineffective drug prescribing. Generally speaking, then, when it comes to patient-mediated noncompliance, inadequate medication intake is associated with poor therapeutic outcomes that tend to generate more drugs, almost always to the patient's detriment.

Factors Influencing Compliance. Clearly, noncompliance with medications is an important window of vulnerability when it comes to drug therapy, and interventional strategies designed to improve medication intake are central to the pharmatectural approach. As previously mentioned, many factors influence medication compliance including: patient education, written instructions reinforcing medication intake, cost of the drug, and total pharmacologic burden. Attention to these issues is mandatory for maximizing medication compliance. Studies demonstrate that if patients know the function of the drug prescribed for them, they are far less likely to have another drug added to their regimen (Figure 1-1). No single factor, however, is as important for preserving optimal medication intake as daily dose *frequency*. Many trials have confirmed that both scheduling errors and unnecessary drug additions are significantly reduced when medications are prescribed on a once-daily basis (Figure 1-2).[31,40,42,54,57]

Figure 1-1

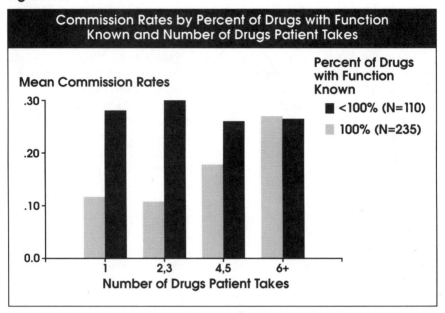

Figure 1-2

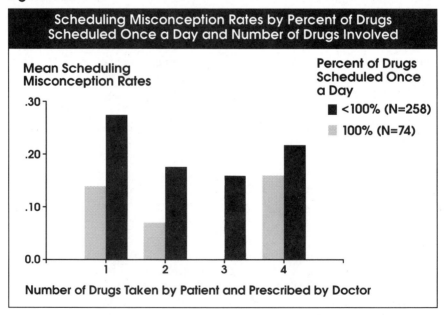

To be sure, the importance of once-daily dosing is much more than a marketing point promulgated by pharmaceutical companies. In fact, there are now "science of compliance" studies demonstrating the undeniable link between daily dose frequency and drug compliance.[31] Eschewing traditional pill counting methods that have characterized previous medication compliance trials, these studies are unique because they rely upon computer microchips to monitor daily medication intake. An accurate chronicle of medication intake is facilitated by microchips that are surreptitiously embedded into the lids of pill bottles. Every time the patient removes the lid to retrieve a pill, the microchip registers, within 15 minutes, the time of day and date the pill bottle is opened. In this manner, a record of pill consumption is silently recorded for a 180-day period, at which time the bottles and microchips are collected, and a computer printout of medication intake is generated for evaluation.

The results of these studies are quite fascinating, and confirm that obtaining a realistic assessment of drug intake requires honesty from patients who, as a rule, are either not very forthcoming, or, occasionally, are frankly delusional about their medication intake. In fact, when the results of the microchip data are compared to written questionnaires, on which patients have documented their perceptions of medication compliance, there is a significant divergence between the computer-generated data and questionnaire results. In other words, when it comes to medication compliance, very nice people lie through their teeth. These studies demonstrate in no uncertain terms, first, that medication intake is closely linked to daily dose frequency and, second, that it is unwise to rely upon patient perceptions to make accurate assessments of medication compliance.[22,23,55] Overall, these investigations show that once-daily dosing is associated with a compliance rate of about 92%, twice-daily dosing with compliance rates of about 85%, and three- and four-times daily dosing with rates of about 50% over the long term.[31,43,58,59]

Based on these and other studies, the most direct pharmatectural approach for addressing the window of vulnerability manifested by poor medication compliance is the use of once-daily medications. Although simplification of dosing schedule is an important strategic maneuver for constructing drug regimens, it should be stressed that once-daily medications represent a *necessary,* but not *sufficient* condition for optimal medication compliance. In other words, simply because a drug can be dosed on a once-daily basis does not give the physician carte blanche for its use. There are, after all, other windows of vulnerability—side effects, drug interaction profiles, cost, etc.—which may require physicians to discriminate among many different medication options dosed on a once-daily basis.

Choosing Once-daily Medications. Within each drug class, there are better and worse once-daily preparations and, for each clinical situation an attempt should be made to identify the safest once-daily preparation with the greatest efficacy and fewest side effects.[5] For example, even though flurazepam (Dalmane®) is dosed on a once-daily basis, it has a prolonged, 120 hour half-life, and therefore, is more likely to cause somnolence, falling,[60] and hip fractures than the intermediate-acting, once-daily benzodiazepines which, in general, are safer and associated with fewer side effects.[12,21,47,61,62] Among the tricyclic antidepressants (TCAs), amitryptiline (Elavil®) can be dosed on a once-daily basis. Unfortunately, it produces more anticholinergic side effects (dry mouth, sedation, orthostatic hypotension) than such once-daily, selective serotonin reuptake inhibitors (SSRIs) as sertraline (Zoloft®), which demonstrates equal efficacy in the treatment of depression but has a much more favorable side effect profile. Even among the once-daily SSRIs, there may be a need for discriminating among the available options. For example, fluoxetine (Prozac®), because of the prolonged half-life of its active metabolites, may be less desirable than a drug such as sertraline, which has a half-life of only 24 hours and causes only minimal to moderate inhibition of the P450 IID6 cytochrome oxidase isoenzyme.[14,35,63,64,65]

Because cardiovascular drugs are associated with a high incidence of side effects,[34,66,67,68] special vigilance is required when choosing among once-daily medications used to treat heart disease. With respect to calcium channel blockers, verapamil (Calan®) is available as a once-daily preparation, but it is more likely to cause sinus bradycardia, congestive heart failure, and conduction inhibition than a calcium blocker such as amlodipine (Norvasc®), which spares both the conduction system of the heart as well as myocardial pump function.[7,32,68,69] The important point is that among the compliance-enhancing, once-daily preparations within a drug class, the physician should attempt to identify those agents with the fewest side effects and safest drug interaction profiles.

Education

From a pharmatectural perspective, there are many opportunities for closing the window of vulnerability associated with medication noncompliance.[1,10,21,70,71] Some of these involve selection of medications based on their pharmacologic properties as discussed above. Other approaches must address informational and behavioral needs.[51,53] To be effective in reducing noncompliance, the health care provider must function as teacher, motivator, and persuader. Accurate information about drug intake should be conveyed and the patient must be motivated to take the drugs as instructed. This requires good patient-pharmacist and patient-physician communication. The risk of noncompliance can be reduced by careful labeling of prescriptions. This entails placing both the name and purpose of each drug on the prescription container. Moreover, regimens should be simplified. Each regimen should be examined periodically to ensure that it is the simplest, safest, and most effective therapy currently available. In addition, efforts should be made to titrate medications against treatment response to determine the smallest amount of medication required. Finally, unnecessary medications should be eliminated.

Windows of Opportunity: Smart Drugs

By windows of opportunity is meant the recognition that optimizing drug selection requires identification of so-called "smart drugs". Smart drugs do not make pharmacists, physicians, or patients smarter, but they do offer an important window of opportunity by reducing overall pharmacological burden (i.e., the number of prescription ingredients required for a long-term drug regimen), which is an important risk factor for noncompliance, as well as drug-drug and drug-disease interactions.

Smart drugs share many of the properties and advantages associated with "smart bombs", in that they do more with less, and at lower overall cost. Smart bombs, of course, travel precisely to their targets and, therefore, obviate the need for dumping several hundred conventional bombs to accomplish a strategic endpoint. Although smart bombs carry a princely price tag—sometimes costing as much as $600,000—it, nevertheless, is more cost-effective to launch one of these so-called, smart, laser-guided, Sidewinder missiles than it is to send up a B-52 and dump a bunch of "dumb" (conventional) bombs in order to accomplish the same mission.

Like smart bombs, smart drugs also have the capacity to target their action against well-defined endpoints. These smart pharmacologic agents, however, go one step farther, insofar as they can be thought of as smart bombs with multiple warheads. The smartest drugs can hit many targets simultaneously. Specifically, from a pharmatectural point of view, smart drugs are "high productivity" medications that possess the uncanny ability to strike all the necessary clinical endpoints with *one* active prescription ingredient. It is as if they have been designed to: (1) survey a disease landscape and identify the entire cluster of pathophysiological derangements—or, in the case of infectious diseases, anticipate all the co-infecting organisms—that characterize the condition; (2) target many endpoints simultaneously; and (3) service many impaired target-organs associated with the condition, and do so with a single pharmacotherapeutic agent.

The specificity and comprehensiveness of targeting afforded by smart drugs *minimizes* dependency on several different drugs to achieve therapeutic end points that once required many agents working in combination. The final result of optimizing drug prescribing through the use of smart drugs is a *reduction in overall pharmacologic burden.* This reduction decreases excessive and unnecessary costs incurred from drug-drug and drug-disease interactions which, studies confirm, are closely tied to the total number of different prescription ingredients in a drug regimen.[15,26,72-75]

Smart Drugs: Patient Specificity

Perhaps more than any other drug class, antibiotics are selected according to their "smartness". To understand the meaning of smartness as it applies to drug therapy, it is helpful to consider the manner in which oral antimicrobials are chosen for the management of infections. In general, when choosing an antibiotic, the physician mentally lists the etiologic organisms most likely to be involved in the infection. Then, whenever possible, an attempt is made to identify a *single* antibiotic that provides antimicrobial activity against *all* the likely offenders. For example, in the case of uncomplicated urinary tract infection, trimethoprim-sulfamethoxazole (Bactrim®) is considered a smart drug, since it will treat the expected species of E. coli and other gram negative organisms usually implicated in such infections. On the other hand, for skin and soft tissue infections, diclox-acillin, azithromycin (Zithromax®) or cephalexin (Keflex®) would represent smart drugs because they cover both streptococcal and staphylococcal species most often implicated in these conditions.

As might be expected, the smartness of a drug *varies* according to the situation. In this regard, it should be stressed that any given antibiotic, antihyper-tensive, or antidepressant will not, in every patient, *always* be smarter than some other drug to which it is being compared. In other words, in one patient, drug A may be smarter than drug B, but in another case, the converse may be true. Drug smartness, from a pharmatectural perspective, is *patient-specific.* The relative wisdom of any pharmacotherapeutic decision depends upon the medication's suitability for the individual patient—with all the attendant demographic, host, and environmental factors—in which the drug's use is being considered.

For example, in a non-immunologically compromised, healthy outpatient with a bacterial exacerbation of chronic obstructive pulmonary disease or a community-acquired pneumonia, azithromycin (Zithromax®) is a smart drug, because it provides *in vitro* activity against the four principal pathogens— *Streptococcus pneumoniae, Hemophilus influenzae, Moraxella catarrhalis,* and mycoplasma—that are most often implicated in these outpatient conditions in-volving the lung. On the other hand, in a community-acquired pulmonary infec-tion occurring in a patient with AIDS, a drug such as trimethoprim-sulfamethox-azole may represent a smarter choice, because it is active against *Pneumocystis carinii* pneumonia (PCP), a common infectious complication of this disease. In general, selecting antibiotics according to their smartness reduces the risk of pharmacologically reservicing (i.e., retreating) patients and, therefore, represents a cost-effective approach to management of infectious diseases.

From a pharmatectural perspective, identifying smart, high productivity drugs plays a critical role in Total Pharmacotherapeutic Quality Management (TPQM™, see below), an approach designed to pharmacologically service pa-tients with the *fewest* number of drugs at the lowest cost. To achieve this goal, smart drugs must be tailored to individual patient needs. Consider the following illustration: Imagine you are faced with the challenge of constructing a drug regimen for an individual who suffers from all of the following conditions simultaneously: migraine headaches, hereditary familial tremor, angina, and hypertension. Moreover, suppose this patient also requires prevention of myocar-dial re-infarction. What would represent a "smart" drug for this particular patient? There are many possibilities and combinations, but, compared to other choices, a beta-blocker would be considered a smart drug because it has the potential capacity to treat all these conditions with a *single* prescription ingredient. In other words, each of the conditions afflicting this patient is potentially improved by a lipophilic beta-blocker such as propranolol. If one had *not* selected the smart drug approach to this patient, the physician might have prescribed ergotamine for the migraine headache, a benzodiazepine to control the tremors, a calcium blocker for angina, an ACE inhibitor for the high blood pressure, and aspirin plus a beta-blocker to prevent secondary myocardial infarction.[76] This six-story "drug house" would probably incur greater cost, increase the risk of drug reactions and interactions, and, possibly, produce more quality-of-life impairment than the single agent construction. Although this is an exaggerated example, it does emphasize the need for identifying single medications with *multiple sites of action* and, whenever possible, matching such drugs with the appropriate clinical profile.

Additional examples of smart drugs include ACE inhibitors, which have the capacity for simultaneously treating congestive heart failure, hypertension, and protecting the kidney in patients with diabetic renal disease.[47,77-81] Among cardiovascular agents, smart medications include calcium blockers that can offer symptomatic relief in angina and treat high blood pressure, and such peripheral alpha-blockers as doxazosin (Cardura®), which can reduce blood pressure, lower serum cholesterol, and provide symptomatic relief in patients with benign prostatic hypertrophy. Among the psychotropics, heterocyclic antidepressants have the capacity to treat depression, induce sedation in patients with insomnia, increase pain threshold, and provide symptomatic relief in patients with diabetic neuropathy. When patients present with this constellation of needs, low doses of antidepressants with reduced anticholinergic side effects should be recommended.

BUILDING MATERIALS: BETTER CHOICES, WORSE CHOICES

When it comes to designing three-dimensional spaces made of glass, wood, steel, and stone, architects bear the responsibility for identifying better and worse materials for the building under construction. Much like a physician trying to select the antiarrhythmic agent that is ideally suited for a patient's heart problem, architects are always faced with the challenge of choosing among many different material options for their projects. For example, maple is a hardwood and, therefore, is far better suited than softer woods such as mahogany or fir for the construction of bowling alley lanes or floors for a basketball court. Among the many materials available for a particular architectural purpose, there are superior and inferior choices depending upon functional needs, climate, durability, and safety considerations.

And so it is with pharmacologic options. *The fact is that all drugs within a drug class are not created equal.* There are better and worse choices, with some pharmacologic building blocks clearly offering advantages over others.[10,11] As a rule, physicians select medications according to cost, efficacy, safety, side effect profile, and their own clinical experience.[4,5,13,14,82] In this vein, the pharmatectural approach to outpatient drug construction stresses the importance of distinguishing among chemical agents (i.e., building materials) *within* a drug class, evaluating their similarities and differences, accounting for the nuances, comparing their relative smartness, and then selecting the medication best suited for a particular therapeutic objective in a specific patient subgroup.[17,27,83,84] For example, among the beta-blockers, lipophilic agents such as propranolol (Inderal®) have greater central nervous system (CNS) penetration than hydrophilic beta-blockers such as atenolol (Tenormin®) which, some studies show, is associated with less fatigue, depression, somnolence, and sexual dysfunction. While atenolol may represent a better choice for the treatment of hypertension, angina, or prevention of myocardial infarction, propranolol is better-suited for the prophy-laxis of migraine headaches because of its CNS penetration.

The necessity for distinguishing between better and worse pharmacologic options is especially important in geriatric patients,[20,85,86] in whom side effects, drug interactions, half-life of medications, and functional considerations play a critical role in pharmacological management.[6,10,71,87] In the treatment of major depression in the elderly, for example, SSRIs have clear advantages over other classes of antidepressants. Although all the SSRIs are free of the myocardial and CNS effects characteristic of tricyclic antidepressants (TCAs), there are still significant differences among the three marketed drugs in this class that indicate sertraline (Zoloft®) may represent a better choice for the management of depres-sion in the elderly.[3,25,88,89] Unlike fluoxetine (Prozac®) and paroxetine (Paxil®), sertraline has linear pharmacokinetics in both young and elderly patients. Thus, special dosing is not required in older individuals. Moreover, unlike fluoxetine, neither sertraline nor paroxetine has metabolites with clinically significant activ-ity with regard to serotonin reuptake inhibition. A final advantage is that ser-traline, as a rule, has a less prominent inhibitory effect on the P450 IID6 isoenzyme than some other drugs in its class. The reduced potential for pharmacokinetic drug interactions with sertraline is especially important in el-derly patients who are likely to be taking a wide variety of medications concurrently.

Although identifying the best choices between and within drug classes is central to the pharmatectural approach, perhaps, even more important, is arriving at the proper *combination* of better drugs. Since many patients require treatment with multiple medications, the enlightened pharmatect not only selects the best agents *within* a drug class, but takes this process one step further and evaluates a drug's suitability for use in combination with other drugs. Many excellent drugs, for example, function well in *isolation* of other agents[83,90,91,92] but, when com-bined with other medications, can produce problems. The key is to identify better drugs that can be combined safely and effectively.[9,15,16,74,93]

This is especially true for cardiovascular drugs. For example, although verapamil may provide good blood pressure control with minimal side effects in some older patients, the addition of a beta-blocker to a regimen that includes verapamil may result in symptomatic bradycardia, AV node conduction distur-bances, or clinically significant myocardial suppression in a significant minority of *susceptible* older individuals. Therefore, other calcium blockers (i.e., amlodipine, felodipine, isradipine) that spare both the conduction system and pump function are considered preferable because they can be used safely in combination with other drugs, such as beta-blockers.[69,94]

Similar considerations are important when prescribing antimicrobials. For example, although erythromycin and clarithromycin (Biaxin®) may produce excellent clinical results when used in isolation of other agents, they have the potential of producing undesirable—even, life-threatening—drug interactions in patients who are on concomitant terfenadine (Seldane®) therapy. Azithromycin (Zithromax®), another antibiotic with similar antimicrobial activity, represents a better choice in these patients, inasmuch as it does not produce clinically significant interactions with this antihistaminic agent. Alternatively, one could use a different non-sedating antihistamine (e.g., loratidine), which is not associated with such interactions.

As far as less-than-optimal drug combinations are concerned, one of the most common pitfalls is routine use of ACE inhibitors in elderly patients with hypertension (Figure 1-3). Although ACE inhibitors represent an excellent choice for many older hypertensive patients, it should be noted that many elderly individuals may be taking other (postassium-sparing) agents that can interact with this class of antihypertensive. Most important among them are the nonsteroidal anti-inflammatory drugs (NSAIDs), which are commonly used for management of chronic arthritic conditions. NSAIDs decrease prostaglandin synthesis in turn, which decreases aldosterone secretion (NSAID-induced inhibition of ACE activity), causing a reduction in renal potassium excretion. When ACE inhibitors are added to NSAIDs, one may observe additive suppression of the renin-angiotensin-aldosterone axis, which can produce clinically significant elevations in serum potassium levels. These are just a few examples of inappropriate drug combinations, most of which can be avoided by prudent drug selection practices.

Figure 1-3

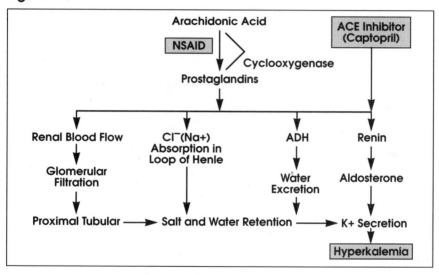

GUIDING PRINCIPLES

Less Is More

For many centuries, the world of architecture was dominated by buildings copiously robed with ornaments, figurines, and decorative embellishments in all shapes and sizes. A prestigious lineage of architectural works, from the Greek Parthenon to Italian Borromini Churches to the Gothic-inspired Woolworth Building in New York City, subscribed to this "more is better" philosophy. In the early 1930s, however, there was a precipitous rebellion against this kind of ornament-rich architecture, and the intellectual driving force behind the Bauhaus movement, Mies Van der Rohe, coined the expression "less is more." With this modernistic pronouncement came a generation of simpler, stylistically straight-forward buildings, stripped bare to their essentials, in which function took precedence over frippery, fanciful forms, and figurative flourishes. This was a conceptual revolution that produced such clean, gleaming skyscrapers as the Seagram's Building, Rockefeller Center, and the Empire State Building. Less became more and, in the process, much more was accomplished with far less.

The pharmatectural approach to drug regimen design strongly supports this "less is more" philosophy. (Figure 1-4) When it comes to drugs, there is beauty in *simplicity*. Pharmacologically speaking, the more that can be achieved using the fewest number of prescription ingredients, at the lowest clinically effective dose, and the lowest daily dose frequency, the better off the patient will be. Support for this position comes from many investigations, all of which confirm that the total number of different prescription drugs in a patient's regimen is the single most important determinant of drug interactions.[16,72,93,95] While using fewer drugs at their lowest effective dose is a virtuous goal, accomplishing this in clinical practice is far more problematic.

Polyphysicians

Achieving therapeutic goals with fewer drugs is especially difficult in older persons, in whom polypharmacy is the norm. Consequently, any approach to reducing pharmacological burden and making good on the "less is more" philosophy must address and moderate the forces that fuel excessive drug prescribing in this population. First, many older patients are afflicted with more than one chronic disease. This fact, coupled with the increased number of hospitalizations that multiple illnesses bring, makes the simultaneous administration of many different medications, frequently prescribed by *different* physicians, common-place. In this regard, when it comes to excessive drug prescribing, it should be emphasized that the problem of more than one clinician managing the pharmaco-logic aspects of a patient's disease is at the root of much polypharmacy. In other words, "polyphysician" is often the precursor to polypharmacy.

Figure 1-4

PHARMATECTURE™: Guiding Principles

- **Less Is More**

- **Pharm Follows Function**

- **Total Pharmacotherapeutic Quality Management (TPQM)**

- **Sequential Construction**

The Elderly

Elderly patients in emotional distress often seek medical attention under the pretense of having a physical illness. Unfortunately, physicians frequently fail to link the patient's perceived physical complaints with their emotional distress, and instead focus on finding a pharmacotherapeutic solution to each symptom. Consequently, there is a tendency for physicians to consummate outpatient visits, especially from the elderly, with prescriptions for an analgesic, diuretic, hypnotic, or sedative—all because their underlying depression may have produced somatic complaints. Accordingly, fewer unnecessary medications will be introduced into a drug regimen if physicians can tame a well-documented compulsion to service vague symptoms of unclear etiology with pharmacologic therapy.[11,21,82,91]

Communication. Compounding the problems caused by somatic complaints is the difficulty elderly patients have with communication. Many elderly patients are intimidated by health care professionals and are uncomfortable communicating information about drug-related side effects. If physicians do not give patients enough time to express their concerns about drug therapy, create a comfortable climate in which patients can express themselves, and question their own attitudes about what the patient is saying, one or more prescriptions of *questionable* value and safety may be the result. Whenever physicians assess patients' progress from histories provided by caretakers, a special note of caution is necessary. Caretakers may feel frustrated or harrassed by elderly persons with dementia, and may pressure physicians to prescribe medications to help them restore their sense of control over such patients. The result may be the introduction of an unnecessary medication for symptomatic relief or a psychotropic medication that is potent enough to neutralize the patient.

Medication Patterns. There are other reasons that the "less is more" approach is difficult to implement in the elderly population. Besides the presence of multiple diseases, somatic complaints, and communication problems, the elderly also may receive an excessive number of drugs because of the way they take pharmaceuticals. These problems arise because of poor compliance patterns, drug interactions, and decreased tolerance to drugs. Although compliance is a major obstacle in many patients, it is a particularly vexing problem in the elderly.[8,22,45,75,85,96] Many elderly patients suffer from diminished hearing, poor vision, and joint disease. These conditions may leave them unable to understand instructions regarding drug intake, make it difficult to swallow large tablets, read labels, and open container lids, especially if they are of the child-proof variety.

Older persons may have cultural attitudes that make taking certain drugs at odds with long-standing beliefs, and others cannot reach the pharmacist or physician because of a lack of transportation. As a result of these problems, a significant percentage of elderly patients do not take medications they need, and this leads to a poor clinical response. Unless noncompliance is recognized as a potential cause of such therapeutic failures, physicians may be prone to *increasing* dosages and frequencies of *existing* drugs, or worse, to prescribe additional medications.[8,97]

Side Effects. In addition, the large number of daily drugs consumed by many older persons, combined with their inability to tolerate the effects of many pharmaceuticals, increases their susceptibility to adverse drug reactions and toxicity.[36,60,64,77,98] This is especially true for gastrointestinal intolerance associated with NSAID use, for CNS depression with benzodiazepines, for anticholinergic effects of diphenhydramine, for the nocturnal cough associated with ACE inhibitors, the depression induced by beta-blockers,[99,100,101] and the somnolence caused by heterocyclic antidepressants. In some cases, physicians may not recognize new symptoms as being due to drug effects, especially if one or more of the problematic drugs was prescribed by *another* physician, or if it is an over-the-counter (OTC) agent.[73] As is the case with poor compliance, physicians may prescribe more drugs to treat the effects of *other* drugs whose side effects are *mistaken* for *disease*-mediated exacerbation of symptoms.

Indications. Finally, many elderly patients come to physicians already taking medications that were initially prescribed *without* adequate indications. Occasionally, a drug may have been introduced into a regimen based on a faulty diagnosis. Unfortunately, the elderly tend to be creatures of habit, clinging to these medications like pharmacologic security blankets and refusing to have them eliminated from their drug lists—or even their dosages reduced—despite the clinical wisdom of such modifications.

There are, however, general principles that make it possible to achieve the pharmatectural objective of "less is more". This requires an emphasis on making *specific* diagnoses, obtaining a meticulous history of drug usage, understanding the pharmacology of drugs, simplifying therapeutic regimens, and identifying drug-induced symptoms. In the end, these approaches will be effective only if the primary drug prescriber communicates openly with consulting physicians who, after only a single encounter with the patient, may have prescribed a drug without a full understanding of the patient's overall clinical picture. Systematic application of these principles will produce less costly, safer, and more manageable drug regimens.

Building a Drug House: Sequential Construction

Architects understand that buildings must follow an ordered sequence of construction. First, the foundation is laid, then the house is framed, then windows are inserted, electrical and plumbing systems installed, and only then, is the finish work begun. The more complicated the house, the more painstaking and specific the sequence of adding these elements. The same is true for drug houses, which also must follow *sequential construction*. What this means is that there are many different options for treating patients and, in general, drug prescribing also should follow a sequential order. From a pharmatectural perspective, this means prescribing as drugs of first choice those agents shown to work most of the time at a reasonable cost while incurring minimal toxicity. Monotherapeutic agents with regimen durability and dose stability are recommended as initial choices, or "foundation" drugs. Only if these medications fail should the next tier of drugs be introduced into the drug regimen. This process continues with the progressive addition of more expensive or toxic medications until therapeutic results are achieved.

There are many diseases for which drug houses are frequently constructed in poor sequence. One common example is the premature use of theophylline for the management of chronic obstructive pulmonary disease. Although theophylline is indicated for the treatment of bronchospastic pulmonary disease, it is associated with more side effects and risk of toxicity than other therapeutic options, such as inhaled beta-agonists or inhaled steroids. In these patients, sequential pharmacologic construction might begin with a trial of an inhaled beta-agonist such as albuterol (Proventil®). If the patient does not seem to be responding to the beta-agonist, the next step is to *teach* the patient once again how to use the inhaler appropriately. Studies show that many patients use inhalers like breath freshener spray or room deodorizers, and poor results may reflect inadequate medication use rather than the failure of the drug. If the patient is adequately instructed and *still* fails therapy, then inhaled steroids should be added. If both inhaled steroids and beta-agonists fail, sequential addition of theophylline (Theo-Dur®) and oral prednisone therapy can be considered.

Sequential construction is an important cost-saving and side effect sparing maneuver that should be employed when building complicated drug houses in patients who seem to require increasingly intensive therapy to produce therapeutic results.

Pharmatectural Substitution

In an era characterized by intense scrutiny of drug costs,[94,102,103] the concept of therapeutic substitution was introduced to permit pharmacy-based substitution of less expensive, but therapeutically equivalent, pharmacologic alternatives. In general, such substitutions are sanctioned only when bioequivalency is demonstrated between less and more expensive alternatives. (i.e., generic versus trade name drugs), or in the case of two different chemical compounds, when the two drugs are shown to produce virtually equivalent therapeutic results.

From a pharmatectural perspective, drug substitution is an extremely simplistic concept and, what is more worrisome, is associated with the risk of using drugs that *appear* to be interchangeable based on their chemical properties but, in fact, yield very different clinical outcomes in the "real world." To address the potential limitations of adherence to this concept, the pharmatectural perspective on therapeutic substitution pays homage to a wide range of parameters—chemical, behavioral, financial, perceptual, toxicological—that influence therapeutic endpoints, and which must be considered when assessing the substitutability of one drug for another.

This approach, called "pharmatectural substitution", acknowledges that many different factors come into play when evaluating whether two drugs are actually substitutable for one another. Pharmatectural substitution stresses that, in the *real world* of pharmacotherapeutic management, two drugs are substitutable only if they overlap on all the following parameters:

- **Smartness.** To ensure equal performance, the drug being considered as a substitute must be as smart as the drug it will replace. In other words, it must have an equally comprehensive range of indications and provide the same degree of pharmacologic efficacy.
- **Daily dose frequency.** To ensure comparable compliance, the drug considered as a possible substitute should be dosed on the same daily basis, or *less frequently* than the drug being considered for replacement.
- **Side effect profile.** The drug considered as a possible substitute should have the same or a more advantageous side effect profile as the drug being considered for replacement.
- **Drug-drug compatibility.** The drug interaction profile of the drug being considered as a possible substitute should be the same or more desirable than for the drug being considered for replacement.
- **Drug-disease compatibility.** The drug-disease interaction profile of the drug being considered as a possible substitute should be the same or more desirable than for the drug being considered for replacement.
- **Cost.** Drugs evaluated for possible exchange must either cost the same, or the potential substitute must cost less than the drug being replaced.

Two drugs are considered candidates for pharmaceutical substitution only if they satisfy *all* the equivalency parameters as outlined above. The importance of satisfying all the aforementioned criteria is easily illustrated. For example, if I have drug A in one hand and drug B in another, and these two agents satisfy all the criteria mentioned, except drug A is dosed *three* times a day and drug B is dosed *once* a day, are these two medications pharmatecturally substitutable? The answer is "No". Why? Because the drug dosed three times daily will be associated with compromised compliance, and therefore, is likely to produce therapeutically less satisfactory results than the once-daily medication. If drug A and B are similar in every respect, except drug B produces inhibition of the p-450 cytochrome oxidase system, are these agents pharmatecturally equivalent? Again, the answer is "No," because drug B, especially in a patient with multiple medications has the potential to produce clinically significant drug interactions. If the two agents meet all the aforementioned parameters, but drug A is likely to cause conduction abnormalities in the heart, but drug B has no such liability, are these two agents pharmatecturally or, for that matter, therapeutically, equivalent? Once again, "No", because one may produce exacerbation of an underlying cardiac condition while the other drug is free of such complications.

It should be stressed that pharmatectural substitution supports drug substitutions for the purpose of cost savings. But it attempts to ensure that two drugs behave in the same way and produce equivalent outcomes in actual clinical practice. The key to any drug substitution or comprehensive prescribing system is flexibility, something pharmatecture encourages.

Pharm Follows Function

The caveat that pharmacology should follow function, or more simply, "pharm follows function," plays a governing role in the pharmatectural approach to drug regimen design. This concept has broad implications for how pharmacists and physicians should think about building safe, cost-effective drug houses. In fact, from these three simple words issue a prescribing directive that occupies the intellectual nexus point of the entire pharmatecture system: Pharmacologic interventions, rather than simply being pegged to *diseases,* should serve the *functional objectives* of specific patients and address their unique constellation of conditions. Not surprisingly, virtually all pharmatectural principles either directly or indirectly flow from this caveat.

Many readers, of course, will recognize that this pharmatectural guidepost is inspired by the time-honored architectural mandate, "form follows function."[1] An understanding of how this conceptual beacon changed the face of modern architecture will help illuminate the strategic importance of applying "pharm follows function" principles to the domain of clinical pharmacology.

Although function has always played an important role in architecture, for many centuries, the final form that buildings took was based as much on ornamental concerns as it was on functional needs. In the early 1900s, however, with the rise of modern architecture, these attitudes changed dramatically, and it was the Chicago architect, Louis Sullivan, who popularized the notion that "form follows function." What this meant, from a practical point of view, was that *functional* objectives now emerged as the major determinants of architectural design, and they became the primary generators of the final form a house or skyscraper would take. Under the auspices of this scheme, buildings no longer would be constructed according to styles, the whims of fashion, or time-pegged preferences for one kind of ornamental flourish versus another. Instead, buildings would be shaped almost exclusively according to the functional needs programmed by the architectural work.

Tailoring Therapy. In a similar manner, functional needs and clinical objectives should also predominate in the design of drug houses. Extrapolation from numerous clinical trials suggests that the most cost-effective, therapeutically specific, and safest drug regimens are constructed around the principle that pharm follows function. This scheme represents a significant departure from the approaches that have governed prescribing practices in the past. For so long, most drug therapy has been symptom- or disease-oriented. In other words, the clinician identified a disease and then prescribed a drug for that condition. If another disease or symptom surfaced, another drug was added, and before long the patient would be taking several different agents, some of which might be redundant or, even worse, conflict with other drugs in the regimen or with underlying conditions.

Generally speaking, redundant, excessive, suboptimal, and costly drug houses are a byproduct of poorly integrated medication regimens that are built around disease states, rather than around functional needs and end-organ requirements. The reality is, diseases are characterized by a range of pathophysiological abnormalities, end-organ disturbances, metabolic alterations, and clinical derangements. Regardless of the disease, each patient has a unique cluster of these abnormalities, and pharmacologic therapy must follow, or service, the specific mix of symptoms and target organ needs.

In short, pharm must follow function. Until recently, this concept was very difficult to apply to clinical practice. Now, however, this approach is very feasible because we are able to characterize, quantify, and analyze many different parameters associated with a disease state, and then generate a composite picture of how these features affect the patient. This permits a better, more tailored fit between drug and patient. In fact, from a pharmatectural perspective, it no longer makes sense, and, therefore, it is not clinically useful to say, "This patient has 'hypertension,' or 'diabetes,' or 'heart disease,' " and then go on to match a drug with the appropriate condition. Sophisticated diagnostic techniques allow a broader and more in-depth characterization of clinical disorders, thus permitting drugs to be chosen that provide a more tailored fit to the patient's functional needs and clinical abnormalities. It follows that, because diseases express themselves in *different* ways in *different* individuals, the pharmacologically integrated approach to drug therapy recognizes that every patient with hypertension, depression, or arthritis, is different from all the other patients in a particular group, despite the fact they may carry the same disease label. Consequently, their pharmacologic needs also will be different.

The Disease Kaleidoscope. The pharm follows function approach to medication prescribing addresses these patient variations and, in the process, suggests an entirely new mechanism for constructing drug regimens. One analogy that is helpful for illustrating how pharm follows function applies to clinical pharmacotherapeutics, is to think of a disease as a kaleidoscope. In this kaleidoscope, the number, shape, and size of the colored glass shards and pieces remain constant. Now think of the colored fragments as different abnormalities associated with a particular disease, such as, say, high blood pressure. In this kaleidoscope of hypertension, imagine red represents renal function, yellow represents left ventricular mass, green represents lipid profile, purple represents cerebrovascular disease, etc. In addition, let's assume the more color a piece transmits, the greater the severity of the problem and vice versa. Now, depending how you turn the tube and how the components fall, they will create a different image, sometimes with one color (disease abnormality) or intensity (severity) predominating, and sometimes with others making a stronger showing.

In other words, each patient exhibits a different face of a particular disease state. In fact, there are as many faces as there are kaleidoscopic arrangements. Accordingly, one individual may have a little bit of this and a lot of that, and another may have a lot of this and little bit of that. For example, one patient with hypertension may have elevated cholesterol, mild kidney dysfunction, a history of a previous heart attack, diastolic hypertension, and diabetes. However, with a slight rotation in the kaleidoscope of hypertension, the colors rearrange themselves and we can see yet another patient—one with primarily systolic blood pressure elevation, no heart or renal problems, and an extremely favorable lipid profile. Drug therapy (the "pharm" component) must address the kaleidoscopic mix of objectives and functional goals. The first patient, for example, may benefit from a drug that is smart enough to improve renal function, prevent secondary myocardial infarction, and has a favorable effect on lipid levels, whereas the second patient will benefit most from a drug with established efficacy in *systolic* hypertension.

What this means is that, in a drug prescribing system in which pharm follows function, physicians no longer use drugs primarily to treat symptoms or diseases. They use drugs to treat individual patients! In other words, drug therapy is integrated—it is linked and targeted to the entire complex of issues requiring attention in a specific patient. As strange as this may seem, if you ask the practicing pharmatect what drug he or she would use to treat diabetes, depression, high blood pressure, pneumonia, or virtually any other disorder, he or she could not give you an answer. This is because pharmatects do not focus their attention on diseases, per se, but rather they direct their drug therapy at the kaleidoscopic *mix of disease-generated abnormalities and endpoints* as visualized in the *individual* patient.

This is a much different way of approaching drug therapy than has been traditionally practiced. The physician attuned to pharmatectural principles will tailor drug choices and combinations according to the unique mix of needs for a specific patient. To achieve this goal physicians and pharmacists, in collaboration with patients, should list and prioritize the *entire constellation* of functional needs, metabolic abnormalities, pathophysiological derangements, symptom-relief objectives, and prevention goals pertaining to the patient's condition. This detailed list of functional and clinical end points will then generate a drug regimen, and if pharmatectural principles are applied, this regimen will feature either a single smart drug, or the fewest number of drugs, best suited to pharmacologically service the patient's needs. If the diagnoses are accurate and the drugs carefully prescribed with the patient's goals clearly in mind, pharmacology will inevitably follow function, and the result will be a cost-effective, clinically targeted drug house in which pharmacologic redundancy is eliminated and therapeutic efficacy is maximized.

There are numerous clinical examples that testify to the wisdom of this approach. Consider, for example, the myriad therapeutic options available for the treatment of major manic-depressive disorders. The pharmacopiea includes heterocyclic antidepressants, MAO inhibitors, lithium, SSRIs, carbamazepine, and valproic acid. How does one apply the "pharm follows function" concept to help choose among these options? The first step is to identify the functional objectives of the patient. For example, it should be recognized that some patients suffer from debilitating insomnia as a result of depression. In these patients, the functional objectives for pharmacologic intervention include not only alleviation of their depressive symptoms (feelings of sadness, crying spells, low self-esteem, etc.) but also management of sleep dysfunction. In this subset of patients, an SSRI antidepressant such as fluoxetine (Prozac®), with its propensity to cause tremulousness, edginess, and hyperkinesis, might exacerbate the insomnia, whereas a sedating antidepressant such as trazodone (Desyrel®) might be better suited to meet the entire cluster of functional needs.

Other patients may require a different pharmacologic solution. For example, consider the patient with a bipolar manic-depressive disorder, in whom the *manic* component of the illness is the most problematic aspect of the patient's clinical picture. Again, an SSRI might be less desirable than lithium. On the other hand, a depressed patient who must perform job-related duties is prone to sessile behavior, and hypersomnia might benefit from an SSRI, because of its ability to enhance alertness and minimize sedation.

Similar examples illustrating the importance of linking pharmacology with function can be offered for diabetes, heart failure, and hypertension. For example, the patient who has insulin-dependent diabetes mellitus complicated by proteinuria, high blood pressure, and congestive heart failure will have these functional needs best managed by an ACE inhibitor. On the other hand, a diabetic with hypertension whose physical exertion is limited by angina pectoris precipitated by coronary artery disease is best serviced by a slow release calcium channel blocker. And finally, the diabetic hypertensive with a mild elevation of serum cholesterol and benign prostatic hypertrophy might benefit most from a peripheral alpha-blocker such as doxazosin. In every patient, regardless of the disease entity, the most cost-effective, integrated approach to drug therapy will emerge if pharm follows function and if other pharmatectural principles also are applied to the patient's overall therapeutic program.

Total Pharmacotherapeutic Quality Management (TPQM™)

One important aspect of architectural design is Total Quality Management (TQM), a quality-assurance, maintenance, and improvement process that is incorporated into a number of disciplines under similar banners, including continuous quality improvement (CQI), continuous quality management, and other variations. From an architectural point of view, TQM is devoted to producing state-of-the-art buildings that combine the durable and visually pleasing materials into structures that meet the ever-expanding and increasingly complex, range of human and technological needs that contemporary buildings must serve.

Much like the evolving relationship between building materials and architectural design, the relationship between drug therapy and disease states also is in a state of constant flux. In this regard, *new* indications for established drugs are constantly being approved, unexpected drug interactions are reported in postmarketing surveillance studies, and newer agents with less toxicity and expanded indications continually are being introduced. In addition, chronic diseases present an ever-expanding list of associated abnormalities that are either amenable to drug therapy, or, on occasion, even exacerbated by medications once thought to represent drugs of choice.

In the world of pharmatecture, TPQM™ (See Figure 1-5) plays a central role in ensuring that drug regimens and medication choices are periodically reviewed by the physician. Specifically, therapeutic programs should be evaluated and reviewed on a regular basis to ensure that: (1) they have kept pace with newer drugs, developments, and therapeutic options as they surface in the pharmaceutical marketplace; (2) they continue to provide the full range of pharmacologic servicing required by the patient; and (3) they still represent the most cost-effective, compliance-enhancing approach to drug therapy for the patient's clinical needs.

Quality Choices. The power of TPQM as an assessment and quality assurance tool is best explained using an historical example. For example, consider a disease such as hypertension which, it is estimated, afflicts as many as 50 million Americans. When it comes to drug therapy, this is just one of many common diseases that has witnessed dramatic changes over the past 20 years. More information is available than ever before to guide clinicians in managing this important public health problem. Unfortunately, this increase in information has made the pharmacotherapeutic choices increasingly complex.

In fact, most of the advances in drug therapy for hypertension can be explained simply by analyzing the shifting emphasis on various clinical aspects and functional end points of this disease. This is where TPQM plays a valuable role in drug therapy. The usefulness of TPQM in building and maintaining state-of-the-art drug houses for common diseases such as hypertension is best illustrated by taking a journey in Jules Verne's time machine. Imagine, for a moment, that we travel back to the year 1975 and find ourselves transported to a doctor's office in St. Louis, Missouri. There, we encounter a family physician who has just recorded an elevated blood pressure reading in a patient and, therefore, is faced

Figure 1-5

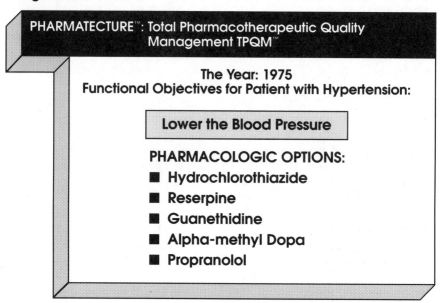

with initiating drug therapy. (Figure 1-5) Let's assume for a moment that the physician is interested in providing TPQM for this patient. To meet this goal, the clinician will ask the following question: "What functional objective(s) am I trying to achieve in this patient?".

Remember, this is 1975! The functional goals for treatment of high blood pressure were limited then. What's more, the full range of therapeutic, functional, preventive, and drug-disease interaction concerns was poorly characterized at this time. In fact, there was only one well-accepted end point in 1975—to lower the diastolic blood pressure to reduce the risk of stroke. In other words, in 1975, applying TPQM in a patient with high blood pressure, required little more than the selection of a drug that would reduce diastolic blood pressure to less than 90 mm Hg. For all practical purposes, this was the only therapeutic goal physicians had during this era.

Consequently, to achieve TPQM almost two decades ago, physicians felt perfectly comfortable selecting from among a smorgasbord of what, in retrospect, are relatively barbaric medications (reserpine, guanethidine, hydralazine, propranolol, alpha-methyldopa, etc.) to accomplish this very limited end point. In other words, these drugs successfully lowered diastolic blood pressure, but they also produced a wide range of undesirable side effects, quality-of-life impairments, and drug-disease interactions that, history would eventually show, patients would prefer to live without. Unfortunately, many patients stopped taking their medication. In fact, one can argue that the side effects associated with these agents oftentimes exceeded the discomfort of hypertension, thus producing an epidemic of noncompliance-induced disease deterioration among Americans with hypertension.

Now let's step back in the time machine and journey to the year 1997. We are transported to an ambulatory care clinic, this time in Portland, Oregon. Here, we encounter a consulting pharmacist and physician discussing options for implementing TPQM in a 70-year old man with newly diagnosed high blood pressure. Things are much different now. In 1997, when these clinicians ask the same question posed by the family practitioner 20 years ago, "What functional end points are we trying to achieve in a patient with hypertension?" something different happens. A new TPQM readout appears (Figure 1-6) There emerges an expanded constellation of target-organ needs, physiological end points, quality-of-life, prevention, and drug-drug and drug-disease interaction issues that must be considered for TPQM in a patient with high blood pressure.

Figure 1-6

PHARMATECHURE™: TPQM™

The Year: 1997
Functional Objectives for Patient With Hypertension:
- Lower blood pressure (J-point curve limits)
- Reduce left ventricular hypertrophy
- Maintain coronary artery perfusion
- Lower blood pressure
- Maintain quality of life: Cognitive function, sexual function, emotional function, sleep function, etc.
- Minimize impairment of cardiac conduction system
- Maintain renal blood flow
- Maintain lipid profile associated with reduced CHD risk
- Preserve myocardial pump function

PHARMACOLOGIC OPTIONS:
Calcium Blocker (Amlodipine, Norvasc®)
Peripheral Alpha-Blocker (Doxazosin, Cardura®)
ACE Inhibitor (Enalapril)

To implement TPQM, for a patient with hypertension in 1997, means satisfying *many different* end points. As in 1975, the diastolic blood pressure still needs to be lowered to less than 90 mm Hg, but studies also demonstrate that caution should be exercised in not lowering diastolic blood pressure too low, especially in frail, older persons with underlying heart disease. In addition, new classifications stress the importance of managing systolic as well as diastolic blood pressure elevations. In addition, TPQM for patients with high blood pressure means recognizing that left ventricular hypertrophy (LVH) is an independent risk factor for morbidity in these patients. Consequently, in persons with this co-existing finding, drugs proven to reduce LVH are preferred.

In addition, drug therapy for high blood pressure also must consider other medical conditions. Abnormalities associated with overlapping disease states—ranging from high blood pressure and heart disease to diabetes, kidney disease, and hyperlipidemia—produce new goals in antihypertensive drug therapy. For example, approximately 40% of patients over the age of 70 who have hypertension also have significant coronary atherosclerosis. Some of these patients may even have coronary artery lesions significant enough to produce silent myocardial ischemia. Hence, the use of antihypertensive agents (i.e., calcium channel blockers, beta-blockers) that can maintain coronary artery perfusion and manage angina should be encouraged, particularly in patients with hypertension and underlying coronary heart disease.[104-109]

Other hypertensive patients, especially those with diabetes, a previous history of myocardial infarction, or congestive heart failure, benefit from ACE inhibitors, which improve outcomes in patients with poor heart function. Still other hypertensive patients have conduction system abnormalities, i.e., they are prone to slow heart rates or disturbances in AV node conduction. Hence, prevention-oriented TPQM would include avoiding drugs that are known to impair impulse conduction in the heart (i.e., verapamil). Finally, about 45% of all hypertensive patients have clinically significant elevations in blood lipid levels. When blood cholesterol levels are elevated or HDL/LDL ratios are low, drugs known to improve lipid profiles and, therefore, reduce coronary heart disease (CHD) risk, are preferable to drug combinations (beta-blocker and thiazide diuretic) that elevate lipid levels.

Although it seems routine now, in 1975, physicians and pharmacists rarely invoked quality-of-life (maintenance and enhancement) issues as essential functional criteria against which to measure the success of their antihypertensive regimens. New attitudes that argue for inclusion of quality-of-life issues in drug therapy are supported by large-scale investigations.[106,110,111,112,113] Clinical trials in recent years confirmed that drugs used for the treatment of high blood pressure can wreak havoc on many cognitive, sexual, and neuropsychiatric parameters (See Figure 1-6).[111,114,115] In the 1990s, quality-of-life maintenance became such a popular cause that pharmacists and physicians became increasingly aware of the importance of including these issues as part of the value-added equation for drug therapy of all kinds. As a result, TPQM for the patient with high blood pressure now means prescribing drugs that meet a wide range of functional needs. It requires drawing upon a different set of pharmacologic options. It means identifying those agents best able to service the *full* set of patient needs—physiological, pharmacological, and functional. Among those options, amlodipine, a calcium channel blocker that is indicated for both high blood pressure and angina, (and has the added benefits of sparing both the conduction system and cardiac pump function), offers a unique window of opportunity for incorporating TPQM in the hypertensive patient. In those hypertensive patients with congestive heart or elevated lipid levels, ACE inhibitors (enalapril) and peripheral alpha-blockers (doxazosin), respectively, also play an important role.

This kind of analysis can be applied to many different outpatient conditions. Regardless of the disease, however, one thing is clear. Periodic reviews of drug regimens that stress TPQM will produce better-tolerated drug combinations that incorporate both prevention and cost-efficacy into the therapeutic program.

Foundations of a Drug Regimen

In the world of building construction, it is well-accepted that a house or skyscraper is only as good as its foundation. It is difficult to expand, remodel, or reconstruct a house with a poor foundation. And so it is with drug regimens. In fact, much of the unnecessary—and, more importantly, avoidable—expenditures fueling drug costs result from the constant reshuffling (adding and subtracting) in polypharmacy drug regimens that is required to keep pharmacologic harmony among different agents. This is called the *pharmacologic "churn factor."* Pharmacologic churning not only incurs direct costs associated with drug discontinuation and initiation, but from adverse drug-related events that produce costly hospitalizations.[36,39,101,116] Most often, these problems arise when pharmacists or physicians initiate long-term drug therapy without considering whether the agent is a good foundation drug, in other words, whether or not it will tend to be *compatible* with the other drugs or diseases that may come into the picture over time. [Please refer to Chapter 3, the Drug-Drug and Drug-Disease Incompatibility Profile (DIP™) System.]

Figure 1-7

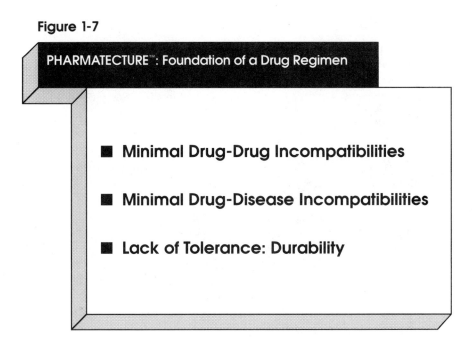

PHARMATECTURE™: Foundation of a Drug Regimen

- ■ **Minimal Drug-Drug Incompatibilities**

- ■ **Minimal Drug-Disease Incompatibilities**

- ■ **Lack of Tolerance: Durability**

Hence, the pharmatectural approach to designing drug regimens, especially those that will require three or more prescription ingredients, stresses the importance of identifying and selecting *centerpiece* drugs as initial therapeutic agents. Centerpiece agents, or foundation drugs (Figure 1-7), should be initiated *early* in the natural history of a chronic disease. These medications are characterized as foundation drugs because they are hospitable to the addition of a wide range of prescription ingredients without incurring drug interactions, and because they can be used safely in the setting of complications that may arise from the primary disease. Centerpiece drugs will be compatible with other *drugs* that are likely to be prescribed over time, as well as other associated conditions or diseases that may evolve as part of the patient's clinical course. The Drug Incompatibility Profile (DIP) system discussed in Chapter 3 provides a practical approach for making drug selections based on these principles.

From a pharmatectural perspective, then, the use of foundation drugs represents an important step in safe cost-effective drug selection. As mentioned, much of the cost associated with long-term drug therapy results from the shuffling of pharmacotherapeutic agents in order to prevent drug interactions. Consequently, one of the most important aspects of constructing safe, cost-effective, long-term drug regimens is selecting agents on a *proactive* basis. Medications with a low-risk for producing drug-drug or drug-disease interactions can serve as a foundation for drug regimens to which additions, alterations, and deletions can be made over time without adversely affecting the natural history of emerging conditions.

Framework

An architectural framework is constructed based on time-honored engineering principles to which the architectural skeleton must adhere. The same is true for pharmatectural constructions, in which compliance, comfort, quality-of-life, and cost-effectiveness constitute important rafters in the framework of all drug regimens. (Figure 1-8) All drug houses must be designed with this framework in mind.

Safety Considerations

All works of architecture must pass a *safety inspection.* Building codes mandate that electrical, heating and cooling, pollution control, and plumbing systems meet basic standards to ensure safety for human use. Safety is an equally important pharmatectural issue. Many safety issues (drug interactions, side effect profiles, polypharmacy, etc.) have already been discussed. But at the root of all safe drug prescribing is the mandate for selecting drugs that have low toxicity and then using these drugs at the lowest effective therapeutic dose. These safety considerations, along with compliance, comfort, quality-of-life, and cost-efficacy constitute the full pharmatectural framework for drug regimen construction.

Figure 1-8

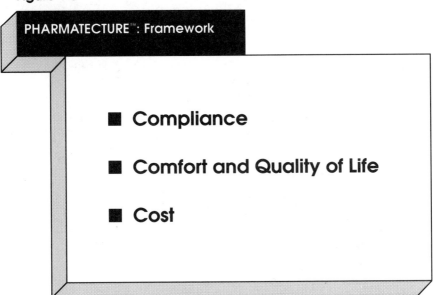

PHARMATECTURE™: Framework

- **Compliance**

- **Comfort and Quality of Life**

- **Cost**

Styles of Pharmatecture

A New York skyline, with its variegated collection of skyscrapers, serves as a vivid testimonial to a wide range of architectural styles. In fact, there may be almost as many styles as there are architects. In the world of drug prescribing, there are also *stylistic* differences in the way pharmacists and physicians select and combine medications. (Figure 1-15) These stylistic variations have important therapeutic and policy implications. The wide range of prescribing styles suggests there is no universally accepted system for designing safe, intelligent, and cost-effective drug regimens. It also suggests that physicians have failed to reach a consensus on what the principal goals should be in drug prescribing, such as what factors (cost, smartness, side effects, convenience, etc.) are most important.

It is staggering to observe just how different drug prescribing styles are. For example, in most of the symposia on drug prescribing that I have conducted, I present physicians and pharmacists in attendance with a patient case study, and ask them to design what they feel is an appropriate drug regimen. It is remarkable how many different drug houses are constructed for the same patient! Some physicians may build their drug house using four prescription drugs, whereas another may prescribe only two drugs. Perhaps, this is the art of drug prescribing. No matter what you call it, and regardless of how tenaciously we may cling to our particular style of drug prescribing, there always are better and worse approaches to drug regimen design.

From a pharmatectural perspective, we say there is Victorian architecture, and there is Victorian pharmatecture. The analogy is very instructive. Victorian houses generally consist of a warren of small rooms, with each room being pegged to a specific human function. Victorian pharmatecture is similar, in that many drugs are prescribed for different conditions in a single patient.

Although a consensus on drug prescribing is difficult to build, we need to move away from traditional drug prescribing approaches toward more contemporary strategies, i.e., those that emphasize simpler, integrated drug regimens that are constructed with an eye towards prevention, enhancing compliance, and minimizing drug interactions.

Kitsch Pharmatecture

The world of architecture is replete with numerous examples of wacky, bombastic, or otherworldly building designs, many of which fall into the category of "Roadside Americana." Architectural critics have dubbed these works, "kitsch architecture," to highlight the fact that they are whimsical, vernacular works.

Unfortunately, pharmacists and physicians acknowledge that there is also "Kitsch Pharmatecture." (Figure 1-9) Kitsch pharmatecture refers to those drug additions, deletions, and alterations made by the *patient,* without pharmacist or physician collaboration. In this regard, OTC drugs may be added to the regimen, medications are exchanged, dosing schedules are altered, and a work of kitsch pharmatecture is created.

Kitsch pharmatecture can take many different forms. For example, a patient taking an anti-Parkinsonism drug with anticholinergic properties may go to the pharmacy and purchase diphenhydramine (Benadryl®) for self-treatment of allergy symptoms. The anticholinergic properties from the two drugs in combination may be enough to produce urinary retention. Another patient may be prescribed an NSAID such as nabumetone (Relafen®), and then purchase OTC ibuprofen, failing to understand that the two drugs in combination may produce serious gastrointestinal side effects.

The widespread prevalence of kitsch pharmatecture emphasizes the importance of obtaining comprehensive drug histories from patients. These histories must be meticulous and make a special effort to identify OTC agents that may be undermining the established drug house constructed by the practitioner. Kitsch pharmatecture will become an increasing problem as more prescription agents gain approval for OTC distribution.

Figure 1-9

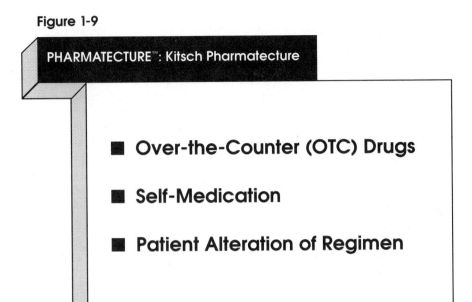

PHARMATECTURE™: Kitsch Pharmatecture

- **Over-the-Counter (OTC) Drugs**

- **Self-Medication**

- **Patient Alteration of Regimen**

Remodeling

Great old buildings frequently don't stand the test of time, unless they have been remodeled to address current needs and stylistic preferences. The same is true for drug houses. The aim of the pharmatecture program is to critically evaluate drug regimens and then, based on good clinical trials, *desconstruct* and *reconstruct* the drug house so it makes use of smart, safe drugs that service all the functional objectives of a particular patient. This deconstruction and reconstruction must be gradual, and is discussed in more detail in the following chapters.

[1]Jordan LK 3d, Jordan LO. Prudent prescribing. Prescribing suggestions for physicians. NC Med J 1992 Nov; 53(11):585-8.

[2]Parrish RH. Understanding physician prescribing behavior. Am J Hosp Pharm 1991 March; 48(3):463.

[3]Reus VI. Rational polypharmacy in the treatment of mood disorders. Ann Clin Psychiatry 1993 June; 5(2):91-100.

[4]Burns LR, Denton M, Goldfein S, Warrick L, Morenz B, Sales B. The use of continuous quality improvement methods in the development and dissemination of medical practice guidelines. QRB 1992 Dec; 18(12):434-9.

[5]Chinburapa V, Larson LN. The importance of side effects and outcomes in differentiating between prescription drug products. J Clin Pharm Ther 1992 Dec; 17(6):333-42.

[6]Kahl A, Blandford DH, Krueger K, Zwick DI. Geriatric education centers address medication issues affecting older adults. Public Health Reports - Hyattsville 1992 Jan-Feb; 107(1):37-47.

[7]Lamy, PP. Adverse drug effects. Clin Geriatr Med 1990; 6:293-305.

[8]Lexchin J. Why are we still poisoning the elderly so often? Canadian Family Physician 1993 Nov; 39:2298-300, 2304-7.

[9]Peck CC, Temple RJ, Collins JM. Drug interactions: The death pen. JAMA 1993 Sept 15; 270(11):1317.

[10]Beers MH, Fingold SF, Ouslander JG, Ruben DB, Morgenstern H, Beck JC. Characteristics and quality of prescribing by doctors practicing in nursing homes. J Am Geriatr Soc 1993 Aug; 41(8);802-7.

[11]Beers MH, Ouslander JG, Fingold SF, Morgenstern H, Ruben DB, Rogers W, Zeffren MJ, Beck JC. Inappropriate medication prescribing in skilled-nursing facilities. Ann Intern Med 1992 Oct 15; 117(8):684-9.

[12]Belitsos NJ. Overprescribing of benzodiazepine hypnotic drugs in the elderly [letter; comment]. Am J Med 1991 Sept; 91(3):321.

[13]Bjornson DC, Rector TS, Daniels CE, Wertheimer AI, Snowdon DA, Litman TJ. Impact of drug-use review program intervention of prescribing after publication of a randomized clinical trial. Am J Hosp Pharm 1990 July; 47(7):1541-6.

[14]Bliss MR. Prescribing for the elderly. BMJ 1981; 282:203-6.

[15]LeSage J. Polypharmacy in geriatric patients. Nurs Clin North Am 1991 June; 26(2):273-90.

[16]Peck CC, Temple R, Collins JM. Understanding consequences of concurrent therapies. JAMA 1993 March 24; 269(12):1550-52.

[17]Thomas DR. "The brown bag" and other approaches to decreasing polypharmacy in the elderly. NC Med J 1991 Nov; 52(11):565-6.

[18]Ungvarski P, Schmidt J. Polypharmacy: dangers of multiple-drug therapy in patients with immuno-deficiency virus infection. Home Healthcare Nurse 1993 March-April; 11(2):68-69.

[19]Valentine C. Use computers to detect inappropriate prescription. BMJ 1993 July 3; 307(6895):61.

[20]Bloom JA, Frank JW, Shafir MS, Martiquet P. Potentially undesirable prescribing and drug use among the elderly. Measurable and remediable. Canadian Family Physician 1993 Nov; 39:2337-45.

[21]Brahams D. Benzodiazepine overprescribing: successful initiative in New York State. Lancet 1990 Dec 1; 336(8727):1372-3.

[22]Weintraub M. Compliance in the elderly. Clin Geriatr Med 1990; 6:445-52.

[23]Roth HP, Caron HS. Accuracy of doctor's estimates and patients' statements on adherence to a drug regimen. Clin Pharmacol Ther 1978; 23;361-70.

[24]Oates LN, Scholz MJ, Hoffert MJ. Polypharmacy in a headache center population. Headache 1993 Sept; 33(8):436-8.

[25]Olfson M, Pincus HA, Sabshin M. Pharmacotherapy in outpatient psychiatric practice. Am J Psychiatry 1994 April; 151(4):580-5.

[26]Ashburn PE. Polypharmacy in skilled-nursing facilities. Ann Intern Med 1993 April 15; 118(8):649-50; discussion 650-1.

[27]Collins TM, Zimmerman DR. Programs for monitoring inappropriate prescribing of controlled drugs; evaluation and recommendations. Am J Hosp Pharm 1992 July; 49(7):1765-8.

[28]Beardon PH, McGilchrist MM, McKendrick AD, McDevitt DG, MacDonald TM. Primary non-compliance with prescribed medication in primary care. BMJ 1993 Oct; 307(6908):846-8.

[29]Berg JS, Dischler J, Wagner DJ, Raia JJ, Palmer-Shevlin N. Medication compliance; a healthcare problem. Ann Pharmacother 1993 Sept; 27(9 Suppl):S1-24.

[30]Botelho RJ, Dudrak R. 2d. Home assessment of adherence to long-term medication in the elderly. J Fam Prac 1992 July; 35(1):61-5.

[31]Eisen SA, Miller DK, Woodward RS, Spitznagel E, Przybeck TR. The effect of prescribed daily dose frequency on patient medication compliance. Arch Intern Med 1990 Sept; 150(9):1881-4.

[32]Jones JK. Assessing potential risk of drugs: The elusive target. Ann Intern Med 1992 Oct 15; 117(8):691-692.

[33]Litchman HM. Medication noncompliance: a significant problem and possible strategies. Rhode Island Medicine 1993 Dec; 76(12):608-10.

[34]Lamy PP. A "risk" approach to adverse drug reactions. J Am Geriatr Soc 1988; 36:79.

[35]Larson EB. et al. Adverse drug reactions associated with global cognitive impairment in elderly persons. Ann Intern Med 1987; 107:169-173.

[36]Col N, Franale JE, Kronholm P. The role of medication and adverse drug reactions in hospitalizations of the elderly. Arch Intern Med 1990 April; 150(4):841-5.

[37]Futrell DP. Drug compliance, Are you getting the most out of your medicine? NC Med J 1993 Oct; 54(10):523-4.

[38]Hood JC, Murphy JE. Patient noncompliance can lead to hospital readmissions. Hospitals 1978; 52:79-82, 84.

[39]McNally DL, Wertheimer D. Strategies to reduce the high cost of patient noncompliance. Md Med J 1992 March; 41(3):223-5.

[40]Steiner JF, Robbins LJ, Roth SC, Hammond WS. The effect of prescription size on acquisition of maintenance medications. J Gen Intern Med 1993 June; 8(6):306-10.

[41]Stewart RB, Caranasos GJ. Medication compliance in the elderly. Med Clin North America 1989; 73:1551-1563.

[42]Sclar DA, Chin A, Skaer TL, Okamoto MP, Nakahiro RK, Gill MA. Effect of health education in promoting prescription refill compliance among patients with hypertension. Clin Ther 1991 July-August; 13(4):489-95.

[43]Deyo RA, Inui TS, Sullivan B. Noncompliance with arthritis drugs: magnitude, correlates, and clinical implications. J Rheumatol 1981; 8:931-36.

[44]Conn VS, Taylor SG, Kelley S. Medication regimen complexity and adherence among older adults. Journal of Nursing Scholarship 1991 Winter; 23(4):231-5.

[45]Lamy PP. Compliance in long-term care. Geriatrika 1985; 1(8):32.

[46]Cochrane RA, Mandal AR, Ledger-Scott M, Walker R. Changes in drug treatment after discharge from hospital in geriatric patients. BMJ 1992 Sept 19; 305(6855):694-6.

[47]Anonymous. Prescription drugs and older consumers issued August 10, 1990. Michigan-Medicine 1991 Feb; 90(2):27-31.

[48]Anonymous. Writing prescription instructions. Can Med Assoc J 1991 March 15; 144(6):647-8.

[49]Coleman TJ. Non-redemption of prescriptions. Linked to poor consultation. BMJ 1994 Jan 8; 308(6921):135.

[50]Ito S, Koren G, Einarson TR. Maternal noncompliance with antibiotics during breastfeeding. Ann of Pharmacother 1993 Jan; 27(1):40-2.

[51]Park DC, Morrell RW, Frieske D, Kincaid D. Medication adherence behaviors in older adults; effects of external cognitive supports. Psychology & Aging 1992 June; 7(2):252-6.

[52]Knight JR, Campbell AJ, Williams SM, Clark DW. Knowledgeable noncompliance with prescribed drugs in elderly subjects—a study with particular reference to nonsteroidal antiinflammatory and antidepressant drugs. J Clin Pharm Ther 1991 April; 16(2):131-7.

[53]Macdonald ET, Macdonald JB, Phoenix M. Improving drug compliance after hospital discharge. BMJ 1977: 2:618-621.

[54]Phillips SL, Carr-Lopez SM. Impact of a pharmacist on medication discontinuation in a hospital-based geriatric clinic. Am J Hosp Pharm 1990 May; 47(5):1075-9.

[55]Green LW, Purrell CO, Koop CE, et al. Programs to reduce drug errors in the elderly: direct and indirect evidence from patient education. Improving Medication Compliance, Reston, Va: National Pharm Council, 1985.

[56]Kucukarslan S, Hakim Z, Sullivan D, Taylor S, Grauer D, Haugtvedt C, Zgarrick D. Points to consider about prescription drug prices: an overview of federal policy and pricing studies. Clin Ther 1993 July-Aug; 15(4):726-38.

[57]Skaer TL, Sclar DA, Markowski DJ, Won JK. Effect of value-added utilities on prescription refill compliance and Medicaid health care expenditures—a study of patients with non-insulin dependent diabetes mellitus. J Clin Pharm Ther 1993 Aug; 18(4):295-9.

[58]Jordan LK. 3d., Jordan LO. Prudent prescribing. Prescribing suggestions for physicians. NC Med J 1992 Nov; 53(11):585-8.

[59]Keen PJ. What is the best dosage schedule for patients? J R Soc Med 1991 Nov; 84(11):640-1.

[60]Granek E, et al. Medications and diagnosis in relation to falls in a long-term care facility. J Am Geriatric Soc 1987; 35:505.

[61]Cormack MA, Howells E. Factors linked to the prescribing of benzodiazepines by general practice principals and trainees. Fam Pract 1992 Dec; 9(4):466-71.

[62]Hamilton IJ, Reay LM, Sullivan FM. A survey of general practitioners' attitudes to benzodiazepine overprescribing. Health Bulletin 1990 Nov; 48(6):299-303.

[63]Bauman JH. Kimelblatt BJ. Cimetidine as an inhibitor of drug metabolism: therapeutic implications and review of the literature. Drug Intell Clin Pharm 1982; 16:380.

[64]Greenblatt DJ, Shader RI. Anticholinergics. N Engl J Med 1984; 288(23):1215-1218.

[65]Nesbit F. Noncompliance with psychotropic drug prescriptions. Am J Psychiatry 1994 May; 152(5):783-4.

[66]Halpern MT, Irwin DE, Brown RE, Clouse J, Hatziandreu EJ. Patient adherence to prescribed potassium supplement therapy. Clin Ther 1993 Nov-Dec; 15(6):1133-45; discussion 1120.

[67]Held P. Effects of beta-blockers on ventricular dysfunction after myocardial infarction: tolerability and survival effects. Am J Cardiol 1993 March 25; 71(9):39C-44C.

[68]Johnston D, Duffin D. Drug-patient interactions and their relevance in the treatment of heart failure. Am J Cardiol 1992 Oct 8; 70(10):109C-112C.

[69]Hussar DA. New drugs of 1993. Am Pharm 1994 March; NS34(3):24-47, 51-6; quiz 57-9.

[70]Huszonek JJ, Dewan MJ, Koss M, Hardoby WJ, Ispahani A. Antidepressant side effects and physician prescribing patterns Ann Clin Psychiatry 1993 March ; 5(1):7-11.

[71]Inman W, Pearce G. Prescriber profile and post-marketing surveillance. Lancet 1993 Sept 11; 342(8872):658-61.

[72]Colley CA, Lucas LM. Polypharmacy: the cure becomes the disease. Gen Intern Med 1993 May; 8(5):278-83.

[73]Holden MD. Over-the-counter medications: Do you know what your patients are taking? Postgrad Med 1992 June; 91(8):191-194, 199-200.

[74]Kroenke K, Pinholt EM. Reducing polypharmacy in the elderly. A controlled trial of physician feedback. J Am Geriatr Soc 1990 Jan; 38(1):31-6.

[75]Montamat SC, Cusak B. Overcoming problems with polypharmacy and drug misuse in the elderly. Clin Geriatr Med 1992 Feb; 8(1):143-58.

[76]Frishman WH. Beta-adrenergic blockers as cardioprotective agents. Am J Cardiol 1992 Dec 21; 70(21):21-61.

[77]Downs GE, Linkewich JA, DiPalma JR. Drug interactions in elderly diabetics. Geriatrics 1986; 36(7):45.

[78]Hood, WB, Jr. Role of converting enzyme inhibitors in the treatment of heart failure. J Am Coll Cardiol 1993 Oct; 22(4 Suppl a):154A-157A..

[79]Khosla S, Somberg J. Mild heart failure: why the switch to ACE inhibitors? Geriatrics 1993 Nov; 48(11):47-8, 51-4.

[80]Pfeffer M. Angiotensin converting enzyme inhibition in congestive heart failure: benefit and perspective. Am Heart J 1993 Sept; 126(3 Pt 2):789-93.

[81]Richard C, Thuillez C, Depret J, Auzepy P, Giudicelli JF. Regional hemodynamic effects of perindopril in congestive heart failure. Am Heart J 1993 Sept; 126(3 Pt 2):782-8.

[82]Chinburapa V, Larson LN, Brucks M, Draugalis J, Bootman JL, Puto CP. Physician prescribing decisions: the effects of situational involvement and task complexity on information acquisition and decision making. Soc Sci Med 1993 June; 36(11):1473-82.

[83]De Santis G, Harvey KJ, Howard D, Mashford ML, Moulds RF. Improving the quality of antibiotic prescription patterns in general practice. The role of educational intervention. Med Aust 1994 April 18; 160(8):502-5.

[84]Reveilleau S, Boissel JP, Alamercery Y. Do prescribers know the results of key clinical trials? GEP (Groupe d'etude do la Prescription). Fundam Clin Pharacol 1991; 5(4):265-73.

[85]Davidson W, Molloy DW, Somers G, Bedard M. Relation between physician characteristics and prescribing for elderly people in New Brunswick. Can Med Assoc J 1994 March 15; 150(6):917-21.

[86]Holt WS Jr., Mazzuca SA. Prescribing behaviors of family physicians in the treatment of osteoarthritis. Fam Med 1992 Sept-Oct; 24(7):524-7.

[87]Hux JE, Levinton CM, Naylor CD. Prescribing propensity; influence of life-expectancy gains and drug costs. J Gen Inter Med 1994 April; 9(4):195-201.

[88]Mant A, Saunders NA. Polypharmacy in the elderly. Med J Aust 1990 June 4; 152(11):613.

[89]Stewart RB, Yedinak KC, Ware MR. Polypharmacy in psychiatry: three case studies and methods for prevention. Ann Pharmacother 1992 April; 26(4):529-33.

[90]American college of Physicians Improving medical education in therapeutics. Ann Intern Med 1988; 108:145-147.

[91]Greenblat RM, Hollander H, McMaster JR, Henke CJ. Polypharmacy among patients attending an AIDS clinic: utilization of prescribed, unorthodox, and investigational treatments. J Acquir Immune Defic Syndr 1991; 4(2):136-43.

[92]Meyer TJ, Van Kooten D, Marsh S, Prochazka AV. Reduction of polypharmacy by feedback to clinicians. J Gen Intern Med 1991 March-April: 6(2):133-6.

[93]Lisi DM. Reducing polypharmacy. J Am Geriatr Society 1991 Jan; 39(1):103-5.

[94]Abernathy DR, Andrawis NS. Critical drug interactions: A guide to important examples. Drug Ther 1993; Cot 15-27.

[95]Safavi KT, Hayward RA. Choosing between apples and apples: physicians' choices of prescription drugs that have similar side effects and efficacies. Gen Intern Med 1992 Jan-Feb; 7(1):32-7.

[96]Nolan L, O'Malley K. Prescribing for the elderly. Part II. Prescribing patterns: differences due to age. J Am Geriatr Soc 1988; 36:245-254.

[97]Poulsen RL. Some current factors influencing the prescribing and use of psychiatric drugs. Public Health Reports - Hyattsville 1992 Jan-Feb; 107(1):47-53.

[98]Gilley J. Towards rational prescribing. BMJ 1994 March 19; 308(6931):731-2.

[99]Medications for the elderly. A report of the Royal College of Physicians. J R Coll of Physicians 1984; 18:7-17.

[100]Montamat SC, Cusak BJ, Vestal RE. Management of drug therapy in the elderly. N Engl J Med 1989; 321:303-309.

[101]Pickles H, Fuller S. Prescriptions, adverse reactions, and the elderly. Lancet 1986; 2(8497):40.

[102]Berger MS. A proposal for using generics. Pa Med 1993 May; 96(5)10.

[103]Ellmers SE. Limiting the drugs list. The trouble with generic prescribing. BMJ 1993 June 19; 306(6893):1687.

[104]Ben-Ishay D, Leibel B, Stessman J. Calcium channel blockers in the management of hypertension in the elderly. Am J Med 1986; (81 Suppl 6a)81:30-34.

[105]Abernethy DR, Schwartz JB, Plachetka JR, et al. Comparison in young and elderly patients of pharmacodynamics and disposition of labetalol in systemic hypertension. Am J Cardiol 1987; 60:697-702.

[106]Ahronheim J. Practical pharmacology for older patients; avoiding adverse drug effects. Mt Sinai J Med 1993 Nov; 60(6):497-501.

[107]Amery A, et al. Mortality and morbidity results from the European working party on high blood pressure in the elderly. Lancet 1985; 1:1349-1354.

[108]Amir M, Cristal N, Bar-On D, Loidl A. Does the combination of ACE inhibitor and calcium antagonist control hypertension and improve quality of life? The LOMIR-MCT-IL study experience. Blood Pressure 1994; Suppl 1:40-2.

[109]Ancill RJ, Carlyle WW, Liang RA, Holliday SG. Agitation in the demented elderly: a role for the benzodiazepines?. Int Clin Psychopharmacol 1991 Winter; 6(3):141-6.

[110]Baxter JD. Minimizing the side effects of glucocorticoid therapy. [Review] Adv Intern Med 1990; 35:173-93.

[111]Bulpitt CJ, Fletcher AE. Drug treatment and quality of life in the elderly. [Review] Clin Geriatr Med 1990 May; 6(2):309-17.

[112]Coons SJ, Kaplan RM. Assessing health-related quality of life: application to drug therapy. Clin Ther 1992; 14(6):850-8; discussion 849.

[113]deBoer JB, van Dan FS, Sprangers MA, Frissen PH, Lange JM. Longitudinal study on the Quality of Life of symptomatic HIV-infected patients in a trial of zidovudine versus zidovudine and interferon-alpha. AIDS 1993 July; 7(7):947-53.

[114]Dimenas E, Wallander MA, Svardsudd K, Wiklund I. Aspects of quality of life on treatment with felodipine. Euro J Clin Pharmacol 1991; 40(2):141-7.

[115]Fletcher AE, Battersby C, Adnitt P, Underwood N, Jurgensen HJ, Bulpitt CJ. Quality of life on antihypertensive therapy: a double-blind trial comparing quality of life on pinacidil and nifedipine

in combination with a thiazide diuretic. European Pinacidil Study Group. J Cardiovas Pharmaco 1992 July; 20(1):108-14.

[116]Gibaldi M. Prescription drugs and health care reform. Pharmacotherapy 1993 Nov-Dec; 13(6):583-9.

2

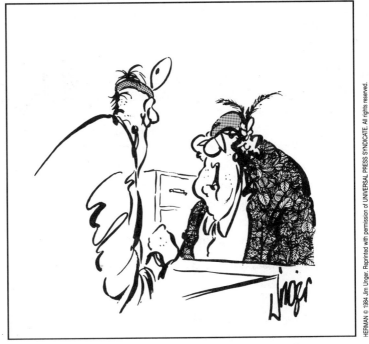

"I feel a lot better since I ran out of those pills you gave me."

Drug House Construction: Principles Put Into Practice

The blueprint for drug regimen construction is now in place. In the preceding chapter, the broad brush strokes for a hands-on approach to designing, building, and maintaining drug regimens were presented. Pitfalls associated with inappropriate drug prescribing were highlighted and general approaches to remodeling regimens were introduced. The purpose of this chapter is more specific—to generate working drawings, that is, to outline specific strategies and drug selection techniques that will optimize therapeutic outcomes and produce more cost-effective drug regimens. While these pharmatectural principles and concepts can be applied to the construction of virtually all outpatient regimens, there are certain patients and specific clinical situations for which this system is especially applicable. These include individuals treated with polypharmacy regimens, those at high risk for noncompliance[1] and drug-related adverse patient events;[2] the elderly;[3] individuals who can benefit from *prevention*-oriented pharmacotherapeutics; patients on chronic drug therapy;[4] persons prone to excessive or poorly monitored over-the-counter (OTC) drug intake; and those suffering from multiple medical conditions.

Figure 2-1

Patient Candidates For Pharmatectural Intervention
• Patients on polypharmacy
• Patients receiving drugs from multiple sources (polyphysicians)
• Patients at risk for medication noncompliance
• The elderly
• Regimens employing drugs with multiple daily dose frequency
• Poorly monitored drug intake
• Patients at risk for over-the-counter (OTC) drug intake
• Regimens with drugs known to produce drug-drug and drug-disease interactions

Many different issues influence the effectiveness, compliance, and tolerability of a drug regimen. As a result, the pharmatectural approach, with its emphasis on the multiple factors that shape drug intake and affect therapeutic results, will always pay therapeutic dividends when designing long-term drug regimens. But the most dramatic impact of this system will be seen in patients who are living in excessive, inappropriate, cost-ineffective, and compliance-compromising pharmacological environments, that is, in those individuals inhabiting *tenement* drug houses. Consequently, recognizing those patients who will benefit from drug reduction, elimination, simplification, and consolidation (DRESC™ program: Please see Chapter 5) is a critical first step before remodeling of therapeutic regimens can begin.

One of the main purposes of this chapter is to help physicians identify those patients who will benefit most from the system. Strategies are presented for recognizing inferior drug houses, i.e., those pharmacologic environments compromised by drug rot (poor drug selection) and poor construction methods (suboptimal regimen design). In addition, approaches to building durable, prevention-oriented drug houses are presented. A step-by-step approach to sequential drug construction is outlined. Because the elderly are at high risk for drug-related complications and excessive pharmacologic burden, troubleshooting pharmacologic environments in this population is emphasized. In addition, medications most likely to cause drug-related side effects are highlighted and approaches to minimizing their toxicity are discussed in detail.

PUTTING PHARMATECTURE TO WORK

Principles Into Practice. Regardless of the patient or pharmacologic dilemma, putting pharmatecture into practice is a challenging, clinically stimulating, and therapeutically rewarding process for both pharmacists and physicians. Fortunately, the opportunities are plentiful in this system for creative problem-solving. Pharmatecture, after all, is driven by a patient-specific approach to regimen design, and therefore encourages flexibility in drug selection and innovative solutions to therapeutic goals. Nevertheless, when pharmatectural intervention is indicated, the step-by-step process of pharmacologic assessment, drug selection, and regimen remodeling always should be conducted in a logical and systematic manner.

The pharmatectural process usually begins with a comprehensive review of the patient's current drug regimen. Because effectiveness of drug therapy is influenced by a variety of factors, the medication list is analyzed from several perspectives (see Figure 2-2). For example, special functional needs, prevention-oriented issues, and compliance problems are identified. This initial assessment is followed by a pharmacologic evauation that includes determination of efficacy, cost, risk for drug interactions, potential side effects, and quality-of-life issues. The prescriber should also assess the impact that these medications may have on concomitant disease states. After this information is gathered, the process of sequential deconstruction and reconstruction of the drug regimen begins. Once started, remodeling is always undertaken with special regard for compliance enhancement, cost control, and with an eye towards drug reduction, elimination, simplification and consolidation.

Figure 2-2

Systematic Analysis of Drug House Construction	
• Functional needs of patient	• Drug interaction profile
• Does pharm follow function?	• Side effect profile
• Prevention-oriented drug therapy	• Cost control
• Medication compliance survey	• Quality of life maintenance

Sequential Construction: A Three-Phase Process. Pharmatectural modifications are most effectively accomplished within the framework of a *three-step* remodeling process. Consequently, whether designing a new drug house or reconstructing an existing regimen, the pharmacist or physician can expect to be building inspector, architect, and general contractor. These roles correspond to three distinct functions—inspection, design, and construction—that comprise a step-by-step approach to sequential drug house reconstruction (See Figure 2-3). Detailed discussions that address drug selection techniques, possible side effects, preventive pharmacology, and design approaches for each phase of pharmatectural reconstruction are presented later in this chapter. Before these specifics are introduced, however, it is helpful to have a rough working sketch of the process that will guide the prescribing practitioner.

Figure 2-3

Sequential Drug House Construction

Phase I:	Inspection of Drug Regimen
Phase II:	Design Review
Phase III:	Construction or Remodeling

Phase I: Inspection. A meticulous and comprehensive inspection of the existing drug regimen, combined with an assessment of its suitability for the patient's unique constellation of clinical disorders and behavioral patterns, is a prerequisite to pharmatectural reconstruction. As part of the initial, drug regimen evaluation phase, the pharmatect will assume the responsibilities of a building *inspector*. For all practical purposes, this inspection phase is a fact-finding mission that sets the stage for subsequent modifications in the drug regimen. Poor drug choices, unnecessary complexity in the regimen's construction,[5,6] pharmacologic redundancy, compliance-compromising features,[1,7-9] omission of prevention-oriented building blocks, and drug-induced side effects related to the drug regimen are identified. Information suggesting possible noncompliance with medications is carefully reviewed, including subtherapeutic serum drug levels, abnormal clinical parameters (elevated blood pressure, cholesterol levels, and/or blood sugar), and patient admission of erratic drug consumption. Information that includes dosage form, preferences, and special administration requirements also should be documented. The patient's existing drug house is examined to ensure that basic safety codes are being met. A review of all the patient's known medications is conducted to confirm that drug dosages, schedules, and interaction profiles are within acceptable guidelines.[10-12]

During this phase, indications for drug use are reconfirmed and potential drug and disease incompatibilities are identified. Comprehensive reference sources, such as *Drug Facts and Comparisons,* are consulted to help make these evaluations. The inspection phase requires time, patience, and understanding on the part of the physician and pharmacist. A careful history is taken from the patient, and the regimen is screened for possible drug-induced, quality-of-life impairments that might render an agent unsafe to the patient's physical, psychological, sexual, or cognitive health.[13,14,15,16,17,18] An accurate count of pharmacologic building blocks is conducted, noting the number of different active ingredients as well as the total daily pill count. Vigilant and aggressive questioning may be required to determine the full range and patterns of drug intake. If the drug house is comprised of more than *five* pharmacologic building blocks, a polypharmacy warning is issued. When the pharmacologic burden is in this range, the environment is considered to be at very high risk for safety code violations, and options for eliminating excessive building materials should be considered.[19-23]

As building inspector, the physician examines the drug house not only from the perspective of safety, but reviews all aspects of the construction to determine whether sufficient attention was given to patient education and preventive pharmacology.[24] Clearly, polypharmacy increases the likelihood that safety violations (e.g., unneccesary medications, drug interactions, etc.) will be uncovered, and, in turn, opportunities should be explored for reducing drug intake while maintaining therapeutic objectives.[25-28] But the regimen must also be evaluated for the possible *omission* of *prevention-oriented* pharmacologic building blocks that might improve long-term clinical outcomes and reduce the need for further pharmacotherapy. The omission of prevention-oriented medication[29-31] is considered to be a flagrant safety violation.[32-36] Other building code violations such as the use of ineffective medications, excessive use of drugs dosed multiple times daily, failure to step-down drug dose for chronic conditions (hypertension, arthritis, asthma, etc.), regimen complexity, duplication of active ingredients, and lack of adequate patient education are also noted.[14] Once identified, possible solutions, alterations, and recommendations are listed that can correct these problems and that will satisfy drug house safety codes.

Phase II: Design. Once inspection of the drug house is completed and potential problems are identified, strategies for regimen reconstruction are developed. During the second phase of sequential reconstruction, the clinician assumes the role of architect. Findings gleaned from the inspection phase are reviewed, and an overall design plan for the drug house is generated. This scheme incorporates a number of specifications: the total number of different drugs, specific pharmacologic ingredients, advantageous drug combinations, and other features. At this point in the process, the pharmatect weighs the advantages and disadvantages of specific medications and combinations of drugs. Accordingly, decisions are made to *eliminate* specific pharmacologic building blocks and/or to add others. Inevitably, empirical data and value judgements about the desirability of one agent over another will come into play. A careful, comparative assessment of possible side effects is made so that the most user-friendly building materials within each drug class can be incorporated into the pharmacologic environment.

Naturally, drug houses are not constructed in an economic vacuum. Consideration is always given to how much the patient, pharmacy, or institution can afford to spend.[5,37-42] Whenever possible, an attempt is made to consolidate therapy with smart drugs that can perform several functions (i.e., symptom-relief and/or target organ salvage) simultaneously with fewer agents and, therefore, will reduce pharmacologic burden and total drug cost. During this design phase, an overall scheme for the final pharmacologic environment is generated. This includes detailed working drawings that reflect: (a) The total number of different drugs that comprise the drug house; (b) a prioritization of preferred agents based on side effect profiles; (c) a plan for preventive pharmacotherapy; and (d) specific drug combinations.

Phase III: Construction. During the third phase, the design is translated into a pharmacologic environment. To achieve this goal, the physician and pharmacist play the roles of general contractors. In other words, the design plans are put into practice and the nuts and bolts of constructing a new pharmacologic environment can proceed in earnest. It should be stressed that the process of altering a drug house requires patience. Several visits with the patient are usually required. Patient education, delivery of accurate information, and reassurance are important at this stage. Substitutions, deletions, and consolidations are made incrementally, usually one drug change or substitution per 12-week period, with progress evaluations conducted at 4-week intervals. In the case of progressive, acute, or high-risk conditions, modifications in the regimen may have to be made more rapidly. The step-by-step approach to deconstructing and reconstructing drug regimens (DRESC™ Program) is presented in Chapter 5.

Pharmatecture™: Design and Structure

Not surprisingly, patients who live in drug houses that are intrinsically *unstable* are likely to benefit most from the application of this drug prescribing system. As might be expected, primary candidates for a pharmatecture-based approach to drug regimen design include the elderly, patients with chronic diseases on multiple medications, and those individuals on long-term drug therapy in whom quality-of-life and economic issues are of major concern.[16,17,43,44] Pharmatectural approaches to drug prescribing also are especially useful in patients prone to medication noncompliance. Because establishing medication compliance is fundamental to the stability of any drug house, this problem plays a special role in the pharmactecture system and deserves special discussion.

It should be stressed that when it comes to pharmatectural remodeling, not all drug houses need to be gutted. Some constructions are basically solid and require only minor, cosmetic changes or minimal structural modifications. Because pharmatecture promotes medication compliance through simplification, it is extremely helpful to identify patients with behavioral, pharmacologic, economic, or therapeutic requirements known to place them at high risk for suboptimal drug intake. These individuals will usually benefit from remodeling approaches. Although pharmatecture can be instrumental in improving therapeutic outcomes in these patients, the full benefits of the system will not be achieved unless the pharmacist or physician also can ensure *adherence* to the drug regimen.

To maximize the usefulness of this prescribing system, it is important to address these issues and to identify specific applications, concerns, and candidates suitable for pharmatecture-based interventions. A number of risk factors, clinical profiles, and therapeutic pitfalls are highlighted below.

Unstable Foundations. The long-term stability and cost-effectiveness of a drug house depends on maintenance of medication compliance. In an era when efficacious drug therapies exist or are being developed at a rapid rate, it is discouraging that one half of patients for whom appropriate medications are prescribed fail to receive full benefit as a result of inadequate adherence to treatment. From a pharmatectural point of view, noncompliance is like having "drug rot," i.e., a house full of termites that are slowly but perceptibly eroding the structural integrity of the construction.

The morbidity and cost of pharmacologically servicing patients who get sicker because of noncompliance-mediated therapeutic failure is staggering. It is now estimated that 125,000 deaths annually can be attributed to noncompliance.

This includes individuals with treatable diseases who either fail to take[5,6,53,54] their medications properly, or fail to take them at all. Thousands more are hospitalized or placed in nursing homes, while others are not well enough to work or enjoy recreational activities, simply because of suboptimal compliance patterns with prescribed medications. Overall, the health care system spends $11 billion annually to mop up poor outcomes associated with suboptimal drug intake.[55,56,57]

In fact, the consequences of medication noncompliance have reached epidemic proportions. Many reviews, involving hundreds of methodologically sound studies, have emphasized the magnitude and pervasiveness of this problem. Some have called medication noncompliance the invisible epidemic.[1,45-47] A report in the *National Council of Patient Information & Education* estimates that 1.8 billion prescription medications dispensed annually are not taken correctly. According to these estimates, only one-third of patients take all their prescribed medications, another third take some fraction of their prescription, and the final third do not take *any* of their prescribed drugs.[48-50] Other organizations have corroborated these findings. For example, the National Pharmaceutical Council reports that up to 90% of all outpatients make an error in their drug intake. Add to this the 21% of all patients who (according to a survey by the American Association of Retired Persons) never get their prescription filled. In summary, noncompliance is arguably one of the most important factors undermining clinical outcomes associated with long-term drug therapy.[24,51,52]

Designing For Compliance. From a pharmatectural perspective, ensuring medication compliance is a necessary, but not sufficient, condition for maximizing effectiveness and cost-efficacy of any drug regimen. In this regard, the most important factors influencing medication compliance include: (a) daily dose frequency, (b) cost of the medication, (c) side-effects, and (d) patient education. Depending on the patient, each of these factors will play a more or less important role in maintaining medication compliance. The pharmatectural approach to the problem of medication noncompliance is relatively straightforward. For each patient, the pharmacist or physician should attempt to prioritize which factors represent the most *significant* deterrents to drug intake, and then modify those features *first* to improve patient compliance. These patient-specific alterations should be made with the understanding that daily dose frequency is the most important factor influencing drug compliance. Consequently, whenever possible, once-daily medications are preferred building blocks for most drug house foundations[58,59] (See Figure 2-4).

This goal notwithstanding, there are unique considerations that come into play for specific patient groups.[8,46,52,60] Maximizing compliance requires striking the appropriate balance between economic and other aspects of drug therapy. For example, in the case of an indigent or elderly patient on a fixed income, drug acquisition cost may, but will not always, be more important than adverse side effects or dose frequency in determining long-term adherence to a drug regimen.[5,57,61] Consequently, the emphasis for selecting pharmacologic building blocks in this subgroup should be on using drugs of *lower cost*. On the other hand,

Figure 2-4

Designing For Compliance	
• Once Daily Medications	• Patient Motivation
• Cost Suitable For Patient	• Medication Monitoring
• Written Instructions	• Livability of Drug House
• Pill Bottle Labeling	• Communication

in the case of an affluent individual for whom medication cost is *not* the principal determinant of drug access, other factors are more important. In these individuals, quietly festering side effects, subtle mood alterations, and the inconvenience associated with multiple daily dose frequency are more likely to stand in the way of long-term medication compliance. Consequently, agents that provide value-added benefits in these areas are preferred in these patients.

In the world of pharmatecture, designing a durable, compliance-promoting framework for drug therapy means recognizing that every patient is different. As a result, making pharmacotherapy *patient-specific,* is the key to optimizing medication compliance. Drug houses should be built around the behavioral and therapeutic needs of their inhabitants. In other words, pharmacology should follow function. The more faithfully a pharmacologic agent addresses the patient's special mix of clinical, perceptual, economic, and functional needs, the better medication compliance will be.

The most durable foundations are produced when pharmacists and physicians make accurate assessments of which factors motivate or deter a patient from adhering to a medication program. In this regard, the benefits of a drug will vary according to the patient's needs. Drug selection should be shaped by these considerations and, in turn, depend on the patient's age, socioeconomic status, occupational requirements, physical activity, cognitive habits, and the severity of the disease. The corresponding factors that govern how a patient responds to a regimen include drug cost, convenience, symptom reduction, sexual function, mood maintenance, and other qualities.

Just how important cost factors are in determining medication compliance is a fiercely debated issue. Clearly, though, cost is a factor, but the effect of cost on noncompliance will *vary* from patient to patient. When barriers to drug intake are primarily economic, cost should take precedence in drug selection, but when cost factors are *not* the principal concern, the focus should be on drug smartness, convenience, quality-of-life maintenance, and preventive pharmacology. Optimizing selection of pharmacologic building blocks means identifying which drug-related feature—cost, comfort, convenience, dose frequency, possible side effects—is most likely to impair compliance, and then choosing the medication that, based on this prioritization, is the least likely to compromise drug intake. When cost factors are not a concern, maximal compliance is achieved with once-daily preparations that have excellent side effect profiles.[19]

Foundation Maintenance. As far as medication compliance, patient-specific drug selection is only part of the picture. Designing foundations associated with good compliance also depends on a number of more general educational and surveillance factors that are independent of the specific pharmacologic agents chosen. For example, the physician or pharmacist may choose an excellent drug with minimal side effects, but the patient may fail to comply because he or she is unclear of its intended purpose, effectiveness, or potential pitfalls.[52,62,67] Regardless of which drugs are selected, certain strategies are useful in preventing and treating noncompliance, and pharmatecture advocates their implementation. For example, to be effective in maintaining consistent medication intake, particularly in those who have chronic illnesses, the pharmacist or physician must function as teacher, motivator, and persuader. As a teacher, the clinician must use communication skills that ensure the patient understands and can recall the drug-related information that is conveyed. To motivate the patient, the physician should employ strategies designed to attract the patient's attention so that the patient listens to instructions about drug therapy. Finally, even if the patient is motivated to listen to the physician's or pharmacist's message, and even if the message is understood and remembered, the patient will not act on it unless he or she accepts its importance to the therapeutic program.

The pharmacist and physician must also be good persuaders. Specific oral and written communication strategies have been developed that physicians and pharmacists can use to improve medication compliance.[63-65] The purpose of these strategies is to break down barriers to noncompliance. When dealing with multiple drug regimens, physicians can reduce the risk of noncompliance by requesting that, not only the name, but also the purpose of each drug be placed on the prescription container. Labeling of this kind reduces chances for error, especially those errors that are made when there are prescriptions from more than one physician or when prescriptions are filled by many different pharmacists. Careful labeling, of course, requires that the physician be willing to take the time to write the purpose of each drug on the prescription and that the pharmacist be willing to talk to the physician if the instructions are not clear to the patient. Such labeling should be simple, direct, and in terminology easily understood by all patients, regardless of age or educational level; for example, "digoxin—heart pill"; "ampicillin—antibiotic for infection"; and "hydrochlorothiazide—water pill."

Additional benefits accrue from *simplifying* the drug regimen. Physicians and pharmacists should examine each regimen and make sure it is the safest, simplest, and most effective therapy available. An effort should be made to titrate medications against treatment response to determine the *smallest* amount of medication required to achieve therapeutic goals. When it is not feasible to simplify a complex regimen, pharmacists may use a patient profile system to question patients about drug use and to determine whether drugs are being refilled promptly.[9] The format of patient profiles can range from file cards to computer-based systems that are available and represent the optimal approach to compliance monitoring. Prescriptions in such computer systems are filed by name as well as number. The system requirements vary, but the basic components involve a brief history of the patient to determine health status, diagnoses, current drug regimen (including both prescription and nonprescription drugs), dates of drug refills, drug allergies, health insurance coverage, and the names and specialties of physicians writing prescriptions for the patient. By maintaining patient profiles, the pharmacist can also proactively guard against drug-drug and drug-disease interactions that can adversely affect therapeutic results.[66]

When prescribed for long durations, even regimens consisting primarily of once-daily drugs with excellent side effect profiles are prone to noncompliance. Two strategies have been shown to be helpful in this situation. First, the physician or pharmacist may monitor for continued compliance by arranging for the patient to make periodic visits and by performing pill counts. Secondly, the physican can periodically assess the patient's status, carefully review the treatment regimen, and discuss the specifics of the treatment plan at each visit. This kind of meticulous review may also uncover medications with dosages that can be tapered, or other agents that are candidates for discontinuation or reevaluation.

A Failure To Communicate. As already mentioned, patient knowledge about their clinical condition and drug regimens influences compliance. Put simply, patients must both have information and understand recommendations to comply with their drug regimen. This is especially true in the elderly. A considerable amount of noncompliance is involuntary and caused by a disparity between patient and provider understanding. Common errors in medication instruction include the following: (1) prescribing but not discussing medications with the patient, (2) lack of information regarding regimen duration, and (3) incomplete and infrequent written instructions. One study demonstrated that among patients who had a poor understanding of their regimen, only 17% complied with physicians' instructions. By contrast, 60% of patients with accurate information cooperated.[57]

Patients already on long-term therapy, especially the elderly, have a tendency not to communicate problems, side effects, or even financial concerns associated with medication intake. These individuals may perceive, sometimes with good reason, that the pharmacist or physician does not have the time to answer specific questions regarding the drug regimen. As a result, side effects associated with drug intake may get overlooked. In addition, it should be stressed that many older patients matured in an era during which a limited number of therapeutic agents were available for many common medical conditions. These individuals may not realize that a wide variety of therapeutic options are now available as alternatives to the initial medication selected by their pharmacist or physician.

When these perceptions govern attitudes toward drug therapy, individuals may respond very stoically to their regimen, accepting drug-associated side effects as unavoidable. They may be reluctant to question the necessity for their existing medications. Some patients may even fear that if they stop their current medications, there will be few options remaining for therapeutic intervention. Unless told otherwise, patients may even think that drugs dosed many times daily are more effective than medications dosed less frequently. These attitudes can make it difficult for many patients to accept and cooperate with attempts at pharmatectural reconstruction. The elderly, in particular, are known to cling persistently to long-standing drug regimens, viewing them as essential to their survival.

Enhancing medication compliance is part of the pharmatectural approach to drug therapy. In addition to specific manipulations that can be made at the pharmacotherapeutic level (e.g., optimizing drug selections, daily dose frequency alterations, simplification, consolidation, and shortening duration), attention should also be paid to modification of social networks, patient education, and supervision.[8,52,56,57,62] Patient adherence to drug regimens improves with more frequent and direct communication. Specifically, compliance increases when frequency of outpatient visits is increased, home visits are added, patients receive negative feedback about noncompliance, a medication monitor is used, and continuity of care is provided.

Accordingly, pharmacists and physicians should provide each patient with information regarding the risks and benefits of proposed medications. Information about adverse drug effects and the efficacy of proposed treatment should be stressed by the physician and pharmacist. Written instructions should be provided. Eventually, computer-based work stations will facilitate the communication of accurate drug-related information between pharmacist and physician.[67,68]

Intelligent Noncompliance. Although pharmatecture stresses the importance of medication compliance, it also recognizes the necessity for *intelligent noncompliance*. In other words, patients should be encouraged to report and act on side effects that appear to be serious enough to warrant discontinuation or dosage reduction of a drug. Patient-activated drug cessation, however, should *always be communicated* to the physician or pharmacist, without fear of penalty or chastisement; it is important to facilitate communication during the patient encounter. A relationship must be established, usually during the inspection phase, that is conducive to obtaining accurate feedback about the livability of a patient's drug house. Pharmacists and physicians should stress that, in the event the first drug prescribed produces undesirable side effects, other equally effective and, perhaps, more user-friendly agents are available. When necessary, intelligent noncompliance should be used as an option of last resort. Flexibility is the key to pharmatectural adjustments. Channels of communication must remain open between pharmacist, physician, and patient, and the opportunity to answer questions regarding medication intake and side effects should be part of every pharmacist- and physician-patient encounter.

BUILDING INSPECTIONS

Detecting Faulty Constructions And Drug House Safety Checks

A comprehensive and detailed inspection of a patient's drug regimen is a critical component of the pharmatectural process. The purpose of this inspection, which is a prelude to reconstruction, is multifold: (a) to detect "cracks" in the pharmacologic foundation of the drug house (i.e., to identify possible *omission* of drugs that are indicated for disease prevention); (b) to assess the livability of the environment from the patient's perspective (i.e., to evaluate quality-of-life, convenience, and possible side effects); (c) to reconfirm original indications for drug use; (d) to analyze existing pharmacologic building blocks to ensure they still represent good choices for the patient's clinical condition; and (e) to determine whether better, smarter drugs are now available that produce superior results.

Because many issues must be evaluated, the inspection process is multidisciplinary in nature. It includes not only a review of the the regimen itself, but an evaluation of compliance with the regimen, its success (or failure) in producing the desired clinical outcome, and patient response to the pharmacologic environment. Moreover, every inspection should include a survey of the patient's active clinical problem list. So-called "silent" diseases should be noted in case of medication noncompliance.

Not surprisingly, there are almost as many ways to inspect a drug house as there are drugs. A pharmacologic environment can be surveyed directly, or by reviewing secondary sources where the blueprints of the patient's drug house are kept on file. Usually, the pharmacist or physician can sketch the rough outlines of a patient's intended drug regimen by consulting such secondary sources as a computerized pharmacy database (if available), the patient's medical records, and hospital discharge summaries, all of which record pharmacotherapeutic treatment plans. Although such clinical documents provide valuable information, unfortunately, these secondary sources frequently reflect little more than planned therapeutic regimens, and may diverge substantially from the drugs the patient is actually taking. These discrepancies should be noted. Occasionally, changes in drug therapy are not recorded, which can create additional confusion.

Given these pitfalls, there is no substitute for examining the patient's pharmacopoeia in a direct, hands-on fashion in the office or pharmacy. Patients should be encouraged to collect all their medicines, whether prescription or nonprescription, and bring them for evaluation to the physician's office or pharmacy. This information is an important part of the database. Based on a review of written records, a thorough history from the patient, and inspection of the pill bottles provided by the patient, the physician or pharmacist should attempt to reconstruct the patient's current drug regimen and pattern of intake. This approach is effective for discovering multiple sources of prescriptions.

Conducting drug house safety checks is a valuable exercise for all patients on long-term drug therapy. They are especially useful, however, when targeted at individuals at high risk for faulty drug house construction. In this regard, there are a number of risk factors that raise red flags and suggest that safety codes are likely to be violated. Predisposing factors that point to faulty constructions include: (a) polypharmacy; (b) kitsch pharmatecture (patient self-medication or unmonitored alterations in drug consumption; (c) OTC drug use (drug reactions and interactions); (d) complex drug regimens (erratic scheduling, multiple dosing); (e) drug prescribing from multiple physicians; (f) the presence of silent diseases such as hypertension; and (g) *excessive* reliance on *generic* medications (which suggests less pharmacotherapeutically advanced drugs are being used). When one or more of these factors is identified, a drug-by-drug analysis for possible complications is indicated.

Inspecting Every Nook and Cranny. Screening for high-risk prescribing patterns is only part of the process required to uncover violations in pharmatectural safety codes. In this regard, the mere presence of risk factors neither guarantees that violations are present nor that adverse consequences have resulted. And conversely, the absence of risk factors does not ensure that the drug house is in good working order. Consequently, the most fruitful inspections of drug houses cover every nook and cranny, and include a review of the medical records, screening for drug interactions, measurement of serum drug levels when indicated, and detailed interviews with the patient and family members.

A Room by Room Search. Cursory investigations produce unreliable assessments that provide little guidance for drug house reconstruction. Hence, there is no substitute for a "room-by-room" search to uncover drug-related problems. The most productive evaluations result when pharmacists and physicians conduct drug house inspections with the zeal of investigative journalists. For example, when a patient is asked about the tolerability of a regimen, he may confide to his physician or pharmacist that, "Everything is going fine." Statements of this kind should be interpreted with caution because, if accepted at face value, a host of drug-related problems may be overlooked. It is important to incorporate use of open-ended questions. So often, we hear physicians say that the patient seems to be tolerating his regimen "without any problems." Assessments of this kind can undermine detection of serious flaws in the way the drug house has been designed. Most patients do not possess the information and experience necessary to make associations between drug intake and side effects, and all too frequently, physicians take patients at their word. From a pharmatectural perspective, it is the pharmacist's and physician's responsibility to make these associations and to paint a realistic picture of just how well (or how poorly) the patient is thriving in a drug environment.

Because the patient's initial impression of how things are going may not account for the full range of drug-related problems, it is important to give the patient a closer look and to ask more probing questions. In this regard, the inspection process must be thorough, detailed, and, when necessary, delve into personal habits and behavior patterns. Drug house inspections rely on gathering and comparing information from several different sources: patient impressions of side effects, known associations between drug intake and side effects, medical records, pill bottle inspections, patient perceptions of drug intake, and family members' accounts of the patient's behavioral and sexual patterns.

Finally, the undesirable consequences of inferior drug houses take many different forms. It is not good enough simply to look for the *recognized* hazards of drug therapy, such as adverse drug reactions. Rather, the full spectrum of problems, drug-related difficulties and safety code violations must be considered.

Stairway To Heaven: The Pitfalls of Polypharmacy. Drug houses constructed from *several* pharmacologic building blocks require a thorough inspection because the likelihood of detecting suboptimal drug combinations, unnecessary medications, and drug-induced adverse side effects increases as the number of prescribed drugs increases. For example, compliance is reduced and the risk of adverse drug reactions increased when the drug regimen is complex, of long duration, dependent on an alteration in the patient's lifestyle, inconvenient, or expensive. Put another way, there is value in simplicity. In patients with diabetes or congestive heart failure, for example, medication errors are observed in less than 15% of patients when only one drug is prescribed; increases to 25% when two drugs are taken; and exceeds 35% when five or more drugs are consumed.[19,20,51,69]

Patients consuming *four or more* drugs are at high risk for *noncompliance-*mediated disease deterioration. Consequently, pharmatectural principles stressing drug reduction, elimination, and simplification can yield significant benefits in this patient population. A number of different strategies should be considered in this high-risk group. First, the regimen should be made less complex by reducing the number of different medications required. If a patient is taking nitroglycerin for angina and a diuretic for hypertension, the pharmacist or physician should consider a substitution such as a calcium channel blocker (e.g., amlodipine, *Norvasc®*) that consolidates drug therapy into a single prescription ingredient.

Reduction of complexity can also be accomplished by avoiding the routine prescription of nonessential medication, and avoiding unnecessary doses or variations in scheduling (such as synchronized doses). Complexity can also be modified by prioritizing the regimen, and by minimizing both inconvenience and the risk of forgetting a dose by matching the regimen schedule to the patient's regular daily activities.

Polypharmacy constructions offer many windows of opportunity for pharmatectural intervention, among them, drug modifications, application of smart drug therapy, and regimen reconstruction. The elderly are especially sensitive to both the intended, pharmacologic effects of drugs and their undesirable adverse reactions. Compounding this problem is the fact that they are frequently innocent victims of a bona fide epidemic of excessive drug prescribing. Put simply, increased sensitivity to drug side effects combined with prescription drug overuse is an unsavory combination that can produce an uninhabitable drug house, especially for the elderly.

Of all prescription drugs, 25% are taken by those over 65 years of age, although the group comprises less than 12% of the population. The average older person fills more than twice as many prescriptions as those under age 65.[38] Polypharmacy, variable compliance, and multiple diseases, combined with altered physiologic response, make the elderly especially prone to adverse drug reactions. In addition, studies now confirm that medication errors may be compounded by acute hospitalization.[2,70] A group of internists at Brooke Army Medical Center evaluated the medical records of 417 consecutive patients discharged from the hospital, noted the discharge drugs and doses on leaving, and then reassessed the patients 1 month later with respect to their current medications, schedules, and dosing. They found that 50% of patients appear to make some kind of medication error after discharge from the hospital. Based on this study, acute hospitalization is an additional risk factor for drug house deterioration. Accordingly, pharmacists and physicians should routinely attempt to confirm that drug regimens after hospitalization are maintained as prescribed and that inadvertent deletions, additions, or changes in dose amount or frequency are not made.[2,47,70]

As would be expected, the human and resource costs of adverse drug effects are substantial in patients taking multiple drug regimens. Considerable morbidity in the elderly, such as syncope, falls, and change in mental status are associated with drugs used to treat high blood pressure and central nervous system disorders.[71,72] Adverse side effects must always be suspected in any elderly patient who presents with new symptoms of confusion or worsening of a pre-existing dementia, and in patients with symptoms related to altered cardiovascular homeostasis, including falls, sleepiness, and syncopal episodes.[4,72,73]

Kitsch Pharmatecture: When Patients Remodel. Too many designers can spoil a drug house, especially when one of the designers is the *patient.* In general, designing and building a drug house should be the responsibility of a single individual, usually the patient's primary care physician. However, this physician must work in collaboration with pharmacists and other prescribers as required and should communicate openly with the patient about the rationale for choices and changes in the regimen. Unfortunately, even the most intelligently designed drug house can be undermined by patients who get into the drug house remodeling business and start taking pharmacologic matters into their own hands. When patients get in the habit of building their own pharmacologic environments, the primary prescriber can anticipate a wide range of undesirable consequences, from unexpected drug interactions to life-threatening side effects.

Although patients of all ages have shown a tendency to design their own drug houses,[2,50] the problem of kitsch pharmatecture is especially prevalent in the elderly. First of all, obtaining accurate information regarding medication intake in the elderly is problematic at best. Up to 60% of all drugs taken by the elderly are OTC medications (See Figure 2-5). Frequently, their consumption of nonprescription drugs is not reported to a pharmacist or physician, despite a careful drug history. The seriousness of this problem is shown by studies from London Hospital, which show that even when elderly patients are interviewed with vigilance, up to 40% of patients fail to acknowledge significant intake of OTC medications. Moreover, a greater percentage of patients provide inaccurate information about their compliance patterns with *prescribed* medications.[56,62]

Figure 2-5

Kitsch Pharmatecture: Patients Remodel Their Regimens	
OTC Drugs	
• Cimetidine	• Phenylpropanolamine
• Diphenhydramine	• Salicylates
• NSAIDs	

Consequently, repeated questioning and probing are required to elicit an accurate pharmacological history, and no drug house inspection is complete without a thorough survey of nonprescription drug intake. Many OTC drugs have the potential for exacerbating the toxic effects of prescribed drugs and worsening existing conditions, especially in the elderly. For example, a patient taking oral corticosteroid medication such as prednisone may then self-medicate with an OTC nonsteroidal anti-inflammatory drug (NSAID) such as ibuprofen, increasing the risk of gastric ulceration by four-fold. NSAIDs also have the potential to cause renal deterioration, especially in older patients with heart disease, diabetes, and pre-existing kidney disease. They are among the most widely used OTC drugs in the world, despite having a number of well-known potential side effects.

Indiscriminate use of common analgesics such as aspirin also can lead to unexpected consequences. In the case of salicylates, which are contained in more than 200 OTC compounds, uncontrolled and nondirected use can lead to subtle signs of toxicity, and result in confusion, irritability, tinnitus (although this is not a good warning signal in the elderly, who are likely to have it already), vision disturbances, sweating, nausea, vomiting, and diarrhea. Since many of these symptoms may be inappropriately ascribed to old age, toxicity may be over-looked by both patient and provider.

The antipyretic action of aspirin can also cause subnormal temperatures in the elderly. Elderly patients receiving aspirin sometimes complain of shivering. Combined use of aspirin and other drugs can jeopardize the effectiveness of the thermoregulatory mechanisms and may lead to accidental hypothermia. With respect to drug interactions, unregulated salicylate intake can cause impaired hemostasis, hypoprothombinemia, and gastrointestinal bleeding in patients taking oral anticoagulants. At higher doses, aspirin can displace protein-bound first generation oral hypoglycemics such as chlorpropamide (Diabenese®) from their binding sites, placing patients at risk for increased hypoglycemia. Although nondirected aspirin intake clearly poses a risk to older patients, it should be stressed that failure to prescribe aspirin for secondary prevention of myocardial infarction is a certifiable sin of *omission*.[30,34,35]

Among drugs whose actions are potentiated by concomitant aspirin intake is methotrexate. Decreased clearance of methotrexate and increased methotrexate toxicity is reported with aspirin doses of greater than 2 g/day. Although not a drug interaction, it should be stressed that aspirin and NSAIDs can also precipitate asthma in patients with asthma, idiosyncratic asthma sensitivity, and nasal polyps or sinusitis. Greater awareness of the potential adverse effects of aspirin, particu-larly in the elderly, has led to a substantial increase in the use of acetaminophen, which, with its analgesic and antipyretic properties, is often a suitable and desirable substitute.

Other classes of OTC drugs, such as antihistaminic hypnotics, have anticho-linergic effects that may precipitate acute confusion or worsen dementia.[74-77] In addition, a number of common allergy/decongestant preparations contain anti-cholinergic drugs in conjunction with alpha-adrenergic agonists, a combination that can easily precipitate urinary retention or incontinence. Cold remedies containing phenylpropanolamine, a potent peripheral vascoconstrictor, can cause significant elevations in blood pressure, especially when patients self-medicate with quantities that exceed 150 mg of phenylpropanolamine, twice the maximum recommended dose. Finally, the availability of OTC cimetidine, which is a known inhibitor of the p-450 cytochrome oxidase system, can produce drug-drug interactions with theophylline and other medications.

Silent Diseases: Drug Houses That Crumble. The purpose of drug house inspections is not only to uncover drugs that are potentially problematic, but to identify diseases that, because of their relatively *silent* and quiescent nature, predispose to poor medication intake over a long duration. For example, among chronic medical conditions, such relatively silent conditions as hypertension are associated with an unusually high risk of noncompliance. Consider these discouraging observations: up to 50% of patients with hypertension fail to follow referral advice; over 50% fail to follow-up on a long-term basis, and only two-thirds of those who remain under care consume enough medications to adequately control their blood pressure.[78-80]

Overall, only 30% of identified patients with hypertension outside of special care programs are under good control. These findings suggest that the patient with a relatively *silent* condition such as hypertension may value very differently the statistical probability of *future* health benefits from drug therapy relative to the present reality of the inconvenience and side effects associated with prescribed medications. This predisposes the individual to poor medication compliance. Consequently, patients with hypertension, hyperlipidemia, diabetes, and similar chronic conditions, in which the *noise level of the drug tends to be greater than the noise level of the disease,* are ideal candidates for compliance-enhancing approaches.

When drug house inspections uncover the presence of one or more relatively silent diseases, the pharmacist and physician should attempt to assess the noise level of the diseases as well as the noise level of the medications that are used to manage these conditions. The noise level of the disease is defined as the severity of symptoms, changes in daily activity patterns as a result of the disorder, patient perceptions about the risks of not taking medications, and their perceptions about the seriousness of their condition. The noise level of the drug is defined as its side effect profile, cost, convenience of dosing, perceptions about the value of the drug in treating the patient's disorder, and duration of therapy.

When the noise level of the drug is *greater* than the noise level of the disease, patients will have a tendency to take refuge in the silence of the disease rather than tolerate the noise level of the medication. The result is therapeutically significant noncompliance. To avoid this problem, drug reconstructions should attempt to identify medications with noise levels *lower* than the diseases at which they are directed. This will increase the likelihood of maintaining long-term medication compliance and improve therapeutic outcomes. It follows that for highly symptomatic diseases that are perceived as a significant threat to the patient's well-being, there is more flexibility in selecting pharmacologic building blocks. In general, these individuals are much more likely to tolerate medications that make the disease more bearable, even if their potential side effects are less than ideal.

Figure 2-6

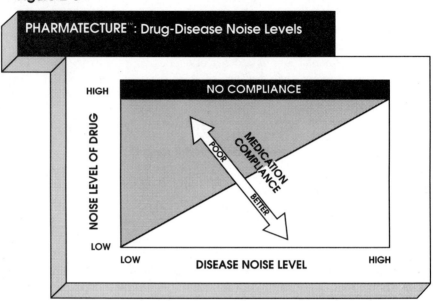

PHARMATECTURE™: Drug-Disease Noise Levels

Housecleaning: Frequency and Duration: Drug house inspections should include a medication review that evaluates drugs from the perspective of dosing frequency and duration of therapy. Frequency and duration are critical factors influencing medication compliance for both short-term and long-term drug regimens. When patients are committed to long-term therapy, the risk of compromised drug intake is high, and adjustments should be made to minimize the negative impact of chronic therapy. For example, one study found a 30% incidence rate of dosage errors in patients with diabetes for 1 to 5 years, but an 80% dosage error rate in patients who had the disease for 20 years. Even estimates of less-than-perfect compliance for short-term courses dosed four times daily are reported to be as high as 92%, and average about 50% for chronic diseases.[20,58,59]

Consequently, compliance issues and pharmatecture-based simplification strategies should be considered for short-term, as well as long-term drug regimens. Patients whose regimens include drugs that are dosed multiple times daily will benefit from pharmatectural modifications. In general, significant compliance-enhancing benefits will be achieved by reducing daily dose frequency of prescribed medications. When available and financially feasible, once-daily medications are almost always preferred. Modifying *duration* of drug therapy usually is more problematic, although many infectious diseases can now be treated successfully with single-dose regimens. Clinically important examples of one-dose therapies include: 2 g of metronidazole (Flagyl®) orally for nonspecific bacterial vaginosis; 1 g of azithromycin (Zithromax®) orally for uncomplicated chlamydial cervicitis and urethritis; and 400 mg cefixime (Suprax®) orally for gonococcal urethritis. (See Chapter 5)

Accordingly, single-dose therapeutic regimens should be identified and incorporated into clinical practice when appropriate. Short-term drug therapy, or at least the perception of it, also can be accomplished by scheduling follow-up visits in quick succession especially when progress and clearcut goals from therapy can be shown. If drug regimens or lifestyles must be altered, these changes should be introduced gradually over the course of several visits. Ideally, these modifications should be introduced one at a time to permit adjustment to new patterns of medication intake.

Polyphysicians: The Road to Polypharmacy. A drug house inspection should not only make note of the medications themselves, but should identify the prescribing sources (physicians, pharmacists, nurse practitioners, etc.) for these therapeutic agents. When inspections reveal *more* than one prescribing source, the drug house should be carefully scrutinized for medication duplications, drug interactions, and drug-disease incompatibilities. The road to polypharmacy is usually paved with good intentions, but when a number of different subspecialists play the role of consulting pharmatects, the drug house needs a thorough going-over. Because subspecialists frequently focus on just one aspect of the patient's pathophysiological or pharmacologic landscape, drug houses designed by multiple sources are frequently unstable or are built with redundant materials. Polyprescribers are an important risk factor for polypharmacy, and when multiple prescribing sources are identified, drugs in the regimen should be re-evaluated to ensure that they are still indicated and compatible with other agents that might have been added by other sources. Whenever possible, all the building blocks in a patient's drug house should originate from a *single* prescribing source.

Mortgage Payments: Expensive Drug Houses. No drug house inspection is complete without a basic, no-holds barred cost-analysis of the mortgage payments required to service the regimen on a month-to-month basis. When drug houses become too expensive, patients attempt to save money by skipping drug doses, consuming medications only in response to symptomatic deterioration, and failing to fill prescriptions for the more expensive drugs in the regimen. The end result is noncompliance-mediated disease deterioration and, down the road, the necessity for even greater expenditures to mop up therapeutic failures.

Drug costs are an important element of pharmatectural construction. To get a handle on this aspect of building maintenance, a total monthly budget for the existing drug regimen should be generated, and should include a careful cost itemization on a drug-by-drug basis. The patient's, instititution's, or health plan's capacity for maintaining these costs should be evaluated. (If costs are deemed excessive, opportunities for making pharmatectural substitutions should be considered.) However, rarely should drug acquisition cost be the *only* factor in drug house design. In other words, if patients are able to afford more effective but expensive agents, these building blocks should be retained in the regimen.

In general, when trimming down mortgage payments for drug houses, budgetary allocations should favor medications used to treat life-threatening conditions such as coronary heart disease, stroke, chronic obstructive pulmonary disease, cardiac arrhythmias, renal disease, and diabetes. From a cost-benefit standpoint, more expensive drugs are justified in these conditions because the risks and costs of poor therapeutic outcome are substantial. On the other hand, when treating diseases that are primarily symptomatic in nature, such as ulcer disease or arthritis, it may be useful to reduce costs by incorporating into the regimens drugs of lower cost that have proven efficacy. As mentioned, symptomatic diseases are characterized by high noise levels, which are a powerful inducement to compliance, regardless of possible side effects.

Shaky Foundations: Building Blocks That Do Not Stand The Test of Time. Some materials simply don't stand the test of time. Drug houses should be inspected for medications that are obsolete and can be replaced by better agents, or are being used beyond their window of therapeutic opportunity. Examples of drugs that have the potential for elimination or substitution in selected patients include dipyridamole (Persantine®), H_2 blockers, NSAIDs, benzodiazepines, misoprostol, theophylline, and many others.[11,12,81-83] (See Chapter 5.)

This Old House: Generic Constructions. From a pharmatectural perspective, old drug houses that feature a *preponderance* of generic pharmacologic building blocks may be cheap and charming, but they deserve inspection for safer and more effective building codes. A pharmacologic environment of this kind may have been created with cost as the top priority, rather than "if all else is equal, choose the less expensive agent." In many instances, generic drugs are appropriate and effective, e.g., aspirin, atenolol, cephalexin. The proper pharmacologic agent should first be chosen; then determine if it is a multi-source drug.

There are two issues: (1) Therapeutic Applicability (Is it the best building material?); and (2) Generic Substitution (Is it the best building material available from several suppliers, and, therefore, is a cost choice available?). Without question, the first issue, therapeutic applicability, should be addressed and answered. Once determined, then investigate if generics are available.

The advantages of the newer (and, usually, single source, more expensive) agents should not be overlooked since improvements in drug delivery systems, reductions in daily dose frequency, improved side effects profiles, or improved antimicrobial coverage may be available and justify increased cost. Any of these advantages may save money in the long-run by increasing compliance and reducing future hospitalizations or therapy.

In summary, a drug house built with a preponderance of generic building blocks deserves close inspection to determine if optimal therapy is being given. Newer therapy may be available that is safer or more effective. However, the reverse also may be true, i.e., that a trade name drug is being appropriately used and that a cheaper equivalent agent is available.

THE PHARMATECTURAL SAFETY CODE

Drug-Related Adverse Patient Events (DRAPEs). No drug house inspection is complete without assessing the risk of incurring drug-related adverse events. The key to making this inspection useful, however, is recognizing the full range of potential pitfalls associated with drug therapy. The detection of drug-related complications is essential because one of the principal objectives of pharmatecture is constructing drug regimens that reduce the risk of (a) adverse side effects, (b) primary drug reactions, and (c) drug interactions in patients on polypharmacy. The ultimate goals are to improve quality of life, maintain work performance, and reduce the unnecessary costs associated with managing medication side effects and drug-induced hospitalizations. Therefore, once medication compliance is maximized, the pharmacist or physician should focus attention on constructing safe regimens, which minimize drug side effects and interactions.

Detecting Drug Rot. Until recently, drug-related adverse consequences were viewed in rather simplistic terms. Traditionally, pharmacists and physicians were on the lookout for run-of-the-mill, adverse drug reactions (ADRs): e.g., diarrhea associated with ampicillin, a rash from a sulfa antibiotic, confusion from cimetidine, or depression after beginning therapy with a beta-blocker. Although these primary drug reactions must be recognized and appropriately managed, there is a wide spectrum of drug-related liabilities that must be considered in order to construct safe, cost-effective drug regimens.[21,51,84,85] To achieve these objectives, pharmatecture focuses on drug-related adverse patient events (DRAPEs), which include any undesired, less than optimal effects of drug therapy.[86,87]

The DRAPE approach is especially useful as a guide to pharmatectural reconstruction because it reflects the *full* spectrum of drug-related difficulties and poor outcomes associated with pharmacotherapy. Accordingly, it includes not only recognized hazards of drug therapy, such as adverse drug reactions, drug interactions, effects of OTC drugs, and potential hazards of combining alcohol with prescribed drugs, but also incorporates less direct problems associated with prescription drug use, such as noncompliance and self-medication.

Accordingly, pharmatectural alterations in a drug regimen should be considered when an inspection uncovers one or more of the following categories of DRAPEs:

● **Primary drug reaction.** Any reaction in a patient that is noxious and unintended and that occurs at doses normally used for prophylaxis, diagnosis, or therapy.

● **Drug interactions.** When two or more drugs, prescription or nonprescription, interact in such a way as to potentiate the adverse side effects of one of the agents.

● **Treatment failure.** A failure to accomplish the goals of treatment because of inadequate or inappropriate drug therapy.

● **Intentional noncompliance.** A failure to accomplish the goals of treatment because of deliberate nonadherence to a therapeutic program:

● **Medication error and scheduling misconception.** A failure to accomplish the goals of treatment because of accidental or unintentional nonadherence to a therapeutic program.

● **Alcohol-related problems.** Interactions between alcohol and prescribed drugs, and problems associated with altered drug intake patterns because of alcohol consumption.

Are There DRAPEs In The House? The prevalence, etiology, and risk of incurring DRAPEs is well studied, especially in older patients. In one large Canadian study evaluating 718 patients taking prescribed drugs and admitted through an emergency department, DRAPEs were identified in 162 (23%) admissions. Many patients had more than one category of DRAPE. Overall, adverse drug reactions represented about one half of all DRAPEs, with 25% of individuals within this group experiencing drug interactions. Intentional noncompliance was identified as a cause for admission in about one quarter of patients, and treatment failure was assigned as the reason in about 34% of patients.[86]

When looking for possible DRAPEs, the following observations will help pharmacists and physicians conduct a systematic review of drug-related problems. First, it should be emphasized that age is not an independent risk factor for DRAPEs. The risk of having a DRAPE is linked to the number of diseases a patient has and the number of drugs being taken. As it happens, older patients are afflicted with more diseases, tend be on more medications, and, therefore, are more likely to suffer from DRAPEs. These risk factors have important implications for preventing drug-related problems. Because most diseases are managed but not eliminated, the most effective way to reduce the risk of DRAPEs is by reducing the *number* of different prescription ingredients in the regimen.[66,88-90]

Figure 2-7

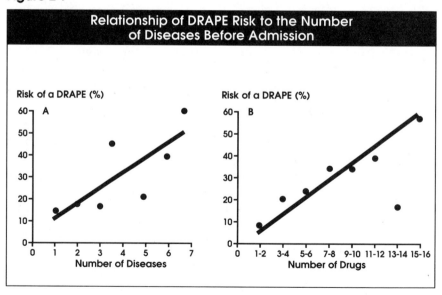

Relationship of DRAPE Risk to the Number of Diseases Before Admission

A comprehensive review of systems, signs, and symptoms is fundamental to uncovering DRAPEs. Of special diagnostic importance is the fact that 50% of all DRAPEs affect the cardiovascular system.[82,86,88] Congestive heart failure is the most common DRAPE in this category, affecting nearly 40% of patients with drug-related cardiac problems, followed by angina, hypotension, and atrial fibrillation. The unusually high incidence of DRAPEs affecting the cardiovascular system should be considered a warning. When building pharmacologic structures to treat hypertension and cardiovascular conditions, special vigilance is required. Drug classes used to treat these disorders represent a high-risk category for causing DRAPEs, and, therefore, drug house inspections should focus on all the possible pitfalls associated with these agents.[91-96]

Figure 2-8

Clinical Manifestations of the 193 Drug-related Adverse Patient Events (DRAPEs)	
CLINICAL MANIFESTATIONS	**NUMBER (%)**
CARDIOVASCULAR: TOTAL	**103** **(53%)**
Congestive Heart Failure	41 (21%)
Angina	9 (5%)
Hypotension	8 (4%)
Atrial Fibrillation	7 (4%)
CENTRAL NERVOUS SYSTEM: TOTAL	**68** **(35%)**
Confusion	16 (8%)
Fatigue/Lethargy	6 (3%)
Dizziness	5 (3%)
Cerebrovascular Accident	5 (3%)
GASTROINTESTINAL: TOTAL	**40** **(21%)**
Nausea/Vomiting	12 (6%)
Anorexia	6 (3%)
RENAL AND GENITO-URINARY: TOTAL	**36** **(19%)**
Hypokalemia	10 (5%)
Dehydration	4 (2%)
ENDOCRINE	17 (9%)
RESPIRATORY	15 (8%)
HEMATOLOGICAL	12 (6%)
DERMATOLOGICAL	8 (4%)
OTHER MANIFESTATIONS	16 (8%)

*There were 315 clinical manifestations associated with the 193 DRAPEs; therefore, total is more than 100%.

One third of all DRAPEs affect the central nervous system.[82,86,88] Confusion is the most common manifestation followed by fatigue, lethargy, dizziness, and syncope.[75,97-99] About 60% of these adverse reactions are caused by drugs used to treat neurological disorders, about one third are caused by cardiovascular agents, and the remainder by drugs used to treat other disorders.

About 20% of all DRAPE events are associated with a gastrointestinal problem or a metabolic abnormality. Drugs most often associated with DRAPEs include systemic steroids, digoxin, NSAIDs, calcium blockers, beta-blockers, theophylline, diuretics, and benzodiazepines.[92,100-105]

Figure 2-9

Drugs Most Often Implicated in Drug-related Adverse Patient Event (DRAPEs)			
Drug or Drug Group	Incidence in Users	Total Number	Number as ADR*
Systemic Steroids	27%	19	11
Digoxin	22%	38	10
NSAIDS	20%	10	7
Alphamethyldopa	20%	9	1
Calcium Channel Blockers	19%	8	6
Beta-Blockers	18%	18	12
Theophylline	17%	12	0
Furosemide	16%	31	7
Sympathomimetics	14%	10	0
Thiazides	12%	19	10
Benzodiazepines	10%	10	5

*ADR: Adverse Drug Reactions

PHARMATECTURAL TROUBLESHOOTING

Putting The Rafters and Girders Into Place

Because complex factors influence drug intake and therapeutic efficacy in the older patient, pharmatectural surveillance and drug prescribing strategies play a central role in the geriatric age group. Many co-existing issues must be addressed simultaneously and pharmatectural reconstruction can have a dramatic impact on clinical outcomes. On the other hand, sketching a pharmatectural blueprint for these patients can be difficult. The problems associated with drug regimen design in the elderly include deciding whether to prescribe fewer drugs or more drugs.

Unfortunately, the answer to this question is not as straightforward as it may seem. In the previous discussion of DRAPEs, the necessity for reducing pharmacologic burden was stressed. And while this strategy is almost always the most prudent course, there simply is no consistently optimal plan for constructing a drug house, even when it comes to the number of pharmacologic building blocks. Every patient is different, and sometimes the *addition* of a drug represents the optimal therapeutic strategy.

Pharmacologic Building Blocks—More or Less. One of the principal objectives of this system is to reduce the risks and therapeutic pitfalls associated with both over- and under-prescribing of medications. Excessive drug prescribing is one of the principal causes of DRAPEs. Medications frequently are used without adequate indications. Common examples include dipyridamole (Persantine®), theophylline (Theo-Dur®), cimetidine (Tagamet®), triazolam (Halcion®), digoxin (Lanoxin®),[103] and pentoxyphylline (Trental®). In other cases, drugs are maintained in the regimen long after their window of therapeutic opportunity has closed. Nonsteroidal anti-inflammatory drugs (NSAIDs), sedative-hypnotics, and narcotic analgesics are common offenders. On the other hand, there are very useful and, occasionally, relatively inexpensive drugs—e.g., aspirin, estrogen, calcium, pneumococcal vaccine (Pneumovax®), beta-blockers, and warfarin—with well-documented, prevention-oriented benefits that, frequently, are inappropriately *omitted* from the therapeutic regimen.

Pharmatecturally speaking, the *exclusion* of prevention-oriented, health-maintaining pharmacologic building blocks from a drug house can compromise its structural integrity and long-term durability. Pharmacologic *underservicing* may result from a number of factors. For example, the physician or pharmacist may fail to identify patients whose risk factors and clinical history mandate the need for a *prevention*-oriented medication. And even when such patients are identified, the pharmatect may be unaware of the role, existence, appropriate dose, or benefits of specific drugs for these conditions. Finally, underservicing can result from patient noncompliance.

With these issues in mind, evaluating patients for possible benefits associated with *prevention-oriented* drug therapy plays an important role in Total Pharmacotherapeutic Quality Management (TPQM™). Implementing TPQM means surveying drug houses to ensure that clinically indicated, prevention-oriented pharmacologic building blocks are in place. This pharmatectural strategy can improve clinical outcomes, delay progression of many chronic diseases, and reduce overall drug costs. In this regard, it should be stressed that the failure to implement prevention-oriented drug therapies—e.g., aspirin for prevention of myocardial reinfarction, stroke, and for thromboembolism prophylaxis associated with chronic atrial fibrillation; dietary calcium supplementation for prevention of osteoporosis; estrogen replacement therapy for cardioprotection; beta-blockers for prevention of reinfarction; and angiotensin converting enzyme (ACE) inhibitors to delay progression of diabetic renal disease—may actually *increase* long-term pharmacologic expenditures. Consequently, a systematic approach to solid foundation-building is the most practical way to ensure the durability and reduce long-term maintenance costs of drug houses for patients with chronic disease.

Building Codes For Preventive Maintenance. A significant percentage of patients have chronic diseases that can deteriorate if pharmacologically underserviced. From a pharmatectural point of view, these patients can be seen as having structural defects in the foundations of their drug houses and are at high risk for incurring increased drug-related expenditures over the long term. A cycle occurs in which more costly agents (thrombolytics, heparin, erythropoietin, intravenous antibiotics, etc.) and procedural interventions (angioplasty, surgical repair of hip fractures, rehabilitation) are used to treat acute illnesses (stroke, myocardial infarction, pneumonia, renal disease, hip fractures, etc.) that might have been delayed, or avoided entirely, with less costly, prevention-oriented pharmacotherapy. As you might expect, balancing sins of commission (drug overuse) with sins of omission (drug underuse) is a formidable challenge and an important component of the pharmatectural approach to drug house design.

It should be stressed that both over- and under-prescribing of drugs are responsible for generating excessive costs, especially in the elderly. Therefore, the total outcome costs associated with pharmacotherapy can be reduced not only by eliminating unnecessary drugs, but by including agents that are useful in disease prevention. Of course, the financial and clinical toll of excessive drug prescribing is readily apparent—more drugs mean greater cost, increased risk for drug interactions, and noncompliance-mediated therapeutic failures. Although the liabilities of under-prescribing are far more subtle to detect, they are every bit as devastating, both financially and clinically. In this regard, pharmatecture advocates a prevention-oriented, quality assurance check-up to ensure that pharmacologic rafters and girders are in place to prevent premature disease deterioration. Specific therapeutic approaches to reducing long-term pharmacologic maintenance costs are discussed in the next section.

Preventive Pharmacology: Designing a Solid Foundation

Building a solid infrastructure for drug houses inhabited by patients with chronic diseases is an important pharmatectural objective (See Figure 2-10). To ensure the structural integrity of pharmacologic environments constructed for these patients and to reduce long-term costs, the following medications with prevention-oriented properties should be considered for possible inclusion in the drug regimens of appropriate patient subgroups.

Calcium Supplementation for Osteoporosis. The picture has finally solidified for the role of calcium in preventing postmenopausal osteoporosis. Until recently, the optimal treatment for prevention of osteoporosis was fiercely debated. Estrogen replacement therapy has been shown effective in preventing the rapid loss of bone that accompanies the early postmenopausal years.[106] Calcium supplementation also retards postmenopausal bone loss, especially in older women (who have a slower rate of bone loss than women in their immediate postmenopausal years). One important study[107] of modest calcium supplementation in women taking less than 400 mg of dietary calcium per day showed significant benefit in slowing osteoporosis. However, the broader ques-

Figure 2-10

Designing A Solid Foundation: Preventive Maintenance
• Calcium supplementation
• Estrogen replacement therapy (ERT)
• Aspirin prophylaxis and myocardial infarction
• Warfarin and stroke
• Beta-Blockers for cardioprotection
• Pneumococcal vaccine
• ACE inhibitors for CHF and diabetes
• Misoprostol and NSAID-induced GI tract ulceration

tion is the efficacy of calcium supplementation in normal women who are not deficient in dietary calcium. In other words, should calcium therapy be a structural component of every drug house occupied by a postmenopausal woman?[108]

Australian investigators shed important new light on this question. In a study designed to evaluate the benefits of providing an additional 1000 mg/day of supplemental calcium to postmenopausal women who were already consuming an average of 750 mg/day of dietary calcium, results indicated that the rate of bone loss density was reduced by 43% in those taking the calcium supplement compared to controls. In the femur the rate of loss was reduced by 35%, and bone loss was eliminated in the trunk. These benefits were not influenced by the amount of dietary calcium, and they were sustained for 2 years following entry into the study.[107-110]

The pharmatectural implications of this study are clear. To prevent premature bone loss, drug houses for postmenopausal women should include at least 1500 mg of calcium per day (diet plus supplements). Those who do not get sufficient exposure to sunlight should also include a vitamin D supplement (400 to 800 U/day). At present, it is not certain that calcium and vitamin D supplementation alone are sufficient to halt the rapid reduction in bone mass that characterizes early menopause. For this reason, hormonal replacement therapy with estrogen (see below) is, at present, the foundation of treatment for prevention of osteoporosis during the first 3 to 5 years of menopause.[107,111]

Estrogen Replacement Therapy (ERT), Osteoporosis, and Cardioprotection. Estrogen replacement therapy (ERT) should be a foundation building block for virtually all drug houses constructed on behalf of postmenopausal women. The appropriate role and method for ERT still remains somewhat controversial in clinical practice, but the evidence supporting its routine use has rapidly mounted in recent years.[106,112-114] On the beneficial side, ERT significantly reduces the rate of postmenopausal bone loss, thereby decreasing the number of hip fractures related to osteoporosis by as much as 60%. Furthermore, although conflicting results are reported, the consensus of existing epidemiologic data strongly suggests that ERT can reduce the risk of ischemic heart disease in postmenopausal women by as much as 40% to 50%. On the downside, although again results conflict, epidemiologic data suggests that ERT may increase the risk of breast cancer in postmenopausal women; a recent study suggested the increase in risk may be as high as 30%.[114] Other studies fail to confirm the link between ERT and breast cancer. Furthermore, there is clear evidence that ERT increases the risk of endometrial cancer sixfold, although this increase can largely be prevented by the concomitant use of progestins.[106,114]

Proponents of ERT argue, however, that even if the rates of endometrial and breast cancer are increased, these detrimental effects are largely outweighed by the substantial beneficial effects ERT has on osteoporosis, cardiovascular disease, and, perhaps, stroke. Nevertheless, concerns about the more immediate potential increases in cancer compared to the long-term protective effects on cardiovascular disorders and osteoporosis deter many patients and clinicians from intitiating ERT. In addition, the inconvenience of the resumption in menstrual bleeding that sometimes occurs with combined estrogen-progestin treatment, and the subsequent increased cancer surveillance procedures (endometrial biopsy) also tend to discourage patients from using ERT.

Despite these barriers to ERT, and because cardiovascular disease is the leading cause of death in women, ERT is important for postmenopausal women. The most compelling evidence for including ERT as an essential part of the drug house in postmenopausal women comes from the Harvard Medical School and Harvard School of Public Health, Nurses Health Study, initiated in 1976. In 1985, this research group reported a beneficial effect of ERT in reducing cardiovascular disease, based on 4 years of follow-up examination in 48,470 women. More recently, the 10-year follow-up data were reported and are equally impressive.[114] Overall, the risk for current users of estrogen, adjusted for age and other risk factors, was reduced by approximately 50% in comparison to women who never used estrogen. The risk was reduced in women who experienced either natural or surgical menopause. These benefits were also present in a subgroup of patients otherwise at low risk for cardiovascular disease.

Even when patients with diabetes, hypertension, hypercholesterolemia, smoking, or obesity were excluded, ERT conferred a 47% reduction in study end points, which include nonfatal myocardial infarction, fatal and nonfatal stroke, total cardiovascular mortality, and deaths from all causes.[114] The degree of protection associated with estrogen use did not differ based on the duration of estrogen therapy, independent of the patient's age. The only effect of dosage noted was an apparent increase in risk for coronary disease among women using more than 1.25 mg/d estrogen.

Although estrogen replacement therapy in postmenopausal women has been shown to reduce the risk of osteoporosis and coronary heart disease, the effects of estrogen on the risk of stroke is somewhat more controversial, but evidence is mounting that it is protective against this disease as well.[112] In addition, data regarding estrogen-progestin combinations and stroke risk are rather limited. This is an important issue because stroke is one of the leading causes of death in the elderly population, as well as a major cause of disability and morbidity. To clarify these issues, and to further solidify the benefits of ERT, a group from Harvard and the University of Upsala in Sweden evaluated 23,008 women, who were followed over a 6-year period. Depending on the form of estrogen used, the results demonstrated a 25% to 40% overall reduction in first-time strokes. Of special interest is the fact that concomitant use of progestational agents that minimize the risk of endometrial cancer did not seem to counter the benefits of estrogen on stroke risk.[112]

Based on these two studies[107,112] evaluating the risks and benefits of ERT, the following therapeutic approach appears pharmatecturally sound. Virtually all postmenopausal women should be considered candidates for ERT; the final decision should be made by the patient and her physician after weighing all relevant medical and nonmedical (e.g., fear of breast cancer) risks for that individual. A history of breast cancer or other estrogen-sensitive malignancy should be the primary consideration used to evaluate inclusion of estrogen in the drug regimen of a postmenopausal woman. When these risk factors are absent, but one or more risk factors for cardiovascular disease are present, ERT is almost always indicated. In women who have had a hysterectomy, the benefits of ERT generally outweigh the risks because there is no risk of endometrial cancer or recurrence of menstrual bleeding. These women should be treated with unop-posed estrogen at a daily dose of 0.625 mg conjugated estrogen (Premarin®) or an equivalent oral or transdermal preparation.

In women without hysterectomy, progestins should be added to the drug house to minimize the risk of endometrial cancer. The addition of progestin is important because, as recent studies demonstrate, cardiovascular protection is conferred even when progestin is added to the standard dose of conjugated estrogen. The potential blunting by progestin of beneficial effects on lipid levels associated with estrogen use do not seem to have a major impact on clinical cardiovascular goals. Hence, combination therapy will both provide cardioprotec-tion and decrease risk of endometrial cancer. The standard recommended cyclical estrogen/progestin regimen (0.625 mg conjugated estrogen days 1 to 25 each month, along with 10 mg medroxyprogesterone) frequently results in withdrawal bleeding, which can affect long-term compliance. The use of continuous low-dose progesterone (2.5 mg per day medroxyprogesterone) along with estrogen use can greatly reduce the frequency of bleeding and thereby improve tolerability of ERT. Doses greater than 1.25 mg of conjugated estrogen (or its equivalent) should be avoided. Finally, once a decision to institute estrogen therapy is made, it should be started as soon as possible after the onset of menopause.

Aspirin: Prevention of Stroke and Heart Disease. There's nothing like having an aspirin in the house. Although aspirin therapy can cause undesir-able side effects (gastric ulceration, gastrointestinal bleeding), it is now clear that, in low doses, salicyclates confer protection from many serious conditions, includ-ing recurrent myocardial infarction, embolic stroke associated with chronic atrial fibrillation (in patients who are not candidates for warfarin therapy), and ischemic stroke.[32,33,35] These conditions are so prevalent, especially among the elderly— and the necessity for their prevention so urgent—that few individuals in this age group will fail to benefit from inclusion of low-dose aspirin in their drug regimens.[30,31,35,115,116]

When considering aspirin prophylaxis, it should be stressed that, depending on the condition for which protection is being contemplated, different doses of aspirin are required. For prevention of recurrent myocardial infarction, 80 mg aspirin orally each day (or, alternatively, 160 mg orally every other day) was demonstrated to substantially decrease adverse cardiovascular everfts. In the absence of contraindications, this dose of aspirin should be used in all patients who have sustained a myocardial infarction. The role of aspirin in primary prevention of heart attacks is less clear, although data points in the direction of using low-dose aspirin for primary prevention of myocardial infarction in all male patients over 50 who have at least one coronary risk factor and no contraindications to aspirin use. Its value for primary prevention in elderly women is not confirmed. A smaller Dutch TIA Trial Study Group has compared two doses of aspirin (30 mg vs. 283 mg) in patients after a transient ischemic attack (TIA) or minor stroke and found that extremely low doses (i.e., 30 mg) can be effective for stroke prevention.[32,34,35]

Aspirin is shown to reduce the risks of death from vascular causes, stroke, and nonfatal myocardial infarction in patients with a previous stroke or TIAs. The need for stroke prevention in elderly patients with history of TIA or stroke is especially pressing, since the annual risk for a serious vascular event is about 10% per year. The Dutch group followed 2,000 elderly patients for about 2.6 years and found that low-dose aspirin (30 mg) equaled standard dose (283 mg) aspirin in ability to prevent death from vascular causes, nonfatal stroke, and nonfatal myocardial infarction. The incidence of major bleeding complications was reduced only slightly, compared with patients taking 283 mg/day, whereas the incidence of minor bleeding complications was reduced by almost 50%.

Based on these studies, there should almost always be an aspirin in the drug house. From a pharmatectural perspective, aspirin is an important foundation drug in all older patients who have had a previous stroke, myocardial infarction, or TIA. The question remains, exactly how much aspirin is enough to acheive prevention, yet minimize side effects. At present, aspirin doses should be tailored to the specific patient. When the secondary prevention of stroke or TIA is the objective, the 30 mg dose is also justified based on results of the aforementioned Dutch Trial. When prevention of recurrent myocardial infarction is the goal, the accepted dose of 80 mg aspirin/day is appropriate. When aspirin therapy is being considered to prevent stroke in patients with chronic atrial fibrillation, higher doses (325 mg/day) are recommended.[117] (For additional information, see Chapter 4, Section on Clinical Guidelines for Antithrombotic Therapy.)

Stroke Prevention and Warfarin (Coumadin®). It should be stressed that stroke prevention in chronic atrial fibrillation is best managed with low-dose warfarin (Coumadin®) therapy, which produces a 74% reduction in systemic and cerebrovascular embolization over 1 year compared with placebo. However, occasionally patients are poor candidates for warfarin, and aspirin should be considered as a substitute. When prevention of stroke associated with chronic atrial fibrillation is the goal, the only dose of aspirin shown to be consistently protective is 325 mg/day.[31,117,118]

Individuals with atrial fibrillation who are ideally suited for warfarin prophylaxis include those without a history of gastric or peptic ulcer disease, patients who are not at risk for traumatic injuries due to falls, patients with no previous history of hemorrhagic stroke, individuals with well-controlled blood pressure, and persons who are likely to be compliant with their medications and participate responsibly in long-term follow-up care. Warfarin should be administered at a dose sufficient to achieve an INR of 1.5 to 2.0. Those patients who, because of their risk and/or compliance profiles, are unsuitable candidates for warfarin prophylaxis in atrial fibrillation, are likely to benefit from aspirin prophylaxis (325 mg aspirin/day), which has been shown to reduce the rate of systemic and cerebral embolization by about 49% per year. It should be stressed that either warfarin or aspirin should be selected for thromboembolic prophylaxis, and that, as a rule, the two agents should not be used in combination unless the increased risk of gastrointestinal hemorrhage is justified (e.g., recurrent thromboembolic events during adequate warfarin therapy).[33,34]

Beta-Blockers for Prevention of Myocardial Reinfarction. It is well-known that some patients do not tolerate beta-blocker therapy and, therefore, are at greater risk for experiencing myriad side effects associated with this drug class, including depression, cardiosuppression, conduction disturbances, and bradycardia. For these reasons, many older patients simply are never even considered to be candidates for long-term, prevention-oriented therapy with this drug—a pattern of underuse that is emphasized in medical and pharmacological literature.[29,36] This is unfortunate, because in older patients with coronary heart disease, the potential side effects of the drug are outweighed by the proven benefits associated with reduction of arrhythmias and recurrent myocardial infarction.[70,119,120]

Beta-blockers have been shown to reduce blood pressure, lower heart rate, and decrease threshold for ventricular arrhythmias, which appears to explain their documented efficacy in reducing mortality and sudden death following myocardial infarction. Initiation of intravenous beta-blocker therapy (when not contraindicated) shortly after myocardial infarction and then continuing long-term outpatient beta-blocker therapy will reduce cardiovascular mortality by 22% to 27% over a 2-year period.[36] Consequently, beta-blockers should be considered a fundamental building block in the drug regimens of all patients who have myocardial infarction, have no contraindications to the drug's use, and who demonstrate a willingness to tolerate this agent's potential side effects. With respect to drug choice and dose, atenolol (Tenormin®) 25 mg to 50 mg/day, is an acceptable initial dose for secondary prevention in coronary heart disease.

Pneumococcal Vaccine for Prevention of Pneumonia. Some prevention-oriented building blocks (e.g., aspirin, estrogen) are used on a daily basis, and can be viewed as a permanent part of a patient's drug house. In contrast, other agents, such as the polyvalent pneumococcal vaccine (Pneumovax®), are introduced in the pharmacologic environment every six years to provide seasonal reinforcement for prevention of high-risk diseases. Based on recent studies evaluating the efficacy of the vaccine in selected populations, it seems prudent to recommend vaccination of all elderly individuals with a high-risk condition (e.g., coronary heart disease, diabetes, congestive heart failure, pulmonary disease, alcoholism, rheumatoid arthritis, stroke, chronic hepatic disease, and renal insufficiency) that places them at high risk for complications of pneumococcal pneumonia and associated infectious complications.[121]

ACE Inhibitors to Prevent Complications of Congestive Heart Failure. Many older patients suffer from cardiovascular disease and, consequently, live in drug houses that reflect chronic therapy directed at preventing recurrence and/or deterioration of heart-related conditions. In this vein, the rationale for including aspirin, estrogen, and/or beta-blockers as part of the permanent foundation for selected geriatric patients has been discussed in detail above. Now, it appears that ACE inhibitors also should be considered for their preventive properties in patients with heart disease. Initially, ACE inhibitors were introduced for management of hypertension. However, in recent years studies have confirmed their usefulness in prolonging longevity and decreasing morbidity (including the need for hospitalization) in patients who have symptomatic congestive heart failure (CHF) and for improving their exercise tolerance and functional status. Accordingly, this drug class has become the mainstay of patients with early, symptomatic CHF, especially when it is part of a regimen that also includes digoxin and diuretics.[122-124]

The role of these agents in *asymptomatic* patients is less clear. However, recent trials now confirm that ACE inhibitors such as enalapril and captopril may play an equally important therapeutic and prevention-oriented role in patients with asymptomatic left-ventricular dysfunction following myocardial infarction. In particular, the evidence confirms that long-term administration of captopril (25 mg to 50 mg by mouth three times daily) is associated with a reduction in morbidity and mortality from major cardiovascular events.

Based on these studies, then, it is reasonable to prescribe ACE inhibitors for patients who have ejection fractions lower than 0.40, a symptomatic LV dysfunction, and are recovering from myocardial infarction. Benefits are observed when ACE inhibition is instituted within 3 to 16 days after myocardial infarction and are independent of the advantages conferred by use of beta-blockers and aspirin, as discussed above. To summarize, these agents should not be used routinely after myocardial infarction but, at present, are reserved for patients with left ventricular dysfunction—even if it is asymptomatic—who are recovering from a myocardial infarction. When ACE inhibitors are indicated for inclusion in a prevention-oriented regimen, a dose of 25 mg to 50 mg captopril by mouth three times daily or 20 mg enalapril every day is usually required.

ACE Inhibitors for Prevention of Diabetic Renal Disease. There is increasing evidence that ACE inhibitors (i.e., captopril, enalapril) should also be considered essential pharmacologic building blocks for type II normotensive diabetics with microalbuminuria and *normal* renal function. Although the exact mechanism of the beneficial effects of ACE inhibitors on preservation of renal function is unclear, it most likely relates, at least in part, to the ability of these drugs to dilate the efferent arteriole of the glomerulus, decrease intraglomerular capillary pressure, and reduce capillary membrane permeability. Studies with such calcium channel blockers as nifedipine GITS have suggested these agents also reduce protein excretion and improve renal function in diabetics, but these results have been less uniform than those with ACE inhibitors.[123-125]

Most of the evidence regarding the benefits of ACE inhibitors on preserving renal function in diabetics have accrued from relatively short-term studies primarily involving patients with type I diabetes. Although approximately 40% of type I diabetics eventually develop nephropathy compared with 20% of type II patients, there are 10 times as many patients with type II disease as there are with type I. Consequently, the absolute number of patients with end-stage renal disease with type II diabetes far exceeds those with type I.

That ACE inhibitors help slow the progression of nephropathy in type II diabetes is confirmed by a very carefully conducted Israeli study that demonstrated amelioration of proteinuria and preservation of renal function in normotensive patients with type II diabetes. This relatively long trial consisted of type II diabetics whose blood pressure was normal at entry and was controlled as necessary during the study. Normotensive patients were given enalapril 10 mg/day. Every 3 to 4 months over a period of 5 years, blood glucose, creatinine, electrolytes, glycosylated hemoglobin, and 24-hour urine protein excretion were determined. During the course of the study, if elevated blood pressure (systolic blood pressure > 145 mm Hg or diastolic blood pressure > 95 mm Hg) was detected on two separate occasions (i.e., enalapril *alone* was not able to control blood pressure), treatment with long-acting nifedipine (Procardia XL®) was instituted. Over the study period, albuminuria essentially remained stable in the enalapril group, while increasing significantly in patients on placebo. Renal function declined by only 1% in the enalapril group, whereas in the placebo group renal function steadily deteriorated by 13% overall between the initial evaluation and 5-year follow-up.[125]

This study provides compelling evidence for inclusion of ACE inhibitors to prevent renal disease in patients who have had type II diabetes for a period of less than 10 years and who demonstrate microalbuminuria. Although similar findings were noted in the past, studies were generally of shorter duration and/or included type I diabetics.[125]

Tight blood pressure control is clearly the most effective means of slowing the progression of nephropathy in diabetic patients with hypertension and renal insufficiency. ACE inhibitors have become important agents for these patients because they have the most consistent effects on reducing proteinuria and preserving renal function in this population. It may still be premature to prescribe this drug uniformly to all patients with type II diabetes, at least until longer-term trials using more precise measurements of renal function are available. Nevertheless, ACE inhibitors are probably justified routinely in type I diabetics, in whom microalbuminuria and a positive family history for cardiovascular disease or hypertension or both are known to be risk factors for nephropathy. In patients with type II diabetes, only microalbuminuria was shown to predict nephropathy and increased morbidity associated with renal deterioration. Based on recent studies, then, it seems justified to consider the routine, prophylactic use of low-dose ACE inhibitors (e.g., enalapril 10 mg every day) in patients with type II diabetes and microalbuminuria, even in the *absence* of hypertension. When hypertension is present with microalbuminuria, ACE inhibitors can be considered smart drugs because they service two target organs (peripheral vasculature and kidneys) with a single prescription ingredient. This prevention-oriented approach to drug house construction is likely to reduce the long-term costs of servicing renal deterioration and related complications associated with this common clinical disorder.

Misoprostol (Cytotec®) and Prevention of NSAID-Induced Peptic Ulceration. Although necessary for many older patients with severe osteoarthritis, chronic use of NSAIDs compromises the safety of geriatric drug houses. Not surprisingly, one of the most controversial areas in the area of preventive pharmacologic maintenance concerns the use of misoprostol in countering the adverse gastrointestinal effects of NSAIDs. The debate as to whether and when misoprostol should be used to prevent NSAID-induced gastrointestinal hemorrhage continues. This is a very important issue because NSAIDs are widely used, the associated risks are significant, and the cost of prevention could be staggering. Almost 100 million prescriptions are written annually in the United States for NSAIDs, exposing about 8% of the population to its side effect risks and complications, which are estimated to cost $3.9 billion per year for the arthritic population alone.[83,126,127]

Although NSAIDs are associated with a wide range of problems that include gastrointestinal tract bleeding, renal dysfunction, and central nervous system changes, this important drug class is highly effective in reducing pain, minimizing functional impairment, and improving quality of life for several million elderly individuals with chronic osteoarthritis and other inflammatory disorders. As a result, balancing the therapeutic properties of NSAIDs against their potential liabilities is an important clinical issue.

Not surprisingly, most attempts at reducing the risk of NSAID-mediated gastrointestinal tract hemorrhage focused on prophylaxis against the development of gastric erosions and ulceration. Many pharmacists and physicians recommend traditional antiulcer therapies, such as histamine-2 receptor antagonists, antacids, and sucralfate, even though these drugs are not effective in preventing ulcerations, nor are they approved by the FDA for this purpose. A more aggressive approach advocates the use of misoprostol, a synthetic prostaglandin E1 analogue that reduces the risk of NSAID-induced ulcers, and perhaps their complications. At issue is its efficacy in patients on long-term NSAID therapy.

The debate surrounding misoprostol use for prevention is especially fierce, and in response to an aggressive marketing campaign launched by the drug's manufacturer, clinicians are divided. One group, which responds with great sensitivity to medico-legal concerns, advocates universal prophylaxis with misoprostol in all elderly patients who are committed to long-term therapy with NSAIDs for primary prevention of gastrointestinal tract hemorrhage. Another faction recommends misoprostol prophylaxis in all patients with a history of "gastric symptoms or complaints" and in all patients 60 years and older requiring chronic NSAID therapy. Still another group suggests that misoprostol use should be limited to a select population of patients who have had radiographically or endoscopically proven gastric or peptic ulceration (secondary prevention). Still another group offers this consensus: the risk of gastrointestinal tract hemorrhage in those patients with a previous history of bleeding gastric ulcer is so great that the more prudent course is to avoid NSAIDs altogether and consider other forms of therapy.

Two approaches are used to answer the question as to whether or not misoprostol should be considered a mandatory pharmacologic building block in drug houses that incorporate long-term NSAID use: clinical trials and cost-analytic models. With respect to clinical trials, one of the largest and most meticulously designed was conducted by the multi-center Misoprostol Study Group.[127,128] In this investigation of almost 650 patients with a mean age of 60 years, misoprostol prophylaxis (200 mcg four times daily) was evaluated in individuals using one of eight commonly prescribed NSAIDs on a daily basis for 3 months. The investigators found that duodenal ulcer developed in 0.6% of misoprostol patients and 4.6% of controls. Gastric ulcer developed in 1.9% of misoprostol patients and 7.7% of controls. However, among those patients with a previous history of ulcer disease, misoprostol-treated patients showed a 3.7% rate of ulceration versus 16.9% for those treated with placebo. Diarrhea due to misoprostol was the most common adverse effect, affecting 33% of misoprostol patients and 18% of controls. There was no difference in upper gastrointestinal symptoms between the misoprostol patients and controls. The rate of serious adverse events was about 3% for both groups.[128]

This study, although short in duration, sheds light on the value of misoprostol prophylaxis for GI ulceration. Although efficacy was demonstrated in the ability to reduce the rate of endoscopic ulceration, there were no differences in frequency of upper GI symptoms or *severe* complications of NSAID use. Moreover, it is important to note the marked increase in diarrhea frequency with the use of misoprostol. Although the study does demonstrate efficacy, using a sensitive test such as endoscopy, it says very little about reducing risk of ulcer pain, hemorrhage, and perforation.

Other investigators at Harvard[127] used a decision-analytic model to evaluate the monetary benefits versus cost of misoprostol prophylaxis, with a special emphasis on the costs incurred with various patient subgroups for saving a year of life. The objective of this pharmaco-economic study was to weigh the increase in costs against the increase in benefits of misoprostol prophylaxis compared with no prophylaxis, by estimating the cost-effectiveness of primary and secondary prophylaxis with misoprostol against NSAID-induced gastrointestinal tract bleeding during a 1 year period in three populations of NSAID users: (1) the general population; (2) persons 60 years of age or older; and (3) individuals with rheumatoid arthritis. Based on their analysis, the incremental cost-effectiveness of misoprostol as primary prevention (all NSAID users) was $667,400 per year of life saved; $186,700 for users aged 60 years of age or older; and $95,600 for users with rheumatoid arthritis. The costs per fatal gastrointestinal bleed prevented in these three respective populations were $3.6 million, $862,900, and $381,500. In those NSAID users with a previous history of gastrointestinal tract bleeding, the cost-effectiveness improved dramatically. Misoprostol used as secondary prevention for those who continued to take NSAIDs despite having a history of gastrointestinal tract bleeding in the previous year was associated with an incremental cost-effectiveness ratio of less than $40,000 per year of life saved.[104,126]

From a pharmatectural and pharmaco-economic perspective, this decision-analytic model generates some very important implications regarding misoprostol prophylaxis. First, it highlights the public policy consequences of inappropriate drug-prescribing practices. In particular, it emphasizes the dismal cost-effectiveness of misoprostol in those individuals with *no* previous history of documented gastrointestinal tract bleeding. In the three populations of long-term NSAID users considered, the prophylactic prescription of misoprostol as primary prevention against gastrointestinal tract hemorrhage is very costly, ranging from $95,600 to $667,400 per year. This is compared to prevention measures such as pneumococcal vaccine for the elderly ($2,200), antihypertensive therapy with beta-blockers ($12,400), or secondary prevention of myocardial infarction with beta-blockers ($14,800).[104]

Based on both clinical trials and decision-analytic models, primary prevention against NSAID-induced gastrointestinal tract hemorrhage cannot be recommended as a cost-effective strategy. Sometimes clinical decisions regarding the preventive value of this drug may be influenced by unusual circumstances and preferences surrounding the individual patient. The use of this drug in individuals with a previous history of peptic or gastric ulceration, who might be willing to tolerate diarrhea associated with full-dose misoprostol use in return for being able to take NSAIDs chronically, shows more promise. A lower dose of misoprostol (100 mcg by mouth four times daily) is associated with less diarrhea but is also less effective. At present, it should be stressed that most study endpoints have been anatomic (i.e., endoscopic manifestations), with very little data on risk of bleeding, pain, hospitalization, or impairment of daily activity.

In conclusion, then, prophylactic misoprostol is cost-effective and pharmatecturally justifiable only in patents who absolutely require NSAID therapy for their condition and who also have a documented history of gastrointestinal ulceration or hemorrhage. It cannot be recommended for *routine* prophylactic use in patients whose only risk factor is age. Finally, it must be emphasized that the use of NSAIDs in any patient with a previous history of gastrointestinal tract hemorrhage or ulceration carries a risk that, even with misoprostol prophylaxis, is formidable enough to warrant consideration of therapeutic options other than NSAIDs.[126]

Preventive maintenance, but not necessarily with misoprostol, is required for all drug houses in which NSAIDs are used as a building material in order to prevent complications associated with NSAID therapy. Based on many studies evaluating the risk, prevention, and epidemiology of NSAID-induced gastrointestinal tract hemorrhage, the following recommendations should be incorporated into drug house construction and surveillance practices: (1) Because there is a significant association between increasing doses of NSAIDs and the risk of developing peptic ulcer disease and complications requiring hospitalization, pharmacists and physicians are advised to use the lowest dose of NSAID possible to achieve acceptable functional status and pain control in patients with osteoarthritic disorders; (2) because the risk for developing NSAID-induced complications is observed during the first 30 days of drug therapy, patients should be followed very carefully during this vulnerable period. The presence of gastrointestinal complaints, weakness, melena, or other symptoms referrable to the gastrointestinal tract or cardiovascular system necessitate immediate follow-up; and (3) monitoring for occult blood is strongly recommended in older patients requiring standard or greater doses of NSAIDs.[129,130]

When It's Time To Remodel: Designer Drug Houses

Once a prevention-oriented foundation is in place, DRAPEs are eliminated, and routine safety checks are completed, it is time to evaluate the structural integrity of the drug house, taking into consideration both the level of craftsmanship and choice of specific materials. This means a drug-by-drug evaluation of the pharmacological environment. It means reassessing the indications, schedules, and dosages for specific agents and classes of drugs that are commonly misused in this population. In this regard, cardiovascular agents, antidepressants, sedative-hypnotics, and antipsychotic drugs deserve the greatest scrutiny. Based on such parameters as safety, half-life, and smartness, there are generally better and worse building blocks within each drug class, and there are inferior and superior remodeling strategies. Not infrequently, it is preferrable to educate and evaluate, rather than medicate.

Home Is Where The Heart Is: Designing Cardiovascular Drug Houses

Drugs with cardiovascular effects must be used with special care, especially in the older age group, in which one-half of all DRAPEs are associated with medications used to treat coronary artery disease, high blood pressure, and congestive heart failure. The pitfalls associated with cardiovascular drugs come in many different forms. For example, digoxin half-life may increase by 40% in normal elderly patients, and even levels of digoxin in the therapeutic range may produce nonspecific symptoms (such as anorexia or changes in mental status) normally attributed to chronic illness. Elderly hypertensive patients have impaired homeostatic mechanisms and are prone to postural hypotension. Diuretics can produce hypokalemia, hypovolemia, fatigue, and hypotension, especially in combination with potent vasodilators and anticholinergic antidepressants. The cost-savings associated with using diuretic agents as initial therapy in hypertension must be weighed against the resulting quality-of-life disturbances which, although usually not life-threatening, can be irksome and irritating over the long term. Other antihypertensive agents, such as ACE inhibitors, can cause cough, especially in elderly females. Among the calcium channel blockers, verapamil should be noted for its propensity to cause bradycardia, conduction disturbances, and myocardial suppression, especially when used in combination with cardioprotective beta-blockers. In general, vigilance is required when selecting drugs used to treat cardiovascular disorders. Special design considerations with respect to prescribing for cardiovascular conditions apply to the following therapeutic agents and drug classes:[3,91,92,94,131,132]

Digoxin: Cost-Effective Maintenance. For no single drug is the application of TPQM™ more important than it is for the time-honored cardiac glycoside, digoxin (Lanoxin®). Digoxin is the sixth most commonly prescribed drug in the United States, it has a long and distinguished history that dates to antiquity, and yet, debate still rages concerning its appropriate use for long-term therapy of cardiovascular conditions. Because of its widespread use and narrow toxic/therapeutic ratio, many pharmacists and physicians have started questioning indiscriminate digoxin use in the outpatient setting and are attempting to identify more precisely those patients most likely to benefit from its long-term use. Although a number of studies have questioned the appropriateness of digoxin therapy for patients with congestive heart failure, as well as its relative efficacy compared to ACE inhibitors, most experts still agree that at least one of the following indications must be met to justify inclusion of digoxin in the drug house of patients with cardiovascular disease: (1) control of rapid ventricular rate in patients with chronic atrial fibrillation; and (2) improvement of myocardial performance in patients with congestive heart failure associated with left ventricular systolic dysfunction.[133]

As a rule, prescribing digoxin to patients with rapid ventricular rates precipitated by atrial fibrillation is usually straightforward and rarely poses a clinical dilemma. When chronic atrial fibrillation is present, and attempts at pharmacologic or electrical cardioversion are unsuccessful, digoxin is indicated for rate control. Lower doses (0.125 mg digoxin daily) should be tried first to achieve rate control and should be increased only if lower doses are unsuccessful. Although digoxin should be included in the pharmacologic environment of patients with atrial fibrillation and a rapid ventricular rate, the drug regimen should also include either coumadin or aspirin to prevent thromboembolic stroke associated with this cardiac arrhythmia.

If the use of digoxin in atrial fibrillation is rather straightforward, selecting patients with ventricular systolic dysfunction, or those patients with congestive heart failure who are appropriate candidates for digoxin therapy, is much more problematic. The fact is, digoxin is still *overused* to treat congestive heart failure. Interestingly, digoxin is overused in this patient population not because it isn't useful for the management of congestive heart failure—it is extremely effective for the symptomatic treatment of systolic dysfunction—but because congestive heart failure is *overdiagnosed* in the *outpatient* setting. Studies suggest that up to 42% of patients presently receiving digoxin are taking the drug for questionable reasons and that digoxin can be discontinued in these individuals without compromising their clinical status.[35] Further, a significant number of elderly patients have diastolic dysfunction, which is not effectively treated.

Because digoxin is a widely prescribed agent known to cause drug-related side effects, both the pharmaco-economic and clinical consequences of inappropriate prescribing are significant. To determine what clinical criteria must be satisfied to justify cost-effective use of digoxin in patients with normal sinus rhythm, a Veterans Administration Hospital Study in San Francisco evaluated

242 patients in order to identify potential pitfalls associated with digoxin use. To reduce the risk of unnecessary prescribing for this drug, they attempted to determine whether noninvasive testing (i.e., echocardiography) is indicated in outpatients to establish the diagnosis of congestive heart failure. In this investigation, patients with documented atrial fibrillation and confirmed left ventricular systolic dysfunction (ejection fraction less than 45%) were classified appropriate candidates for digoxin therapy. With respect to establishing guidelines for digoxin use, the two most important observations were: (1) the finding that 18% of patients receiving digoxin for congestive heart failure and normal sinus rhythm had *preserved* systolic function; and (2) the finding that detection of an S3 gallop on physical examination was neither specific nor sensitive for decreased ejection fraction.

Based on these findings, it was concluded that the major problem associated with excessive use of digoxin in this population is the *difficulty of assessing left ventricular systolic dysfunction.* Because a substantial percentage of patients with normal sinus rhythm are at risk of being inaccurately diagnosed as having systolic dysfunction, and consequently being started on digoxin therapy, the investigators recommended that all patients in whom digoxin therapy is contemplated undergo noninvasive left ventricular assessment to ensure that appropriate criteria are met for institution of digoxin therapy.

This well-designed study is helpful because it illuminates the risk factors associated with over-prescribing digoxin in patients who have normal sinus rhythm (those with atrial fibrillation are almost always appropriate candidates for the drug). The pro-arrhythmogenic potential, narrow therapeutic-to-toxic ratio, and central nervous system side effects of digoxin therapy are widely appreciated. This investigation is important from a pharmaco-economic and drug house maintenance standpoint because it identifies a subset of patients (i.e., those with normal sinus rhythm) who, in the absence of noninvasive echocardiographic studies, are at especially high risk for being inaccurately diagnosed as having systolic ventricular dysfunction. Because of the potential hazards associated with long-term digoxin use, it is prudent to recommend that all outpatients in whom the drug is being considered undergo noninvasive assessment of myocardial function.[133-136]

Although the cost of this diagnostic evaluation is approximately $330, a 1-year supply of digoxin costs only $85. But when the costs of monitoring drug levels ($70 per digoxin level) and additional office visits are considered over time, noninvasive confirmation that digoxin is indicated can prove cost-effective. Even more important, perhaps, is the fact that echocardiographic assessment can provide valuable information that enhances patient management, suggest clinical conditions not appreciated on physical examination, and spare a large number of patients the unnecessary risks and subtle toxic effects of long-term digoxin therapy.[134-136]

At present, patients who are in normal sinus rhythm and living in drug houses that include digoxin as a basic building block should be evaluated for the possibility of digoxin discontinuation. Noninvasive assessment of cardiac function is the best method for evaluating a patient's suitability for digoxin cessation.

In this regard, if echocardiographic assessment demonstrates normal left ventricular systolic function, and the patient is not taking an ACE inhibitor, the dose of digoxin can be gradually decreased over a 12-week period. The patient's progress should be monitored every 4 weeks to ensure that clinical deterioration does not result from the drug's discontinuation.

Digoxin and ACE Inhibitors. Whether digoxin can, or should, be discontinued in patients already taking an ACE inhibitor is another matter altogether. Although digoxin has been the traditional choice for treatment of congestive heart failure, in recent years ACE inhibitors have been shown to improve clinical status and survival in patients with congestive heart failure. Not surprisingly, they have become increasingly popular for management of this common condition. With more and more patients being treated with ACE inhibitors, an important issue is whether the use of ACE inhibitors obviates the need for digoxin therapy. In other words, can digoxin be eliminated from a drug house that contains an ACE inhibitor as one of its structural elements? This is an important issue from a pharmatectural perspective because it suggests an opportunity to streamline drug therapy in patients with cardiovascular conditions.

To answer this question, a multi-center group conducted a study[103] on the effect of withdrawing digoxin from patients with chronic congestive heart failure. The patients had class II or III heart failure, with a left ventricular ejection fraction of less than 35%, and were clinically stable on a program of digoxin, diuretics, and ACE inhibitors. Heart failure worsened severely enough in 23 of the 93 patients randomized to withdrawal of digoxin to warrant their dropping out of the study, compared to 4 of the 85 patients who continued to receive the cardiac glycoside. The risk of increasing the severity of heart failure was six times greater in the group in whom digoxin was discontinued. Similar deteriorations in quality of life, ejection fraction, heart rate, and body weight were also noted. Of interest, many of the changes did not occur until several weeks after discontinuing digoxin therapy.[103]

What this study demonstrates is that discontinuing digoxin in patients *known* to have congestive heart failure, even if they are on an ACE inhibitor, is a potentially treacherous plan of action. For patients with chronic congestive heart failure who have systolic dysfunction and an ejection fraction less than 35%, digoxin can be an important component of the medical regimen. Patients responding favorably to a program of digoxin, diuretics, and ACE inhibitors should not have their digoxin withdrawn because there is a significant risk of functional deterioration. Unfortunately, there are insufficient data at present comparing the relative benefits and adverse effects of digoxin and ACE inhibitors in chronic congestive heart failure to determine which drug should be used first—an important clinical decision. Given the proven efficacy of ACE inhibitors in diastolic ventricular dysfunction, their relatively well-tolerated side effect profile, and their improvement of survival in patients with congestive heart failure, many pharmacists and physicians advocate that initial therapy for congestive heart failure include this drug class. Whether they are the drugs of choice is still to be determined, although patients with documented congestive heart failure who live in drug houses that already contain digoxin, diuretics, and ACE inhibitors are not ideal candidates for elimination of agents directed at improvement of cardiac function.

The Pressure Is On: Design Competition for Antihypertensive Therapy. Optimal therapy for high blood pressure remains an extremely controversial issue. As recently as 15 years ago, state-of-the-art management of patients who had mild to moderate elevations in blood pressure and who required drug therapy for their disease was relatively simple, and consisted of merely selecting an agent that would lower diastolic blood pressure to a range between 80 and 90 mm Hg. Because the primary emphasis was on lowering diastolic blood pressure, with minimal concern for other metabolic, renal, cardiovascular, and quality-of-life parameters associated with hypertension, it is not surprising that pharmacists and physicians prescribed reserpine, guanethidine, hydralazine, alphamethyldopa, hydrochlorothiazide, and propranolol.

In 1993, the Fifth Report of the Joint National Committee on Detection, Evaluation, and Treatment of High Blood Pressure (JNC V) attempted to set standards based on a consensus analysis of leaders in the field and contributed to progress in the primary prevention and control of high blood pressure. Despite a number of recommendations and an overwhelming amount of information, pharmacotherapeutic choices for management of hypertension have become increasingly complex and controversial.

The JNC V Report introduced some new recommendations that appear to be motivated primarily by drug acquisition cost issues, rather than by concerns for quality of life, compliance maintenance, comprehensive pharmacologic servicing, smart drug therapy, and reduction in total outcome costs accruing from preventive pharmacologic maintenance. Although JNC V appropriately expanded the list of agents suitable for initial monotherapy to include the alpha-1-receptor blockers (e.g., doxazosin, Cardura®) and the alpha-beta-blocker (labetalol), the report also made recommendations that, from a pharmatectural and TPQM™ perspective, signal a return to stylistic approaches to drug house design that are associated with many pitfalls. With respect to initial monotherapy for high blood pressure, JNC V argued that because beta-blockers and diuretics are the only classes of drugs shown to reduce cardiovascular morbidity and mortality in controlled clinical trials, these two classes of drugs are preferred for initial drug therapy. The alternative drugs—calcium antagonists, ACE inhibitors, alpha-one receptor blockers, and alpha-beta blockers—are equally effective in reducing blood pressure. The report argued that, although these alternative drugs have potentially important benefits, they have not been used in long-term controlled clinical trials to demonstrate their efficacy in reducing morbidity and mortality and, therefore, should be reserved for special indications, or when diuretics or beta-blockers are unacceptable or ineffective.

From a pharmatectural perspective, this design strategy represents a very rigid position that ignores comprehensive pharmacologic servicing of the patient with hypertension. Specifically, JNC V failed to account sufficiently either for the well-documented pitfalls associated with diuretic and beta-blocker therapy, or for the technological advances and clinical outcome studies that document multifactorial improvements—delayed progression of diabetic renal disease, improved survival in congestive heart failure, enhanced exercise tolerance in angina, lipid lowering effects, 24-hour blood pressure maintenance with once-daily dosing, and quality-of-life improvements—associated with more recent, post-Framingham additions (calcium antagonists, ACE inhibitors, and alpha-blockers) to the antihypertensive pharmacopoeia. Given the present fiscal belt-tightening in health care, the reality is that large-scale, long-term investigations such as the Framingham Study, will probably never be implemented again, and therefore the incentives for using agents other than beta-blockers and diuretics must be based on clinical trials of shorter duration.[137-139]

The alternative to JNC V's primarily cost-driven approach to drug selection is pharmatecture's *value*-driven design strategy for pharmacologic servicing of high blood pressure. It takes into account not only direct acquisition costs and time-honored clinical studies (the primary design generators for JNC V), but also drug interactions, subjective side effects, sexual function, mental acuity, exercise tolerance, preventive maintenance, and compliance enhancement.[93,140]

Drug Selection Systems. Pharmatectural approaches to a medication prescribing in heart disease are designed to account for all the "real world" factors that go into the equation for drug selection. These "real world" factors include the cost of drug, the compliance profile, side effects, drug-drug incompatibility, drug-disease incompatibility, regimen durability, the smartness of a medication, and dose stability. This comprehensive approach is necessary because the journey between the prescription pad and optimal clinical outcomes can be impeded by several resistance barriers including prescription resistance, patient resistance, and drug resistance.

Cardiovascular Drug Therapy. *STEP (Sequencing Therapy for Emerging Pathology) Therapy,* represents a pharmactectural strategy used for constructing long-term regimens for chronic cardiovascular conditions. Because treatment for chronic conditions is usually not curative, but prevention-oriented or symptom-reducing in nature, the parameters used to evaluate the usefulness of these agents are different from those used for short-term courses (cure-directed).

The landscape of drugs used to treat hypertension, angina, congestive heart failure and cardiac arrhythmias is congested, complex, and constantly changing. In addition, achieving therapeutic objectives for *chronic* conditions requires identification of medications that can be used over the *long term* to manage such diseases as angina, hypercholesterolemia, high blood pressure, and prevention of recurrent myocardial infarction. Complicating the selection of drugs used to treat these conditions is the fact that cardiovascular agents must frequently be used in *combination* with other drugs in order to achieve therapeutic endpoints. Because combination drug therapy increases the cost of drug regimens, the risk of drug interactions, and the likelihood of adverse side effects, pharmatecture emphasize *monotherapeutic* approaches, whenever possible.

By using pre-determined parameters and criteria, the pharmatectural approach guarantees that "better" drugs will rise to the surface. Moreover, these approaches can be applied to a broad range of agents and to a wide variety of clinical settings including managed care environments, primary care clinics, teaching institutions, HMO physicians, and fee-for-service, office-based practitioners.

Although many drug selection approaches have been offered to guide initial therapy for common cardiovascular diseases, few of these schemes offer a logical, systematic approach that accounts for the *multiplicity* of variables that determine how successful the journey will be from the prescription pad to an optimal therapeutic outcome.

From a pharmatectural perspective, the variables that must always be considered include the following: (1) compliance; (2) side effects; (3) drug-drug interactions; (4) drug-disease interactions; (5) smartness of the drug (a single agent that is able to salvage, treat, or appropriately modify more than one target organ simultaneously within the context of a single prescription ingredient); (6) regimen durability; (7) dose stability; and (8) cost. When drug therapy options are analyzed against *all* these parameters, the most cost-effective, compliance-promoting, therapeutically targeted agent will emerge. Finally, selection of antihypertensive/cardiovascular agents also must be "in step"—matched with, targeted to, and sequenced—for emerging pathology and clinical problems that are likely to unfold on the cardiovascular morbidity continuum.

Cardiovascular Therapy: Optimizing Clinical Success Profiles

In general, cardiovascular drugs associated with optimal clinical success profiles will satisfy the following parameters: (1) they will demonstrate *regimen durability,* i.e., they can be used as monotherapy over the long term with a low probability of discontinuation because of side effects, and without the necessity for add-on drugs; (2) the agent will have *cardiokindness,* i.e., it will not have negative inotropic effects, it will not adversely affect the conduction system, it will not cause bradycardia or tachycardia, and it will not produce adverse metabolic effects; and (3) the agent will have dose stability, i.e., it will achieve its therapeutic objectives over the long term at the original starting dose, thereby reducing the toxicity and cost increases associated with higher dose ranges.

Regimen Durability. Treatment of hypertension and cardiovascular disease is a long-term affair. Drugs must be evaluated not only by their capacity to produce short-term results in clinical trials, but according to their capacity for "standing the test of time" as *monotherapy* over the long haul. These drugs represent a *cost-effective* choice because expenditures associated with having to introduce pharmacologic reinforcements—i.e. "add-on" drugs—into the regimen can be prevented. In addition, the long-term use of a *single* agent also is associated with a decreased risk of drug-drug and drug-disease interactions.

Cardiovascular Morbidity Continuum (CMC). Initiation, targeting, and selection of specific antihypertensive medications should be tailored to disease states, target organ-dysfunction, and specific conditions that unfold over time on the CMC. With a great degree of predictability, the Cardiovascular Morbidity Continuum (CMC) unfolds according to the following sequence: (1)

Hypertension Ischemia, Angina, Myocardial Infarction, Conduction Disturbance, Diabetes/Nephropathy, Congestive Heart Failure, Recurrent MI.

The fact is, different age groups tend to manifest specific clinical disorders on this continuum and, as a result, require treatment with those agents best able to address these endpoints. For example, the younger hypertensive patient most likely will occupy a point on the CMC characterized by hypertension, silent ischemia, angina, or MI. On the other hand, if the patient is 85 years old, the spectrum of target organ dysfunction will also include congestive heart failure, and perhaps diabetic nephropathy. Accordingly, calcium blockers might reasonably constitute initial therapy (at the beginning and middle portion of the continuum), followed by ACE inhibitors, which should be introduced into the regimen at a later position on the CMC at which time they are likely to do the most good (i.e., provide treatment for congestive failure and diabetic nephropathy)

Figure 2-11

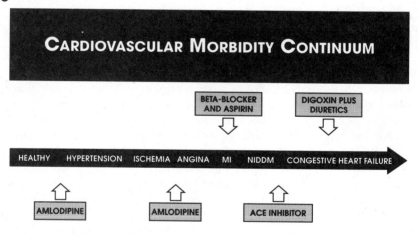

Generally speaking, those conditions (i.e., hypertension, ischemic burden-related issues) which occur early in the CMC, are best-served by a calcium blocker such as amlodipine, which does not suppress pump function, does not impair conduction system, does not decrease sinoatrial node rate, and has long-term regimen durability as monotherapy. In contrast, the disease states such as diabetic nephropathy and congestive heart failure are best-served by an ACE Inhibitor such as lisinopril or enalapril, which are most appropriately introduced later in the CMC, at a point on the age time-line when their therapeutic effects are likely to do the most good. When patients enter the CMC with pre-existing conditions, sequencing of therapy will have to be modified accordingly.

The Prescription Pen and The Pendulum: A Matter of Style.
Over the past several years many new agents for the treatment of high blood pressure were introduced. While the choices are plentiful, calcium channel blockers and ACE inhibitors are preferred by many pharmacists and physicians for the treatment of hypertension. In fact, when quality of life issues and treatment of comorbid conditions are the primary factor, the critical pharmacotherapeutic issue is whether to prescribe an ACE inhibitor or a calcium blocker. It should be stressed that in selected patients, a peripheral alpha-blocker, beta-blocker, diuretic, or an alpha-beta-blocker may be used as initial therapy for mild to moderate hypertension, but most pharmatects will use either a calcium blocker or ACE inhibitor.

Given that both drug groups are highly efficacious and well-tolerated, it is interesting to explore what factors influence prescribing practices. There are many impulses, documented clinical advantages, and subjective perceptions that cause pharmacists and physicians to favor the use of ACE inhibitors. They like to prescribe ACE inhibitors as first-line agents for hypertension because this class does not adversely affect the conduction system or heart rate and because they have therapeutic effects in patients with congestive heart failure. Moreover, ACE inhibitors delay development and progression of renal disease in patients with diabetes and proteinuria. And finally, we perceive the ACE inhibitors, especially captopril, as being quiet and smooth drugs with quality-of-life enhancing profiles.

Fueling the preference for ACE inhibitors are concerns about potential pitfalls with the first generation calcium channel blockers such as verapamil and diltiazem, which are potentially disruptive to the conduction system of the heart and to pump function. Other concerns included constipation, myocardial suppression, possible bradycardia, peripheral edema, and headaches.

Although use of ACE inhibitors predominates in clinical practice, the calcium blockers are used about 30% of the time. The calcium channel blocker amlodipine has the potential to be catapulted to the performance level of an ACE inhibitor. Amlodipine is unique in its versatility as a pharmacologic building block because of its ability to combine many of the advantages that characterize both calcium blockers and ACE inhibitors, while avoiding the majority of side effects and pitfalls associated with these classes.

Specifically, amlodipine is a smart drug with "cardiokindness" that has the capacity for combining the effects of different drug classes within the context of a single prescription ingredient. In the past, TPQM for mild-to-moderate hypertension required crossing over into several different drug classes. Now, this is more effectively accomplished with a single drug.

Although ACE inhibitors, as the JNC V report indicates, have not come under Framingham study-like scrutiny, they are nevertheless the preferred antihypertensive agent in: (1) patients who have high blood pressure and congestive heart failure; and (2) patients with type I and II diabetes and documented proteinuria. And when patients do not meet criteria for ACE inhibitor use, amlodipine can be considered the preferred agent for many individuals who have mild to moderate hypertension.

Psychoactive Drugs

Psychoactive drugs are often a vital part of medical therapy in the elderly. Unfortunately, they also pose unique problems. The benzodiazepine sedative-hypnotic drugs exemplify a group of drugs that have similar therapeutic effects but vary considerably in their pharmacokinetic properties in the elderly. While death due to overdose with benzodiazepines is rare, these drugs can cause excessive sedation, lethargy, short-term memory impairment, falls, and a decrease in attention and reaction time in the elderly.

Sedatives and Hypnotics: Avoid Safety Violations. Although a recent consensus panel of the National Institutes of Health discouraged the use of hypnotics for chronic insomnia, benzodiazepines may be appropriate for short-term therapy of anxiety or insomnia associated with specific situations.[141] If this class of drug is used, it should be stressed that long-acting agents such as flurazepam hydrochloride (Dalmane®) with a half-life of 150 hours—as well as diazepam (Valium®) and chlordiazepoxide (Librium®)—should be avoided. A rational approach would be to consider nonpharmacologic therapies first. If this proves unsuccessful, and a benzodiazepine must be used, those agents with relatively short half-lives such as lorazepam (Ativan®, 12 hour half-life); temazepam (Restoril®, 10-hour half-life); and triazolam (Halcion®, 3.3 hour half-life) are preferred.[142-147] Prescribers should attempt to tailor the half-life of the benzodiazepine to clinical objectives.

There is considerable debate regarding the safe use of triazolam in older patients, in whom such drug-related side effects as short-term memory loss, addiction potential, and confusion are reported. Triazolam is one of the most widely prescribed hypnotics in the United States. Its relatively short serum half-life reduces the risks of daytime and cumulative sedation compared with longer acting hypnotics such as flurazepam. However, behavioral disturbances and impairment of memory have been reported, with particular concern for the elderly who seem to be more sensitive to the medication. The mechanism and severity of susceptibility to the adverse effects of triazolam remain incompletely defined and the subject of considerable research.[145]

A study at the New England Medical Center in Boston,[100] however, clarified a number of prescribing and pharmacokinetic issues regarding triazolam use in the elderly. Using both 0.125 mg and 0.25 mg doses of the drug, elderly subjects manifested higher serum levels than did younger participants because of a 50% reduction in drug clearance. Degree of sedation and psychomotor retardation were greater in the elderly and paralleled increases in serum triazolam levels.

Post-marketing surveillance studies, which showed many potential problems with triazolam, are widely publicized. These side effects were more frequent at the initial recommended dose of triazolam (i.e., 0.5 mg to 0.75 mg by mouth at bedtime) although, they can also occur with lower doses of the drug. Inasmuch as the dosing range for triazolam has been modified considerably since the drug was introduced into the market, new prescribing practices are possible. When used at the currently recommended dose range of 0.0625 to 0.125 mg triazolam orally, this sedative-hypnotic is well-tolerated in the elderly and has a side effect profile similar to other short- and intermediate-acting benzodiazepines. The issue of an idiosyncratic behavioral disturbance triggered by triazolam remains a concern, and the literature must still be followed carefully for more details about its occurrence and identifying patients at risk.

Despite the short-term value of intermediate- and short-acting benzodiazepines, these drugs are still grossly overused and inappropriately prescribed for many individuals in the geriatric age group. From a pharmatectural perspective, reduction and/or elimination of benzodiazepine use in the elderly is a remodeling priority. When it comes to insomnia, it is oftentimes preferable to evaluate rather than medicate the patient. Reduction in hypnotic use can be facilitated by characterizing suboptimal prescribing patterns and diagnostic pitfalls associated with overuse of these agents for patients with insomnia.

A study performed by Jerry Avorn at Harvard Medical School has shed light on the diagnostic, assessment, and prescribing patterns that underpin excessive hypnotic use in the elderly.[102] Using an interview format, the study compared the decision-making process of 500 primary care physicians and 300 nurse practitioners when managing a hypothetical 77-year-old patient with insomnia. In this study, fewer than half of all physicians asked for any information about the patient's sleep pattern, and less than one quarter inquired about the patient's evening caffeine consumption. Furthermore, two thirds of physicians recommended the use of a hypnotic, most often triazolam, followed by flurazepam.

Approximately one in three adults in the United States has some trouble sleeping during a given year. Patients clamor for sedatives as sleep aids. Despite the pressures to prescribe, insomnia should always be regarded as a symptom rather than a diagnosis. A basic but thorough history to elucidate underlying medical or psychological illnesses, sleep apnea syndrome, or behavioral patterns that may be responsible for the sleep disturbance is essential for proper diagnosis and therapy. Initially, nonpharmacologic approaches to insomnia should be tried in most patients. Hypnotics are widely, and often inappropriately, prescribed despite a plethora of evidence that they lack long-term efficacy and are associated, in the case of long half-life agents, with an increased risk of falls and hip fractures.

Up The Down Staircase: Minding The Drug House

When drug therapy is needed for an affective disorder such as depression, antidepressants can provide dramatic improvements in quality-of-life, mood, sleep behavior, cognitive function, and pain perception for many patients. In fact, numerous studies confirm that depression is under-diagnosed and antidepressants may actually be underused. The fact is, when used appropriately, this drug class occupies a unique position in the geriatric pharmacopoeia.[148,149]

Antidepressants. From a pharmatectural point of view, antidepressants give pharmacists and physicians the opportunity to *consolidate* many different drugs into a single active agent that is capable of pharmacologically servicing a wide range of symptoms. In particular, they are useful for simplifying and reconstructing the foundations of drug regimens oriented toward management of insomnia, somatization disorders, chronic pain, and recurrent panic attacks. With respect to reduction of pharmacologic burden, these agents are smart drugs that can (a) provide sedation to induce sleep in patients with chronic insomnia; (b) treat depression; (c) reduce the frequency of panic attacks; (d) manage pain associated with diabetic mononeuropathy; and (e) decrease amplification of bodily sensations. All of these benefits are possible with a single prescription ingredient. These multiple actions may be especially helpful in managing older patients with sleep disturbances.

Despite the potential advantages of low-dose antidepressant therapy, care is needed in selecting the most appropriate agent and dose schedule. Geriatric specialists and consulting pharmacists are moving away from tertiary amines such as amitryptiline chloride (Elavil®), with its sedating, hypotensive, and anticholinergic properties, and toward use of once-daily, serotonin-specific reuptake inhibitors (SSRIs) such as sertraline (Zoloft®), which has a neutral psychomotor profile in the elderly, a low risk of drug interactions, and minimal anticholinergic toxicity. When sedative properties are deemed desirable for the management of affective disorders, therapy with low-dose trazodone hydrochloride (Desyrel®) is effective.[150-152]

Antipsychotics: A Sane Approach To Drug Selection. The antipsychotic/neuroleptic drugs, which are useful in the management of behavioral and psychiatric disorders, have similar pharmacokinetic and antipsychotic properties. However, their hypotensive, anticholinergic, and extrapyramidal side effects vary substantially. For example, drugs such as haloperidol (Haldol®) and trifluoperazine (Stelazine®) should be avoided in patients in whom induction of extrapyramidal side effects would be especially worrisome, e.g., those with gait disorders and Parkinson's disease. On the other hand, in patients with postural hypotension, gait instability, or patients with conduction disorders, drugs such as chlorpromazine (Thorazine®) and thioridazine (Mellaril®) are not recommended, because of their propensity to cause sedation, hypotension, and anticholinergic toxicity.[145,153,154] It should be stressed that there is currently little evidence that neuroleptics offer any therapeutic benefit to patients with Alzheimer's dementia, although their judicious use is still appropriate when managing the behavioral consequences of the disease. In general, this category of drugs should be given only to severely behaviorally disturbed, elderly patients or patients previously stabilized on neuroleptics who are at risk of harm to themselves or others; moreover, a clear therapeutic end point must be closely monitored.[146,155,156]

The House That Pharmatecture Built

The working drawings for drug house construction are now in place. Specific strategies are outlined for drug selection, compliance enhancement, and construction of prevention-oriented drug houses. Patient groups at high risk for inhabiting or creating suboptimal drug houses have been highlighted. In particular, strategies for conducting a thorough drug house inspection have been discussed in detail and the importance of identifying and characterizing the full spectrum of DRAPEs before pharmatectural reconstruction is stressed. From a pharmatectural perspective, the safest and most durable drug houses are the product of a systematic, three-phase process consisting of drug house inspection, design, and reconstruction. When consistent with pharmatectural guidelines, this process will produce cost-effective pharmacologic constructions associated with optimal therapeutic outcomes and quality-of-life maintenance.

[1]Berg JS, Dischler J, Wagner DJ, Raia JJ, Palmer-Shevlin N. Medication compliance; a healthcare problem. Ann Pharmacother 1993 Sept; 27(9 Suppl):S1-24.

[2]Col N, Fanale JE, Kronholm P. The role of medication noncompliance and adverse drug reactions in hospitalizations of the elderly. Arch Intern Med 1990 April;150(4):841-5.

[3]Riegger GA. Lessons from recent randomized controlled trials for the management of congestive heart failure. Am J Cardiol 1993 June 24;71(17):38E-40E.

[4]Pickles H, Fuller S. Prescriptions, adverse reactions, and the elderly. Lancet 1986;2(8497):40.

[5]Steiner JF, Robbins LJ, Roth SC, Hammond WS. The effect of prescription size on acquisition of maintenance medications. J Gen Intern Med 1993 June;8(6):306-10.

[6]Stewart RB, Caranasos GJ. Medication compliance in the elderly. Med Clin North Am 1989;73:1551-63.

[7]Beardon PH, McGilchrist MM, McKendrick AD, McDevitt DG, MacDonald TM. Primary non-compliance with prescribed medication in primary care. BMJ 1993 Oct 2;307(6908):846-8.

[8]Botelho RJ, Dudrak R 2d. Home assessment of adherence to long-term medication in the elderly. J Fam Prac 1992 July;35(1):61-5.

[9]Hamilton RA, Bricland LL. Use of prescription-refill records to assess patient compliance. Am J Hosp Pharm 1992 July;49(7):1691-6.

[10]Beers MH, Fingold SF, Ouslander JG, Ruben DB, Morgenstern H, Beck JC. Characteristics and quality of prescribing by doctors practicing in nursing homes. J Am Geriatr Soc 1993 Aug;41(8):802-7.

[11]Beers MH, Ouslander JG, Fingold SF, Morgenstern H, Ruben DB, Rogers W, Zeffren MJ, Beck JC. Inappropriate medication prescribing in skilled-nursing facilities. Ann Intern Med 1992 Oct 15;117(8):684-9.

[12]Beers MH, Ouslander JG, Rollingeer I, Reuben DB, Brooks J, Beck JC. Explicit criteria for determining inappropriate medication use in nursing home residents. [Review] Arch Intern Med 1991 Sept;151(9):1825-32.

[13]Nolan L, O'Malley K. Adverse effects of antidepressants in the elderly. [Review] Drugs Aging 1992 Sept-Oct; 2(5):450-8.

[14]Willcox SM, Himmelstein DU, Woolhander S. Inappropriate drug prescribing for the community-dwelling elderly. JAMA 1994 July 27;272(4):292-6.

[15]Abernethy DR, Schwartz JB, Plachetka JR, et al. Comparison in young and elderly patients of pharmacodynamics and disposition of labetalol in systemic hypertension. Am J Cardiol 1987;60:697-702.

[16]Amir M, Cristal N, Bar-On D, Loidl A. Does the combination of ACE inhibitor and calcium antagonist control hypertension and improve quality of life? The LOMIR-MCT-IL study experience. Blood Press 1994;Suppl 1:40-2.

[17]Bulpitt CJ, Fletcher AE. Drug treatment and quality of life in the elderly. [Review] Clin Geriatr Med 1990 May;6(2):309-17.

[18]Coons SJ, Kaplan RM. Assessing health-related quality of life: application to drug therapy. Clin Ther 1992;14(6):850-8; discussion 849.

[19]Conn VS, Taylor SG, Kelley S. Medication regimen complexity and adherence among older adults. Image J Nurs Sch 1991 Winter;23(4):231-5.

[20]Downs GE, Linkewich JA, DiPalma JR. Drug interactions in elderly diabetics. Geriatrics 1986;36(7):45.

[21]Lamy PP. A "risk" approach to adverse drug reactions. J Am Geriatr Soc 1988;36:79.

[22]May FE, Stewart B, Cluff LE. Drug interactions and multiple drug administrations. Clin Pharmacol Ther 1970;2:705.

[23]Ouslander JG. Drug therapy in the elderly. Ann Intern Med 1981;95:711-22.

[24]Knight JR, Campbell AJ, Williams SM, Clark DW. Knowledgeable noncompliance with prescribed drugs in elderly subjects—a study with particular reference to nonsteroidal antiinflammatory and antidepressant drugs. J Clin Pharm Ther 1991 April;16(2):131-7.

[25]Ballenger JC. Medication discontinuation in panic disorder. J Clin Psychiatry 1992 March;53 Suppl:26-31.

[26]Ballenger JC, Pecknold J, Rickels K, Sellers EM. Medication discontinuation in panic disorder. J Clin Psychiatry 1993 Oct;54 Suppl:15-21; discussion 22-4.

[27]Dichter MA. Deciding to discontinue antiepileptic mediation. Hosp Pract (Off Ed) 1992 Oct 30;27(10A):16, 21-2.

[28]Gherpelli JK, Kok F, dal Forno S, Elkis LC, Lefevre BH, Diament AJ. Discontinuing medication in epileptic children: a study of risk factors related to recurrence. Epilepsia 1992 July-Aug; 33(4):681-6.

[29]Held P. Effects of beta-blockers on ventricular dysfunction after myocardial infarction: tolerability and survival effects. Am J Cardiol 1993 March 25;71(9):39C-44C.

[30]Hennekens CH, Jonas MA, Buring JE. The benefits of aspirin in acute myocardial infarction. Still a well-kept secret in the United States. Arch Intern Med 1994 Jan 10;154(1):37-9.

[31]Kanter MC, Sherman DG. Strategies for preventing stroke. Curr Opin Neurol Neurosurg 1993 Feb;6(1):60-5.

[32]Barnett HJ. Aspirin in stroke prevention. An overview. Stroke 1990 Dec;21(12 Suppl):IV40-3.

[33]Bower S, Sandercock P. Antiplatelet and anticoagulant therapy. Curr Opin Neurol Neurosur 1993 Feb;6(1):55-9.

[34]Couch JR. Antiplatelet therapy in the treatment of cerebrovascular disease. Clin Cardiol 1993 Oct;16(10):703-10.

[35]Dalen JE, Goldberg RJ. Prophylactic aspirin and the elderly population. Clin Geriat Med 1992 Feb;8(1):119-26.

[36]Frishman WH. Beta-adrenergic blockers as cardioprotective agents. Am J Cardiol 1992 Dec 21;70(21):21-61.

[37]Anonymous. Clinton team works with drug companies to expand access, restrict costs. Am J Hosp Pharm 1993 March;50(3):388, 391.

[38]Anonymous. Prescription drugs and older consumers. Report of the Governor's task force on prescription drugs and older consumers issued August 10, 1990. Mich Med 1991 Feb;90(2):27-31.

[39]Cooling H. Non-redemption of prescriptions. Homeless people miss out on prescribed treatment. BMJ 1994 Jan 8;308(6921):135-6.

[40]Gibaldi M. Prescription drugs and health care reform. Pharmacotherapy 1993 Nov-Dec; 13(6):583-9.

[41]Kucukarslan S, Hakim Z, Sullivan D, Taylor S, Grauer D, Haugtvedt C, Zgarrick D. Points to consider about prescription drug prices: an overview of federal policy and pricing studies. Clin Ther 1993 July-Aug;15(4):726-38.

[42]Shulkin DJ, Giardino AP, Freenock TF, Jr., Henriksen DS, Richman C, Friedlander MS, Pandelidis SM, Heywood TJ. Generic versus brand name drug prescribing by resident physicians in Pennsylvania. Am J Hosp Pharm 1992 March;49(3):625-6.

[43]Ahronheim J. Practical pharmacology for older patients; avoiding adverse drug effects. Mt Sinai J Med 1993 Nov;60(6):497-501.

[44]Bailey RA, Ashcraft NA. Pharmacist-physician drug fair for educating physicians in cost-effective prescribing. Am J Hosp Pharm 1993 Oct;50(10):2088-9.

[45]Berger MS. A proposal for using generics. Pa Med 1993 May;96(5):10.

[46]Emrys-Jones G. Dispensing in general practice. Dispensing improves compliance. BMJ 1993 June 26;306(6894):1749.

[47]Macdonald ET, Macdonald JB, Phoenix M. Improving drug compliance after hospital discharge. BMJ 1977;2:618-621.

[48]Coleman TJ. Non-redemption of prescriptions. Linked to poor consultation. BMJ 1994 Jan 8;308(6921):135.

[49]Futrell DP. Drug compliance. Are you getting the most out of your medicine? N C Med J 1993 Oct;54(10):523-4.

[50]Ito S, Koren G, Einarson TR. Maternal noncompliance with antibiotics during breastfeeding. Ann Pharmacother 1993 Jan;27(1):40-2.

[51]Deyo RA, Inui TS, Sullivan B. Noncompliance with arthritis drugs: magnitude, correlates, and clinical implications. J Rheumatol 1981;8:931-6.

[52]Litchman HM. Medication noncompliance: a significant problem and possible strategies. R I Med 1993 Dec;76(12):608-10.

[53]Skaer TL, Sclar DA, Markowski DJ, Won JK. Effect of value-added utilities on prescription refill compliance and Medicaid health care expenditures—a study of patients with non-insulin dependent diabetes mellitus. J Clin Pharm Ther 1993 Aug;18(4):295-9.

[54]Tilson HH. Social policy and drug safety. Clin Geriatr Med 1987;2(1):165.

[55]McEvoy G. American hospital formulary service drug information. Bethesda, Md: American Society of Hospital Pharmacists, 1985;12-13.

[56]McNally DL, Wertheimer D. Strategies to reduce the high cost of patient noncompliance. M Med J 1992 March;41(3):223-5.

[57]Phillips SL, Carr-Lopez SM. Impact of a pharmacist on medication discontinuation in a hospital-based geriatric clinic. Am J Hosp Pharmacy 1990 May;47(5):1075-9.

[58]Eisen SA, Miller DK, Woodward RS, Spitznagel E, Przybeck TR. The effect of prescribed daily dose frequency on patient medication compliance. Arch Intern Med 1990 Sept;150(9):1881-4.

[59]Keen PJ. What is the best dosage schedule for patients? J R Soc Med 1991 Nov;84(11):640-1.

[60]Anonymous. Writing prescription instructions. Can Med Assoc J 1991 March 15;144(6):647-8.

[61]Sclar DA, Chin A, Skaer TL, Okamoto MP, Nakahiro RK, Gill MA. Effect of health education in promoting prescription refill compliance among patients with hypertension. Clin Ther 1991 July-Aug;13(4):489-95.

[62]Park DC, Morrell RW, Frieske D, Kincaid D. Medication adherence behaviors in older adults; effects of external cognitive supports. Psychol Aging 1992 June;7(2):252-6.

[63]Green LW, Purrell CO, Koop CE, et al. Programs to reduce drug errors in the elderly: direct and indirect evidence from patient education. In: Improving medication compliance. Reston, Va: National Pharm Council, 1985.

[64]Kahl A, Blandford DH, Krueger K, Zwick DI. Geriatric education centers address medication issues affecting older adults. Public Health Rep 1992 Jan-Feb;107(1):37-47.

[65]Roth HP, Caron HS. Accuracy of doctor's estimates and patients' statements on adherence to a drug regimen. Clin Pharm Ther 1978;23:361-370.

[66]Abernathy DR, Andrawis NS. Critical drug interactions: A guide to important examples. Drug Ther 1993;Cot 15-27.

[67]Fox GN. Drug interactions software programs. J Fam Pract 1991;33(3):273-80.

[68]Valentine C. Use computers to detect inappropriate prescriptions. BMJ 1993 July 3;307(6895):61.

[69]Johnston D, Duffin D. Drug-patient interactions and their relevance in the treatment of heart failure. Am J Cardiol 1992 Oct 8;70(10):109C-12C.

[70]Cochrane RA, Mandal AR, Ledger-Scott M, Walker R. Changes in drug treatment after discharge from hospital in geriatric patients. BMJ 1992 Sept 19;305(6855):694-6.

[71]Granek E, et al. Medications and diagnosis in relation to falls in a long-term care facility. J Am Geriatr Soc 1987;35:505.

[72]Larson EB, et al. Adverse drug reactions associated with global cognitive impairment in elderly persons. Ann Intern Med 1987;107:169-73.

[73]Nolan L, O'Malley K. Prescribing for the elderly I. Sensitivity of the elderly to adverse drug reactions. J Am Geriatr Soc 1988;36:142-49.

[74]Greenblatt DJ, Shader RI. Anticholinergics. N Engl J Med 1984;288(23):1215-18.

[75]Blazer DG, Federspiel CF, Ray WA, et al. The risk of anticholinergic toxicity in the elderly: a study of prescribing practices in two populations. J Gerontol 1983;38:31-5.

[76]Chan CH, Ruskiewicz RJ. Anticholinergic side effects of trazodone combined with another pharmacologic agent [letter]. Am J Psychiatry 1990 April;147(4):533.

[77]Jue SG, Vestal RE. Adverse drug reactions in the elderly: a critical review. Medicine in Old Age-Clinical Pharmacology and Drug Therapy, London, 1985.

[78]Burris JF. Hypertension management in the elderly. [Review] Heart Disease Stroke 1994 March-April;3(2):77-83.

[79]Flack JM, Woolley A, Esunge P, Grimm RH. A rational approach to hypertension treatment in the older patient. [Review] Geriatrics 1992 Nov;47(11):24-8,33-8.

[80]Furguson RP, Wetle T, Dubitzky D, Winsemius D. Relative importance to elderly patients of effectiveness, adverse effects, convenience and cost of antihypertensive medications. A pilot study. Drugs Aging 1994 Jan;4(1):56-62.

[81]Girgis L, Brooks P. Nonsteroidal anti-inflammatory drugs. Differential use in older patient. [Review] Drugs Aging 1994 Feb;4(2):101-12.

[82]Lamy PP. The elderly and drug interactions. J Am Geriatr Soc 1986;34:586-92.

[83]Anonymous. Drugs for treatment of peptic ulcers. Med Lett Drugs Ther 1991 Nov 29;33(858):111-4.

[84]Gilley J. Towards rational prescribing. BMJ 1994 March 19;308(6931):731-2.

[85]Hood JC, Murphy JE. Patient noncompliance can lead to hospital readmissions. Hospitals 1978; 52:79-82, 84.

[86]Jahnigen D, Cooper D, LaForce M. Adverse events among hospitalized elderly patients. J Am Geriatr Soc 1988;36:65-72.

[87]Black AJ, Somers K. Drug-related illness resulting in hospital admission. J R Coll Physicians Lond 1989;18:40-4.

[88]Beers MH, Storrie M, Lee G. Potential adverse drug interactions in the emergency room. An issue in the quality of care. Ann Intern Med 1990 Jan 1;112(1):61-4.

[89]Brodie MJ, Feely J. Adverse drug reactions. BMJ 1988;296:845-9.

[90]Gosney M, Tallis RL. Prescription of contraindicated and interacting drugs in elderly patients admitted to the hospital. Lancet 1984;2:564-7.

[91]Psaty BM, Koepsell TD, et al. The relative risk of incident coronary heart disease associated with recently stopping the use of beta-blockers. JAMA 1990;263.

[92]Wassertheil-Smoller S, Blaufox DM, et al. Effect of antihypertensives on sexual function and quality of life: The TAIM study. Ann Intern Med 1991;114:613-20.

[93]Testa MA, Anderson RB, Nackley JF, et al. Quality of life and antihypertensive therapy in men: A comparison of captopril with enalapril. N Engl J Med 1993;328:907.

[94]Hine LK, Laird NM, et al. Meta-analysis of empirical long-term antiarrhythmic therapy after myocardial infarction. JAMA 1989;262:3037-40.

[95]Landfeld CS, Goldman L. Major bleeding in outpatients treated with warfarin: incidence and prediction by factors known at the start of oupatient therapy. 1989;87:144-52; Landefeld CS, Rosenblatt MW, Goldman L. Bleeding in outpatients treated with warfarin: relation to prothrombin time and important remediable lesions. Am J Med 1989;87:153-9.

[96]Warram JH, Laffel LMB, et al. Excess mortality associated with diuretic therapy in diabetes mellitus. Arch Intern Med 1991;151:1350-6.

[97]Callahan AM, Fava M, Rosenbaus JF. Drug interactions in psychopharmacology. [Review] Psychiatr Clin North Am 1993 Sept;16(3):647-71.

[98]Ciraulo DA, Shader RI. Fluoxetine drug-drug interactions. II. [Review] J Clin Psychopharmacol 1990 June;10(3):213-7.

[99]Larson EB, Kukull WA, Buchner D, et al. Adverse drug reactions associated with global cognitive impairment in elderly persons. Ann Intern Med 1987;107:169-73.

[100]Greenblatt DJ, Harmatz JS, et al. Sensitivity to triazolam in the elderly. N Engl J Med 1991;324;1691-8.

[101]Sessler CN. Theophylline toxicity: clinical features of 116 cases. Am J Med 1990;88:567-76.

[102]Everitt DE, Avorn J, Baker MW. Clinical decision-making in the evaluation and treatment of insomnia. Am J Med 1990;89:357-62.

[103]Packer M, Gheorghiade M, Young JB, et al. Withdrawal of digoxin from patients with chronic congestive heart failure treated with angiotensin converting enzyme inhibitors. N Engl J Med 1993;329:1-7.

[104]Walt RP. Misoprostol for the treatment of peptic ulcer and antiinflammatory drug-induced gastroduodenal ulceration. N Engl J Med 1992;327:1575.

[105]Lann RF, et al. Low-dose prednisone induces rapid reversible axial bone loss in patients with rheumatoid arthritis. Ann Intern Med 1993;119:963-8.

[106]Felson DT, Ahang Y, Hannan MT, et al. The effect of postmenopausal therapy on bone density in elderly women. N Engl J Med 1993;329:1141.

[107]Dawson-Hughes B, Dallal GE, Krall EA, et al. A controlled trial of the effect of calcium supplementation on bone density in postmenopausal women. N Engl J Med 1990;323:878-83.

[108]Reid IR, Ames RW, Gamble GD, et al. Effect of calcium supplementation on bone loss in postmenopausal women. N Engl J Med 1993;328:460-4.

[109]Aloia JF, Vaswni A, Yeh JK, et al. Calcium supplementation with and without hormone replacement therapy to prevent postmenopausal bone loss. Ann Intern Med 1994;120:97.

[110]Tilyard MW, et al. Treatment of postmenopausal osteoporosis with calcitriol or calcium. N Engl J Med 1992;326(6):357-62.

[111]Dawson-Hughes B, Dallal GE, Krall EA, et al. Effect of vitamin D supplementation on wintertime and overall bone loss in healthy postmenopausal women. Ann Intern Med 1991;115:505-12.

[112]Falkeborn M, et al. Hormone replacement therapy and the risk of stroke. Arch Intern Med 1993;153:1201-9.

[113]Prince RL, Smith M, Dick IM, et al. Prevention of postmenopausal osteoporosis: A comparative study of exercise, calcium supplementation, and hormone replacement therapy. N Engl J Med 1991;325:1189-95.

[114]Stampfer MJ, et al. Postmenopausal estrogen therapy and cardiovascular disease. N Engl J Med 1991;325:11.

[115]McAnally LE, Corn CR, Hamilton SF. Aspirin for the prevention of vascular death in women. Ann Pharmacother 1992 Dec;26(12):1530-4.

[116]Winther K, Husted SE, Vissinger H. Low dose acetylsalicylic acid in the antithrombotic treatment of patients with stable angina pectoris and acute coronary syndromes (unstable angina pectoris and acute myocardial infarction). Pharmacol Toxicol 1994 March;74(3):141-7.

[117]Stroke Prevention in Atrial Fibrillation Study Group. Preliminary report of the stroke prevention in atrial fibrillation study. N Engl J Med 1990;322:863-8.

[118]Nelson E. Current use of antiplatelet drugs in stroke syndromes in the USA. Ann N Y Acad Sci 1990;598:368-75.

[119]Singh BN. Advantages of beta blockers versus antiarrhythmic agents and calcium antagonists in secondary prevention after myocardial infarction. Am J Cardiol 1990 Sept 25;66(9):9C-20C.

[120]Gurwitz JH, Goldberg RJ, Chen Z, Gore JM, Alpert JS. Beta-blocker therapy in acute myocardial infarction: evidence for underutilization in the elderly. Am J Med 1992 Dec;93(6):605-10.

[121]Sims RV, Steinmann WC, et al. The clinical effectiveness of pneumococcal vaccine in the elderly. Ann Intern Med 1988;108:653-7.

[122]Hood WB, Jr. Role of converting enzyme inhibitors in the treatment of heart failure. J Am Coll Cardiol 1993 Oct;22(4 Suppl a):154A-7A.

[123]Lewis EJ, Huniskcer LG, Bain RP, et al. The effect of angiotensin converting enzyme inhibition on diabetic nephropathy. N Engl J Med 1993;329:1456.

[124]Zucchelli P, et al. Long-term comparison between captopril and nifedipine in the progression of renal insufficiency. Kidney Int 1992;42:452.

[125]Ravid M, Savin H, Jutrin I, et al. Long-term stabilizing effect of angiotensin converting enzyme inhibition on plasma creatinine and on proteinuria in normotensive type II diabetic patients. Ann Intern Med 1993;188:577.

[126]Bardham KD, Bjarnason I, Scott DL, Griffin WM, Fenn GC, Shield MJ, Morant SV. The prevention and healing of acute non-steroidal anti-inflammatory drug-associated gastroduodenal mucosal damage by misoprostol. Br J Rheumatol 1993 Nov;32(11):990-5.

[127]Gabriel SE, Campion ME, O'Fallon WM. A cost-utility analysis of misoprostol prophylaxis for rheumatoid arthritis patients receiving nonsteroidal anti-inflammatory drugs. Arthritis Rheum 1994 Mar;37(3):333-41.

[128]Graham DY, White RH, Moreland LW, Schubert TT, Katz R, Jaszewski R, Tindall E, Triadafilopoulos G, Stromatt SC, Teoh LS. Duodenal and gastric ulcer prevention with misprostol in arthritis patients taking NSAIDs. Misoprostol Study Group. Ann Intern Med 1993 Aug 15;119(4):257-62.

[129]Stalnikowicz R, Rachmilewitz D. NSAID-induced gastroduodenal damage: is prevention needed? A review and metaanalysis. J Clin Gastroenterol 1993 Oct;17(3):238-43.

[130]Walt RP. Misoprostol for the treatment of peptic ulcer and anti-inflammatory drug-induced gastroduodenal ulceration [Review]. N Engl J Med 1992 Nov 26;327(22):1575-80.

[131]Alderman MH, et al. Treatment-induced blood pressure reduction and the risk of myocardial infarction. JAMA 1989;7:262.

[132]Akhtar M, Breithardt G, Camm AJ, Coumel P, Janse MJ, Lazzara R, Myerberg RJ, Schwartz PJ, Waldo AL, Wellens HJ, et al. CAST and beyond. Implications of the Cardiac Arrhythmia Suppression Trial. Task Force of the Working Group on Arrhythmias of the European Society of Cardiology. [Review]. Circulation 1990 Mar;81(3):1123-7.

[133]Alegro S, Fenster PE, Marcus FI. Digitalis therapy in the elderly. Geriatrics 1985;38:98.

[134]Dall JLC. Maintenance of digoxin in elderly patients BMJ 1970;2:702.

[135]Forman DE, Coletta D, Kenny D, Kosowsky BD, Stoukides J, Rohrer M, Pastore JO. Clinical issues related to discontinuing digoxin therapy in elderly nursing home patients. Arch Intern Med 1991 Nov;151(11):2194-8.

[136]Stults BM. Digoxin use in the elderly. J Am Geriatr Soc 1985;30(3):158.

[137]Ben-Ishay D, Leibel B, Stessman J. Calcium channel blockers in the management of hypertension in the elderly. Am J Med 1986;81(Suppl 6a):30-4.

[138]Fisher ML, Lamey PP. Special considerations in the use of antihypertensive agents in the elderly patient with coexisting disease. Geriatr Med Today 1987;6(11):47.

[139]Avanzini F, Alli C, Bettelli G, Corso R, Colombo F, Mariotti G, Radice M, Torri V, Tognoni G. Antihypertensive efficacy and tolerability of different drug regimens in isolated systolic hypertension in the elderly. Eur Heart J 1994 Feb;15(2):206-12.

[140]SHEP Cooperative Research Group. Prevention of stroke by antihypertensive drug treatment in older persons with isolated systolic hypertension. JAMA 1991;265:3255-65.

[141]Wysowski DK, Baum C. Outpatient use of prescription sedative-hypnotic drugs in the United States, 1970 through 1989. Arch Intern Med 1991 Sept;151(9):1779-83.

[142]Rickels, Schweizer, et al. Long-term therapeutic use of benzodiazepines: Part I, effects of abrupt discontinuation; Part II, effects of gradual taper. Arch Gen Psychiatry 1990;47:899-915.

[143]Anonymous. Anti-anxiety drug usage in the United States, 1989. Statistical Bulletin-Metropolitan Insurance Companies 1991 Jan-Mar;72(1):18-27.

[144]Gilbert A, Owen N, Innes JM, Sansom L. Trial of an intervention to reduce chronic benzodiazepine use among residents of aged-care accommodation. Aust N Z J Med 1993 Aug;23(4):343-7.

[145]Rothschild AJ. Disinhibition, amnestic reactions, and other adverse reactions secondary to triazolam: a review of the literature [Review]. J Clin Psychiatry 1992 Dec; 53 Suppl:69-79.

[146]Suck JA. Psychotropic drug practice in nursing homes. J Am Geriatr Soc 1988;36:409-18.

[147]Swanteck SS, Grossberg GT, Neppe VM, Doubek WG, Martin T, Bender JE. The use of carbamazepine to treat benzodiazepine withdrawal in a geriatric population. J Geriatr Psychiatry Neurol 1991 April-June;4(2):106-9.

[148]Aguglia E, Casacchi GB, et al. Double blinded study of the efficacy and safety of sertraline versus fluoxetine in major depression. Int Clin Psychopharmacol 1994;8:197-202.

[149]Max MB, Lynch SA, Muir J, et al. Effects of desipramine, amitriptyline and fluoxetine on pain in diabetic neuropathy. N Engl J Med 1992;326:1250.

[150]Heston LL, Garrard J, Makris L, Kane RL, Cooper S, Dunham T, Zelterman D. Inadequate treatment of depressed nursing home elderly. J Am Geriatr Soc 1992 Nov;40(11):1117-22.

[151]Katon W., von Korff M, Lin E, Bush T, Ormel J. Adequacy and duration of antidepressant treatment in primary care. Med Care 1992 Jan;30(1):67-76.

[152]Keller MB, et al. Treatment received by depressed patients. JAMA 1982;248(15):1848.

[153]Ray WA, Taylor JA, Meador KG, Lichtenstein MJ, Griffin MR, Fought R, Adams ML, Blazer DG. Reducing antipsychotic drug use in nursing homes. A controlled trial of provider education. Arch Intern Med 1993 Mar 22;153(6):713-21.

[154]Rovner BW, Edelman BA, Cox MP, Shmuely Y. The impact of antipsychotic drug regulations on psychotropic prescribing practices in nursing homes. Am J Psychiatry 1992 Oct;149(10):1390-2.

[155]Semla TP, Pall AK, Poddig B, Brauner DJ. Effect of the Omnibus Reconciliation Act 1987 on antipsychotic prescribing in nursing home residents. Am Geriatr Soc 1994 June;42(6):648-52.

[156]Shorr RI, Fought RL, Ray WA. Changes in antipsychotic drug use in nursing homes during implementaion of the OBRA-87 regulations. JAMA 1994 Feb 2;271(5):358-62.

3

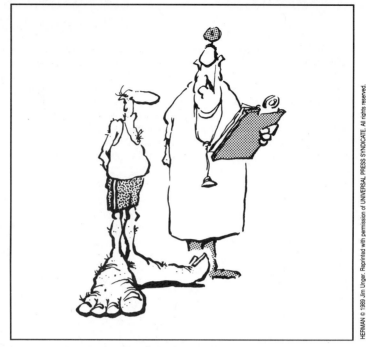

"I warned you about taking steroids with your low blood pressure.'

The Drug and Disease Incompatibility Profile (DIP™) System: Mixing and Matching Pharmacologic Building Blocks

Perhaps it goes without saying that when prescribing drugs, safety comes first.[1-3] Despite the growing recognition that drug reactions and interactions are the nemesis of polypharmacy regimens, few systematic approaches address this problem in a direct manner.[4] The DIP™ system (Drug and Disease Incompatibility Profiles) represents one important solution to these prescribing concerns. Playing a pivotal role in the construction of safe and durable drug houses, the DIP® system is a visually-based, easy-to-use, outpatient practice-oriented drug selection system that pharmacists and clinicians can use to help select commonly used medications based on drug incompatibility profiles.

Identifying centerpiece drugs that are hospitable to the addition of other agents and that do not adversely affect the patient are fundamental clinical and pharmacological priorities. In fact, when it comes to drug interactions, there is a spectrum of pharmacologic issues that must be considered to ensure that drug houses meet pharmatectural safety codes. For example, some drug interactions are very common[5-7] (e.g., the lipid-elevating effects of combining thiazide diuretics and beta-blockers), but their clinical consequences are usually not life-threatening, produce few symptoms, are easily managed, transient, and well-tolerated. However, in other situations, the statistical risk of incurring a drug interaction may be very low (e.g., cardiac arrhythmias produced by the combination of erythromycin and terfenadine [Seldane®]) but the drug-related consequences may be life-threatening.[8,9] Both types of interactions represent potential building code violations, and must be addressed by any system offering guidance for drug selection.[10]

Although there is a tremendous amount of information available regarding drug-drug interactions and drug-disease compatibility profiles, much of it is difficult to access and interpret quickly.[1,2,11,12] This is unfortunate because, in most cases, time is important when making pharmacologic manipulations. Most pharmacists and physicians do not have the time to scan long lists of potential drug-drug and drug-disease interactions for every patient encounter. Even computer-based evaluations and reviews can be cumbersome. The decision to add, combine, or substitute medications is frequently made on the spot, within a limited time framework. Accordingly, prescribing practitioners need a quick approach that weighs the relative risks of combining commonly used pharmacologic building blocks and which also provides quick cross-referencing designed to minimize the other complications of drug therapy.

THE DIP™ SYSTEM

Visually based and stratified according to the relative risk of incurring adverse interactions, the DIP™ system uses a Red-Yellow-Green (i.e., Stop, Caution, Go) drug selection scheme oriented around pie diagrams. Because this pharmatectural approach is based on a color-coded warning system for drug interactions, rather than on a narrative description, the pharmacist or physician can obtain an *instantaneous* reading of potential drug incompatibility profiles. The DIP® system for drug selection is designed to be practical and easy to use. To enhance its day-to-day usefulness, the system emphasizes drugs that are most likely to be used when mixing and matching specific pharmacologic building blocks. Accordingly, the system incorporates and presents information for a wide range of commonly used drug classes including antidepressants, nonsteroidal anti-inflammatory drugs (NSAIDs), corticosteroids, H2 blockers, theophylline, beta-agonists, and oral antibiotics, as well as antihypertensive, antianginal, congestive heart failure-ameliorating, and cardioprotective agents.

With respect to cardiovascular medications, the DIP system provides drug-drug and drug-disease incompatibility profiles for those agents in widest use including, beta-blockers, diuretics, peripheral alpha blockers, ACE inhibitors, calcium blockers, and centrally acting agonists. These drugs deserve special attention because, from a pharmatectural point of view, cardiovascular medications—even those within the same class—can vary slightly from one to another, in subtle but important ways. These variations can be clinically important because these agents frequently are used in many different combinations and in patients who are at high risk for incurring drug-related problems. As a result, these medications must be distinguished from one another in terms of their drug-drug and drug-disease incompatibility profiles. To address these concerns the DIP system evaluates the suitability of specific cardiovascular agents based on drug-drug as well as drug-disease compatibilities.[3]

One of the purposes of the DIP system is to clarify such distinctions in order to optimize drug selection within and between pharmacologic classes. In addition, the patient's underlying disease landscape also must be considered. To enhance its usefulness, the DIP system also evaluates pharmacologic suitability against the backdrop of those diseases most commonly afflicting middle-aged and older Americans (e.g., coronary artery disease, lipid disorders, arthritis, diabetes, congestive heart failure, chronic obstructive pulmonary disease, depression, etc.), as well as against the agents (e.g., beta-blockers, beta-agonists, lipid-lowering agents, calcium blockers, peripheral alpha blockers, nonsteroidal anti-inflammatory drugs, antidepressants, etc.) most likely to be encountered in this patient population.[13-17]

In essence, then, this pharmatectural strategy for optimizing drug selection represents a comprehensive distillation of information gleaned from clinical trials reported in the pharmacologic and medical literature. It also reflects opinions published in expert consensus reports in which the desirability of using different agents for patients on certain drug regimens or with specific disease-cum-risk profiles has been carefully analyzed.[18-21]

GENERAL PRINCIPLES

The DIP system plays a pivotal role in pharmactectural decision-making and should be used to complement a number of other design strategies that are applied to drug house construction. Regardless of which agent or drug class is selected in a given patient or subgroup, adherence to the following drug prescribing principles will help ensure maximal patient compliance and pharmacotherapeutic efficacy: (1) whenever possible, once-a-day drug therapy should be attempted because patient compliance is enhanced significantly by reducing frequency of dosing; (2) adverse side effects must be monitored vigilantly and alterations or substitutions made accordingly; (3) drugs in which the potential for drug-drug interactions are minimized are generally preferable to those associated with one or more possible interactions; (4) drugs should be used only if clinical efficacy has been proven in rigorous scientific studies; (5) drugs shown to improve quality-of-life and minimize functional impairment should be chosen over drugs known to compromise quality of life; and (6) supplementary written instructions to guide patients in their drug use and alert them to potential side effects should be provided because this approach has been shown to enhance patient compliance and overall satisfaction with the therapeutic regimen.

The DIP™ System Color Scheme

For the sake of simplicity, ease of interpretation, and rapid drug analysis, the DIP system is color-based. In this regard, the specific stoplight-scheme colors appearing in DIP profiles are subject to the following interpretations.

Red Designation. Red signifies extreme *caution.* Generally speaking, although there may be unusual exceptions to this rule, the color red in the drug DIP profile suggests that two drugs should never be employed in combination. And when red appears in the disease DIP profile, the drug will almost always adversely affect the underlying disease, and should be avoided in patients who have this clinical disorder.

The red designation, however, is given for a number of different situations and can mean several different things. When this color appears in a drug-incompatibility profile, it indicates the primary drug under consideration has a significant probability of being incompatible (i.e., serious drug interactions are likely to occur) with the other drug in the patient's pre-existing pharmacologic landscape. For example, indomethacin (Indocin®) has a high likelihood for producing hemorrhagic, gastric erosions and, therefore, should not be used with oral anticoagulants, a class of agents which increase bleeding time. Consequently, the drug DIP profile for indomethacin indicates a red color for the pie slice associated with anticoagulant therapy.

It should be emphasized that the red classification also appears when the potential consequences of a drug-drug interaction are severe, even though the probability of its occurrence is very low. In other words, low probability, life-threatening reactions elicit a red DIP designation. For example, the interaction between erythromycin and digoxin is not very common, but erythromycin has the capacity to elevate serum digoxin levels and produce cardiotoxicity, a potentially serious drug-related complication in approximately 10% of patients. Consequently, a red color appears for the erythromycin-digoxin interaction.[6,22]

In the case of pie diagrams devoted to disease incompatibility profiles, the color red indicates the agent has a significant likelihood of worsening the natural history of a common, associated complication of the underlying disease. The red color is used both in situations in which the drug-disease interaction is very common (NSAIDs and peptic ulcer disease) and symptomatically disturbing to the patient, as well as in cases in which the drug-disease interaction is rather uncommon (e.g., amitriptyline-induced cardiac arrhythmias), but has potentially serious clinical consequences.[12,23-25]

Yellow Designation. The color yellow signifies that caution and careful evaluation are required before adding the drug under consideration to the exisiting regimen. From a pharmatectural point of view, yellow represents a permissible, but suboptimal DIP selection. By no means does a yellow pie slice exclude the use of the drug in combination with the drugs or diseases generating this color. But it does mean there are probably better options available (i.e., green designations). Specifically, yellow suggests the drug under consideration usually can be used with safety in conjunction with the drug with which it is being matched. In a significant minority of patients, however, the drug may be either (a) incompatible with the exisiting drug, or (b) another drug combination is preferrable (i.e., a green light combination). For example, NSAIDs usually can be used safely in combination with ACE inhibitors, but in some patients NSAIDs, presumably through prostaglandin inhibition, may compromise the antihypertensive effects of captopril or cause hyperkalemia.[13,17,26,27] Hence, a yellow color is used to suggest caution and the need to reconsider the use of these two agents in combination.[28]

With respect to disease incompatibility profiles, the color yellow suggests that, although the drug can often be used in patients who have this underlying disease, some degree of caution is generally required because the drug may exacerbate the disease, or increase the likelihood of precipitating complications. For example, although digoxin is an excellent choice to treat patients with heart failure caused by left ventricular systolic dysfunction, older patients with advanced congestive heart failure are also more sensitive to potential *toxicity* of digitalis preparations, and therefore, are more likely to experience rhythm disturbances when the drug is used in this setting. Consequently, a yellow pie is used to indicate there is a small, but potentially significant, risk of using digoxin in this patient subgroup.[29,30]

Green Designation. DIP profile pie slices that carry the green color designation represent *optimal* drug-drug and drug-disease combinations. Green pie slices in the drug DIP profile indicate the agent under consideration is almost always compatible with the pre-existing drug. With respect to the DIP profile for drug-disease interactions, green indicates that the newly introduced drug will *not* compromise the natural history of, or produce complications associated with, the underlying disease. Almost without exception, drug-drug and drug-disease matchings that are represented by green pie slices represent optimal pharmacologic management with respect to drug-drug and drug-disease interactions.

Using DIP™ Profiles: Risk, Color, and Compatibility

To maximize its clinical utility, the DIP system uses a "stoplight" color scheme to indicate the relative desirability—or unsuitability—of introducing a specific drug into the regimen of a patient who already is taking one or more other agents, and who has one or more commonly encountered clinical disorders. Consequently, each drug analyzed in the DIP system has two pie diagram profiles: (1) A Drug-Drug Incompatibility Profile and; (2) A Drug-Disease Incompatibility Profile. When contemplating the addition of a drug to a patient's existing *regimen,* the pharmacist or physician should consult *both* DIP profiles.

Two-phase Pharmatectural Evaluation

Step 1: First, consult the drug incompatibility profile (DIP) for the specific drug (i.e., amitriptyline, azithromycin, famotidine) that is being considered for addition to the patient's regimen. The name of the principal drug under evaluation appears in a blue box at the top of each figure. Cross check this drug against the twelve other *commonly* used drugs appearing in the DIP profile. If the drug-drug DIP profile (i.e., the appropriate pie slice) indicates the drug that is being contemplated for inclusion in the drug house is *compatible* with other medications in the regimen with respect to drug-*drug* interactions (i.e., the safety of combined use is confirmed by the presence of a "green" pie, which is optimal—although a "yellow" pie is sometimes acceptable), then proceed to Step 2 (below).

Step 2: During this phase, the drug's suitability with respect to drug-*disease* compatibility is evaluated using the disease DIP profile. If the drug-disease DIP profile demonstrates that the drug under consideration for addition has a low (green) or moderate (yellow) risk for adversely affecting any underlying conditions, then it can be added to the regimen with relative safety. Note: When a yellow color appears in a DIP profile, careful consideration is warranted (see below). Finally, other factors will always come into play and should be considered before a final drug selection is made.

THE DIP™ SYSTEM GUIDE: PROFILES INTO PRACTICE

The drug incompatibility profiles that appear in this chapter incorporate the drug classes and specific agents most often employed in primary care; the disease incompatibility profiles consider the use of these medications against the backdrop of those acute and chronic medical disorders most often managed in the outpatient environment. When using the DIP system, please refer to the color plates of specific DIP profiles appearing in a separate section within this chapter. The following sections provide detailed explanations for why certain drug-drug and drug-disease combinations carry red, yellow, or green designations.

Antidepressants

Amitriptyline (Elavil®), Doxepin HCl (Sinequan®). Because they are relatively inexpensive, tricyclic antidepressants (TCAs), such as amitriptyline and doxepin, are still widely used, despite numerous studies showing that serotonin selective reuptake inhibitors (SSRIs) produce a superior risk: benefit profile for the treatment of depression.[40] There are a number of adverse side effects associated with conventional TCAs, including anticholinergic side effects[31] (dry mouth, urinary retention, visual disturbances, confusion), extrapyramidal movement disorders, disturbances in cognition, and cardiovascular side effects. The cardiovascular profile of TCAs is complex.[32] TCAs and their metabolites are highly concentrated in the myocardium, explaining the vulnerability of the heart to TCA toxicity. For example, TCAs are capable of interfering with heart rate, rhythm, and contractility. Conventional TCAs possess a type Ia antiarrhythmic profile. In contrast, SSRIs are devoid of these properties.

In patients predisposed to cardiovascular disease, therapeutic vigilance is recommended when using TCAs. When the concentration of parent TCA and metabolites exceeds 1000 ng/ml, the risk of cardiovascular toxicity is greatly enhanced. Because of its frequency and potential severity, TCA-induced postural hypotension is another drug-related adverse effect of special concern. Although the mechanism of postural hypotension is not fully understood, blockade of the alpha-adrenergic receptor is the most plausible explanation.[25,33]

Amitriptyline Drug Incompatibility Profile (Tricyclic Antidepressants) (DIP 3-1). In light of these pharmacologic properties, the Drug Incompatibility Profile for amitriptyline and doxepin reveals red warning designations for combined use of these TCAs with alcohol, monoamine oxidase inhibitors (MAOIs) sympathomimetic amines, and antiarrhythmic agents such as quinidine and procainamide. Concurrent use with alcohol is not recommended because TCAs, especially in higher doses, can cause cognitive impairment and sedation, both of which are exacerbated by alcohol intake. There are also studies showing that the combined use of amitriptyline and alcohol can cause additive euphoria, leading to alcohol abuse. Based on these potential interactions, the combined use of TCAs and alcohol should be avoided whenever possible.[6,7,34]

The pharmacologic effects of TCAs such as desipramine and imipramine may be potentiated by the concomitant use of quinidine, which reduces clearance of these antidepressant medications. Although these effects have not been demonstrated specifically with amitriptyline or doxepin, a red warning, nevertheless, is issued. As a group, the combined use of TCAs and Type Ia antiarrhythmic agents has the potential for producing serious adverse effects on cardiac conduction.[7,32]

When TCAs are used in combination with sympathomimetic amines (epinephrine, norepinephrine, phenylephrine, methylphenidate), clinical disturbances such as hypertension and, in rare circumstances, hypertensive crisis may result. These effects are mediated by inhibition of norepinephrine uptake at presynaptic neurons. Because the consequences of acute hypertension can be severe, especially in the elderly, a red warning designation is given for the combined use of these medications. The use of MAOIs in conjunction with TCAs requires extreme therapeutic vigilance. Although these two agents have been used in combination, there are multiple case reports documenting significant adverse consequences when these medications are used together.[1,6,7] A number of deleterious effects are described, including confusion, hyperexcitability, delirium, coma, hyperpyrexia, convulsions, flushing, headache, and death. If for some reason an MAOI and TCA must be used together, the combination is better tolerated when the drugs are started together. When switching from one class to another, a drug-free interval of at least 1 week is recommended when changing from a TCA to an MAOI, and a 2-week drug-free interval is recommended when changing from an MAOI to a TCA. In general, concurrent use is not recommended.[7,35]

A number of drug interactions, although not life-threatening, carry *yellow* DIP® classifications. The anticholinergic side effects associated with TCAs can be exacerbated by combined use with other drugs producing anticholinergic symptoms. These drugs or drug classes include antihistamines (diphenydramine, Benadryl®), muscle relaxants, antipsychotics, anti-Parkinson agents with atropine-like side effects, and scopolamine-containing antidiarrheal agents. The use of cimetidine with TCAs also requires caution because significant anticholinergic side effects (dry mouth, urinary retention, blurred vision, etc.) are produced by cimetidine-mediated elevations in blood TCA serum levels.[22,36-38]

Finally, caution is warranted for combined use of benzodiazepines and TCAs, especially in patients who require maintenance of motor function related to occupational activities. Because both benzodiazepines and TCAs have sedating properties, increased impairment of skills related to driving are observed when these two classes are used in combination.

Amitriptyline Disease Incompatibility Profile (DIP 3-1). For all practical purposes, TCA use is not encouraged in pregnant patients and in individuals with known life-threatening cardiac arrhythmias. Because high doses of TCAs can prolong conduction times, produce arrhythmias, and stimulate sinus tachycardia, this class should be used with great caution in patients[11] with severe coronary artery disease. Orthostatic hypotension may occur in patients with decreased left ventricular function, justifying a yellow classification in individuals suffering from congestive heart failure. Although the mechanism is unclear, both elevated and decreased blood sugar levels have been reported with TCA use, which suggests cautious use in patients with diabetes mellitus.[7]

Because elderly patients are more susceptible to orthostatic hypotension, coronary artery disease, and cardiac arrhythmias, TCAs should be used cautiously in this population. Confusion caused by TCAs is a well-documented side effect in the elderly. Moreover, because elderly patients with arthritis are encouraged to walk, remain active, and exercise their joints, the potential sedating properties of TCAs may be undesirable. Hence, a yellow designation is given for the combined use of TCAs in patients with chronic arthritis.[39,40]

Seizure thresholds can be reduced by TCA use, a finding that dictates cautious use of these agents in patients with a documented seizure disorder or EEG abnormalities. The drug should be used with caution in patients with renal impairment. TCAs also may produce a range of gastrointestinal symptoms, from epigastric distress and cramps to nausea and vomiting. Consequently, selective use in patients with pre-existing ulcer disease is recommended. Finally, the possibility of suicide in depressed patients must always be considered. Although TCAs are used to treat depression, depressed patients should *not* have access to large quantities of the drug. The yellow classification for combining TCAs with depression alludes to this precautionary prescribing practice, which may help reduce the risk of suicide through TCA ingestion. The warning classification and pharmacologic considerations discussed in this section on TCAs (amitriptyline, doxepin) also apply to desipramine. Additional considerations are discussed in the sections below.

The yellow classification for concomitant antihistamine use is downgraded to a red designation because of the potentially severe anticholinergic reaction between desipramine and cyproheptadine. The aggravation of depression that is observed with the combined use of fluoxetine and desipramine also warrants a similar downgrading to a red designation. All other drug interactions are similar to those seen with amitriptyline. Refer to the previous section for an explanation of potential problems associated with use of various TCA-drug combinations.

The disease incompatibility profiles for desipramine would be similar to those generated for amitriptyline. A detailed discussion and explanation of classifications for these drug-disease combinations can be found in the previous section, Amitriptyline-Disease DIP Profiles.

Trazodone (Desyrel®) (DIP 3-2). Trazodone is a commonly used antidepressant, although its precise mechanism of action is not fully understood.

It is not a monoamine oxidase inhibitor, it does not stimulate the CNS, and in animals, it selectively inhibits serotonin uptake. With respect to onset of action, one-half of outpatients responding to trazodone have a significant therapeutic response by the end of the first week of treatment. Three-fourths of responders demonstrate a therapeutic effect by the second week of therapy. As far as drug and disease interactions, trazodone has less anticholinergic toxicity than TCAs, allowing some drugs (e.g., antihistamines, benzodiazepines) to be upgraded to a green designation. On the other hand, there are certain underlying conditions (sexual dysfunction) in which, compared to TCAs, more cautious use is appropriate.[6,7,32]

Trazodone Drug Incompatibility Profile (DIP 3-2). In general, trazodone is less sedating than most TCAs.[41] Although it can cause drowsiness, it can be used in conjunction with alcohol with some degree of caution. Although it is not known how frequently interactions between MAOIs and trazodone occur, a yellow designation admonishes the pharmacist and physician to be aware of possible interactions between these drug classes. Increased phenytoin (Dilantin®) toxicity can be observed with concomitant trazodone therapy, and a yellow cautionary classification is given to create awareness of this possible interaction. Trazodone toxicity may be potentiated by concurrent use with fluoxetine.[41,47] The most common side effect observed in these patients is increased sedation, and therefore, caution is recommended before use with diphenhydramine. Although the interaction between trazodone and warfarin (Coumadin®) is apparently rare, there is a report suggesting that trazodone may reduce the anticoagulant effect of warfarin. Most other commonly used drugs, including NSAIDs, beta-blockers, benzodiazepines, famotidine, and sertraline, can be used in conjunction with trazodone with little risk of adverse interactions. These combinations are given green designations.[1,6,7,12,32,34,35]

Trazodone Disease Incompatibility Profile (DIP 3-2). Many of the same warnings discussed in the section on TCAs also apply to trazodone. It should not be used in pregnancy, and its use is strongly discouraged in this patient subgroup. The risk of using trazodone in patients with severe coronary artery disease appears to be greatest during the initial recovery phase of myocardial infarction. Clinical studies and post-marketing surveillance reports indicate that trazodone may be arrhythmogenic in some patients with preexisting cardiac disease, producing a wide spectrum of disturbances, ranging from PVCs and ventricular bigeminy to short runs of ventricular tachycardia.[32] Occasional reports of sinus bradycardia, shortness of breath, and syncope also have surfaced, suggesting caution (i.e., yellow designation) in patients with known congestive heart failure. The drug's propensity to cause priapism is well-documented, and as a result, it should be used cautiously in men with a previous history of sexual dysfunction, especially those with a history of prolonged or inappropriate erections. Finally, the drug can produce gastrointestinal side effects, a feature that should be considered before use in patients with active peptic ulcer disease.

Serotonin Selective Reuptake Inhibitors (SSRIs).

This class of antidepressants, of which fluoxetine is a member, represents an important advance in the pharmacotherapy of major depression. The SSRIs are comparable in efficacy to the TCAs, but they produce less sedation, are not known to produce adverse cardiac events in therapeutic doses, and carry a category B pregnancy classification. Moreover, the mode of action and side effect profiles associated with SSRIs are different from those seen with TCAs. The DIP® designations for this class of antidepressants reflect these differences.[7,14]

Fluoxetine Drug Incompatibility Profile (DIP 3-3). Although no solid clinical data is presently available to confirm or exclude the possibility of adverse effects from the combined use of MAOIs and fluoxetine, it seems prudent to avoid concomitant use until this issue is settled.[42,43] It is known, however, that depression is aggravated from the combined use of fluoxetine and desipramine, and that fluoxetine's antidepressant effects are reduced by the concomitant use of the antihistamine cyproheptadine. Trazodone toxicity, manifested by excessive sedation, can be precipitated by the introduction of fluoxetine.[41,44] These interactions justify yellow designations. Lithium toxicity is potentiated by the addition of fluoxetine, an observation that necessitates cautious use of these drugs in combination, along with careful monitoring of lithium levels. Fluoxetine, on rare occasions, may produce phenytoin toxicity. Among other commonly used CNS drugs, benzodiazepines such as alprazolam and diazepam interact (i.e., decreased metabolism) with fluoxetine, producing excessive drowsiness and sedation. Finally, the combined use of haloperidol and fluoxetine is associated with increased extrapyramidal symptoms, including one possible case of tardive dyskinesia.[6,7,45-48]

Fluoxetine Disease Incompatibility Profile (DIP 3-3). Fluoxetine can produce agitation, insomnia, and anxiety in a significant minority of patients.[44,49] Hence, cautious use is suggested in patients who have insomnia and in elderly patients with sleep or eating disorders. Although this drug rarely produces seizure,[50] careful use in this patient population is recommended. Careful monitoring is required with chronic use of fluoxetine in patients with significant renal impairment.

Sertraline (Zoloft®) (DIP 3-4). Sertraline is also an SSRI, but it has a shorter half-life (24 hours) than fluoxetine; it may be better tolerated by patients with insomnia, and may be less likely to interact with P450 II D6 than fluoxetine. It has a very favorable DIP profile, both with respect to drug-drug and drug-disease interactions.

Sertraline Drug Incompatibility Profile (DIP 3-4). Although there are no published reports of adverse interactions with MAOIs, the manufacturer's package insert warns of possible adverse events similar to those seen with TCAs. At present, sertraline can be safely used in combination with a wide range of drugs including anticholinergic agents, antihistaminics, famotidine, TCAs, NSAIDs, and theophylline.[1,6,7,32]

Sertraline Disease Incompatibility Profile (DIP 3-4). A yellow designation for pregnancy reflects the drug's category B rating. Caution is also advised when this drug is used in patients with severe renal impairment. In most other common conditions, including cardiovascular disorders, the drug is well-tolerated and, therefore, carries a green DIP designation.

Anti-Inflammatory Agents

Indomethacin (Indocin®) (DIP 3-5). Anti-inflammatory drugs are associated with a wide range of side effects and drug interactions.[6,7,13,18,32,51] Among all NSAIDs, indomethacin probably has the greatest propensity for producing serious drug and disease interactions. Although it can be a useful anti-inflammatory agent in many conditions, including gout and pericarditis, it has a limited role in the pharmatectural approach to long-term therapeutic management of chronic disorders. The significant number of red and yellow DIP designations explains why this drug should be used with therapeutic vigilance.

Indomethacin Drug Incompatibility Profile (DIP 3-5). Because indomethacin can produce gastric erosions, ulcerations, and clinically significant hemorrhage, strong cautionary warnings (red designations) are justified for the combined use of indomethacin with any of the following drugs: alcohol, aspirin, NSAIDs, corticosteroids, and anticoagulants. Because indomethacin is a potent inhibitor of prostaglandin synthesis, it may alter intrarenal hemodynamics, and can precipitate renal failure in patients on triamterene and spironolactone. Consequently, concurrent use with these drugs should be avoided. Although rarely reported, severe hypertension can result from the combined use of phenylpropanolamine with indomethacin. Until more is known about the potential occurrence of this drug interaction, concurrent use is best avoided.[1,6,7]

Even when used alone, ACE inhibitors can produce hyperkalemia and renal deterioration in a small subset of patients. Not surprisingly, NSAIDs such as indomethacin can potentiate these adverse effects. For example, impaired renal function and renal failure can result from the combined use of captopril and indomethacin. Therefore, extreme caution or avoidance of concurrent administration is strongly recommended. A yellow designation is appropriate for these potential drug interactions. Antacids decrease absorption of indomethacin, causing a reduction in its clinical effect. In addition, indomethacin can produce coronary vasoconstriction, blunt the antianginal effects of beta-blockers, and decrease the hypotensive effects of beta-blockers, all of which justify a yellow warning before using these agents together for extended periods in patients with hypertension or severe coronary artery disease. Indomethacin can be used safely with H2-blockers.

Indomethacin Disease Incompatibility Profile (DIP 3-5). The elderly, as well as patients with a history of peptic ulcer disease, renal dysfunction, or congestive heart failure are poor candidates for chronic indomethacin therapy, which can produce fluid retention, congestive heart failure, deterioration of renal function, gastrointestinal bleeding, dizziness, and confusion. Accordingly, red DIP designations warn against the use of this agent in patients who have these underlying conditions. Because many NSAIDs, including aspirin and indomethacin, can produce CNS side effects, including depression, a yellow warning designation appears in the pie slice in this DIP diagram. The capacity of indomethacin to inhibit the antianginal properties of beta-blockers justifies cautious use in the setting of angina and severe coronary artery disease. Finally, indomethacin can produce changes in glucose metabolism, suggesting that its use in diabetic patients should be closely monitored.

Nonsteroidal Anti-Inflammatory Drugs (NSAIDs) (DIP 3-6). Many of the same precautions that are highlighted for use of indomethacin also apply to the use of other NSAIDs such as ibuprofen, naproxen, nabumetone, piroxicam, and many others. In general, the aforementioned NSAIDs are better tolerated than indomethacin and, as a result, many of the red designations are upgraded to cautionary yellow categories for NSAID drug interactions. There are also some important differences between indomethacin and the other classes of NSAIDs, and these differences are reflected in the incompatibility profiles discussed below. Finally, it should be noted that nearly all NSAID-mediated toxicities are dose-related and that reducing the risk for drug-related adverse events can usually be accomplished through decreases in drug dosage.

NSAID Drug Incompatibility Profile (DIP 3-6). The adverse gastrointestinal side effects of NSAIDs are well-known. Consequently, their concurrent use with corticosteroids (i.e., prednisone) and warfarin is discouraged. It should be emphasized that when prednisone is used in conjunction with NSAIDs, the risk of severe gastrointestinal bleeding is increased fourfold. Hence, the concomitant use of these two agents requires strong clinical justification, and whenever possible, alternative therapies should be explored. Because of the significant risk for gastrointestinal tract hemorrhage, the use of anticoagulants is often best avoided in patients on NSAID therapy.[1,7,13,32,52]

Strong cautionary (yellow) classifications apply to the use of NSAIDs with aspirin (additive gastrointestinal toxicity), ACE inhibitors (renal deterioration), alcohol (additive gastrointestinal toxicity), and diuretics (potentiation of NSAID-induced renal failure). Methotrexate-NSAID interactions require special mention. Although the mechanism of this drug interaction is not known, reduced renal clearance is suspected. Several NSAIDs cause severe toxic reactions or delayed methotrexate renal clearance. Renal failure and other clinical effects are observed, prompting experts to recommend that nonsteroidal drugs should be stopped 2 to 3 days before intitiating methotrexate therapy, especially in the elderly and patients with impaired renal function. Most NSAIDs, except sulindac, increase lithium serum levels, an interaction that can be significant and is preventable with careful monitoring of lithium levels. Finally, hypoglycemia occurs when NSAIDs are combined with tolbutamide, an interaction that results from displacement of the tolbutamide from protein binding sites.

NSAID Disease Incompatibility Profile (DIP 3-6). Most of the NSAIDs are given a category B classification for use in pregnancy. Two agents, mefenamic acid and tolmetin are classified category C. Because these agents can inhibit prostaglandin synthesis and produce adverse effects on the fetus, a red designation (i.e., avoidance, if possible) is issued for the use of NSAIDs in pregnancy. Elderly patients are at higher risk for incurring NSAID-induced central nervous system, renal, GI and cardiovascular side effects; consequently, caution and a careful review of the past medical history is advised before initiating therapy with NSAIDs in the older patient.[53] NSAIDs, especially indomethacin, can aggravate depression, mandating cautious use in this subgroup.[54,55] NSAIDs can cause fluid retention and edema, thereby aggravating symptoms of congestive heart failure. Patients with coronary artery disease are at higher risk for developing renal deterioration from NSAID therapy, and as a result, a cautionary yellow designation is applied to this potential drug-disease interaction. Patients with decreased cardiac output and decreased renal blood flow are especially at risk. Finally, NSAIDs can cause disturbances in glucose metabolism and electrolyte elimination, two features that demand prudent administration in patients with cardiac arrhythmias and diabetes.[1,6,18,24,32,56,57]

Corticosteroids (Prednisone, Methylprednisolone) (DIP 3-7). Corticosteroids can produce salutory effects and symptomatic improvement in a number of inflammatory disorders. Despite their proven efficacy, agents from this class must be used cautiously because these drugs also have the capacity for producing a wide range of adverse drug interactions. The drug and disease incompatibility profiles for these agents highlight the most significant clinical concerns when concurrent use is being considered.[58]

Corticosteroid Drug Incompatibility Profile (DIP 3-7). As discussed in a previous section, the concurrent use of NSAIDs and corticosteroids should be avoided when possible because the risk of producing gastrointestinal tract hemorrhage increases dramatically when these two drug classes are used in combination. A red DIP designation warns against this potentially problematic drug combination.

Yellow DIP designations alert pharmacists and physicians to a number of potential drug interactions. For example, many antacids, except those containing a low dose of aluminum phosphate, can interfere with oral corticosteroid absorption, thereby reducing its therapeutic efficacy. Because the combination of corticosteroids and loop diuretics can lead to increased renal potassium losses, careful monitoring of serum potassium concentrations is recommended. Concurrent use of corticosteroids with alcohol, aspirin, and anticoagulants is sometimes unavoidable, although clinicians should be aware of the adverse gastrointestinal effects that can result from these drug combinations. Omeprazole decreases the clinical effects of corticosteroids through a mechanism that is not yet understood. Phenytoin can produce a decrease in corticosteroid effect through increased metabolism. Although the clinical significance of theophylline and sympathomimetic amine-corticosteroid interactions is not well-established, concurrent use should be considered only with careful monitoring of theophylline serum concentrations.

Corticosteroid Disease Incompatibility Profile (DIP 3-7). Corticosteroids can compromise the natural history of many common clinical disorders, which explains why warning designations (red and yellow DIP pie slices) appear for so many conditions. Perhaps the risk of gastrointestinal tract hemorrhage is the most important adverse effect. In this vein, the presence of active peptic ulcer disease virtually contraindicates the use of corticosteroids.[59]

Because corticosteroids can produce alterations in glucose metabolism, predispose to infections, cause neuropsychiatric symptoms (including psychosis), induce fluid retention, and lead to electrolyte disturbances, the use of drugs such as prednisone requires caution in a number of common disorders including diabetes, depression, congestive heart failure, hypertension, coronary artery disease, and renal failure. Many complications can be prevented by using the lowest possible steroid dose necessary to achieve therapeutic effects and by monitoring parameters (e.g., serum potassium, blood glucose) associated with corticosteroid effects.

Aspirin (Salicylates) (DIP 3-8). Widely available and used for their analgesic, anti-inflammatory, cardioprotective, and antirheumatic effects, salicylates are associated with a number of clinically important adverse drug interactions.[6,7,18,24,51,52]

Aspirin Drug Incompatibility Profile (DIP 3-8). The interaction between salicylates and methotrexate is not conclusively confirmed, but the evidence is strong enough to produce a red (i.e., extreme caution,[6,7] avoid concurrent use if possible) designation for their combined use. Either through decreased clearance or reduction in methotrexate protein binding, salicylates can potentiate methotrexate toxicity. Although human data is retrospective and anecdotal, close patient monitoring is mandatory when these agents are used concurrently.

Clearly, the propensity for salicylates to produce gastric erosions and ulceration usually contraindicates their use in combination with anticoagulants. However, there is a subset of individuals with coronary heart disease, a history of myocardial infarction, and thromboembolic disorders who would benefit from the combined use of anticoagulants and salicylate-mediated antiplatelet properties. Studies confirming that low-dose salicylate therapy (i.e., 80 mg orally daily) is sufficient to achieve therapeutic results makes the concurrent use of warfarin-like drugs more attractive. As yet, however, there are no prospective studies demonstrating the degree of safety of this drug interaction. Consequently, a red designation is used for all salicylate-warfarin combinations. (Except as noted, the DIP profiles in this section do not refer to *low-dose* salicylate therapy.)

A number of drug interactions requiring moderate caution are highlighted with yellow DIP pie slices. The risk of gastrointestinal tract hemorrhage is exacerbated by the concomitant use of alcohol, corticosteroids, or NSAIDs with aspirin. In general, concurrent use of aspirin and NSAIDs is to be discouraged. However, elderly patients with a history of both myocardial infarction and osteoarthritis may benefit from low-dose salicylate therapy for cardioprotection and NSAID therapy for symptomatic improvement of their inflammatory disorder. In such cases, the two agents can be used concurrently, but only with careful clinical monitoring. Although the clinical significance of the quinidine-aspirin interaction is not known, there is some suggestion that these two agents have additive antiplatelet effects and, as a result, can significantly increase bleeding time.[6,7] Concurrent use is recommended only with careful clinical surveillance.

A yellow warning designation is used for concurrent use of cimetidine and aspirin because there is a risk of salicylate toxicity as a result of decreased metabolism. Salicylates can displace chlorpropamide from protein binding sites, increasing their effective serum concentration and, in some cases, producing hypoglycemia. High-dose aspirin therapy may also produce hypoglycemic effects. Displacement of valproate from serum binding sites by salicylates can produce valproate toxicity. This reaction encourages the use of alternative analgesic or antipyretic drugs in patients on valproate. Finally, the inhibition of prostaglandin synthesis mediated by salicylates may be responsible for producing a reduction in antihypertensive effects of captopril therapy.

Histamine (H2)-Receptor Antagonists

H2-blockers are used for the treatment of peptic ulcer disease. All four of the currently approved agents—cimetidine, ranitidine, famotidine, and nizatidine—are efficacious, easily taken, and well-tolerated. From the perspective of medication compliance, all four drugs can be taken once a day at bedtime: 800 mg of cimetidine, 300 mg of ranitidine, 40 mg of famotidine, and 300 mg of nizatidine. The potency of these recommended doses is about equal.

Because renal excretion is the major route of elimination of H2-blockers, patients with renal insufficiency should receive reduced doses of agents with dose-related toxicity, e.g., cimetidine. In general, there is little to recommend one H2-blocker over another. There are some subtle but clinically relevant differences, however, that argue for preferential use of one agent over another in specific patient subgroups. All the H2-blockers can produce central nervous symptoms, such as headache and mental confusion. Cimetidine, and to a lesser extent, ranitidine, bind to hepatic cytochrome p-450 microsomal enzymes and may inhibit the catabolism of many drugs metabolized by this system.

These interactions are highlighted in the DIP pie diagrams. Oftentimes, these interactions are not clinically significant, with the possible exception of a few drugs that have narrow therapeutic to toxic ratios, such as theophylline, phenytoin, and some anticoagulants, such as warfarin. Despite the infrequency of serious adverse drug interactions, levels of theophylline and phenytoin and prothrombin times (in the case of warfarin), should be more carefully monitored if cimetidine is used in conjunction with these drugs. Alternately, another H2-blocker such as famotidine can be used to avoid the risk of these interactions.

Recently, all the H2-blockers, with the exception of famotidine, were shown to inhibit gastric alcohol dehydrogenase, an enzyme in the stomach that plays an important role in the first-pass metabolism of oral alcohol. Inhibition of this enzyme by H2-blockers may result in more absorption of oral alcohol, higher blood levels, and greater susceptibility to alcohol toxicity.

These and other distinguishing features are highlighted in the drug and disease incompatibility profiles for the three most commonly used H2-blockers—cimetidine, ranitidine, and famotidine.

Cimetidine (Tagamet®) Drug Incompatibilty Profile (DIP 3-9). Most of the potential adverse drug interactions associated with cimetidine carry a yellow designation. For example, the clinical significance of the increased alcohol effect produced by cimetidine-mediated inhibition of acetaldehyde in

ALDH-1 deficiency is not known, but patients should be warned that they may experience a greater degree of alcohol intoxication when cimetidine is added to their drug regimen. Rarely, the combined use of cimetidine and captopril produces severe neuropathies in patients with renal impairment. The majority of other interactions result from cimetidine-induced inhibition of the hepatic cytochrome p-450 microsomal enzyme system. In this regard, anticoagulants, phenytoin, antidepressants, benzodiazepines, and theophylline must be monitored for toxic side effects when used in conjunction with cimetidine.[60] The clinical effects of beta-blockers and glipizide also should be monitored if this H2-blocker is added to the medication regimen. Concomitant use of cimetidine and narcotics should be avoided, especially in dialysis patients and in individuals with respiratory depression. The clinical significance of a digoxin-cimetidine interaction is questionable, but digoxin concentrations should be routinely evaluated to avoid possible elevations and toxic effects.[1,6,36,61-63]

Cimetidine Disease Incompatibility Profile (DIP 3-9). Cimetidine can be used with a relative degree of safety in most common clinical disorders, but there are some important drug-disease interactions noted in the DIP figures. Cimetidine carries a category B pregnancy rating. Elderly patients are more likely to have renal impairment and central nervous system disorders. Accordingly, cimetidine should be used with some degree of caution in this population. A wide range of reversible central nervous system effects are produced by this H2-blocker, including confusion, agitation, depression, anxiety, and psychosis. Therefore, some degree of caution is required in patients who have pre-exisiting neuropsychiatric disorders, including depression. Rapid intravenous administration of cimetidine can produce cardiac arrhythmias and hypotension. Because cimetidine can affect the serum levels of many antiarrhythmic agents, a cautionary yellow designation is included for use in patients with cardiac rhythm disturbances. Because most arthritic patients are taking either narcotics or NSAIDs, both of which can cause central nervous system side effects, the addition of cimetidine, with its propensity for causing confusion, should be monitored closely.[36,62,64]

Ranitidine (Zantac®) Drug Incompatibility Profile (DIP 3-10). Because ranitidine binds to the p-450 cytochrome oxidase system with *weak* affinity, it can produce some of the drug interactions associated with cimetidine use. In general, however, these interactions are not clinically significant, although on rare occasions, they may be. The effects of alcohol, metoprolol, anticoagulants, oral hypoglycemics, benzodiazepines, and phenytoin may all be potentiated by concurrent ranitidine administration. The clinical significance of these interactions is not yet established, but prudence requires calling attention to their possible occurrence.[6,7,35,62]

Ranitidine Disease Incompatibility Profile (DIP 3-10). Because elderly patients often have reduced renal function, ranitidine use should be monitored in this group. Older patients should also be evaluated for possible central nervous system side effects associated with ranitidine use.[65] Bradycardia, tachycardia, and PVCs are seen with rapid intravenous administration of this

H2-blocker.[37] A yellow designation is issued to alert the clinician of this possible side effect.[50,66]

Famotidine Drug Incompatibility Profile (DIP 3-11). Famotidine can be used safely in combination with most commonly used medications. Probenecid, however, can rarely produce famotidine toxicity, and concurrent use of these two agents is not recommended. Rare cases of famotidine-induced phenytoin and anticoagulant toxicity are reported.[6,7]

Famotidine Disease Incompatibility Profile (DIP 3-11). Famotidine can be used safely in most clinical disorders. It carries a category B pregnancy classification and its use should be monitored in patients with renal impairment.

Benzodiazepines

Benzodiazepines are frequently used to relieve short-term anxiety in middle-aged and older patients.[67] Although all these agents—flurazepam, diazepam, chlordiazepoxide, alprazolam,[68] temazepam, oxazepam, etc.—produce central nervous system effects,[69] those agents with a longer half-life tend to be more problematic, especially in the elderly. Somnolence, confusion, and depression are the most common presenting symptoms of anxiolytic toxicity associated with long-acting benzodiazepines. A number of drug-drug interactions also deserve attention, especially those with agents such as narcotics, alcohol, and diphenhydramine, all of which have the capacity for potentiating central nervous system and respiratory depression associated with benzodiazepine use.[70-74]

Benzodiazepine Drug Incompatibility Profile (DIP 3-12). The use of alcohol with anxiolytics should be strongly discouraged because even small amounts of alcohol may impair driving ability in patients taking benzodiazepines. Because the effects of benzodiazepines and alcohol may be additive, a red (avoid concurrent use) designation is used. Several case reports describe a syndrome of hypotension, stupor, and respiratory distress from the combined use of loxapine and lorazepam. Accordingly, these two agents probably should not be used simultaneously.[6,7]

Yellow classifications are used to indicate a number of interactions in which benzodiazepine toxicity is potentiated by concomitant administration of another drug. For example, propranolol and metoprolol may be associated with increased diazepam and clorazepate toxicity. These combinations can be avoided by use of hydrophilic beta-blockers. When beta-blockers and benzodiazepines *must* be used in combination, the concurrent use of hydrophilic beta-blockers such as atenolol and lorazepam is recommended as an alternative. Drugs that are known to produce central nervous system depression or sedation (i.e., narcotics, sedating antihistamines, antidepressants, etc.) should be used cautiously with benzodiazepines. Even fluoxetine, although it is nonsedating, may cause increased impairment of skills related to driving when used with diazepam or alprazolam as a result of decreased clearance.[6,7,35]

Theophylline produces a decrease in diazepam's sedative effects, probably because of adenosine receptor blockade. In general, concurrent use is not recommended.

Benzodiazepine Disease Incompatibility Profile (DIP 3-12). Long-acting benzodiazepines can produce confusion, respiratory depression,[75] disorientation, hallucinations, and falls in the elderly. Consequently, their use in this population should be avoided if possible. Benzodiazepines should not be used in pregnancy. Finally, benzodiazepines should be used only with caution in conditions requiring mobility (arthritis), mental alertness (depression), and respiratory motivation (chronic obstructive pulmonary disease).[71-73]

Sympathomimetic Bronchodilators

Sympathomimetic bronchodilators are used to produce bronchodilation. This is accomplished by relieving reversible bronchospasm through relaxation of bronchiole smooth muscles in such conditions as asthma, bronchitis, emphysema, or bronchiectasis. The relative selectivity of action of beta-agonists is the principal determinant of clinical usefulness and can predict the most likely side effects. The beta-2 selective agents provide the greatest benefits with minimal side effects. Because sympathomimetics with ∝-agonist properties can produce a number of actions, from pressor effects and nasal decongestion to bronchial dilation and increased myocardial contractility, these drugs should be administered with caution to individuals with unstable vasomotor systems, hypertension, hyperthyroidism, diabetes, prostatic hypertrophy, or a history of seizures. Cautious use is also recommended in elderly patients, in psychoneurotic individuals (who may have a tendency to overuse these drugs), and in patients with long-standing bronchial asthma who have developed degenerative heart disease.

Although generally safe in healthy individuals and well-tolerated, sympathomimetics can cause nervousness, restlessness, and sleeplessness. The presence of these symptoms requires dose reduction. Occasionally, patients develop severe paradoxical airway resistance with repeated, excessive use of inhalants. The precise cause for this is unknown, but when this is observed, the drug should be withdrawn immediately and alternative therapy instituted.

Beta-Agonist (Albuterol, Metaproterenol, Isoetharine) Drug Incompatibility Profile (DIP 3-13). A red warning designation is given for the combined use of beta-blockers and beta-agonists. Beta-blockers antagonize the effects of sympathomimetics, and concurrent use is counterproductive. Moreover, the introduction of a beta-blocker into the drug regimen of a patient with bronchospastic pulmonary disease can produce severe clinical consequences.

A yellow warning for concurrent use of theophylline and beta-agonists reflects the observation that, in children, terbutaline and albuterol may actually decrease theophylline effect by increasing the metabolism of the drug. Theophylline concentrations should be monitored in patients receiving an inhaled beta-agonist in conjunction with oral theophylline. Digoxin toxicity has been observed in patients on digoxin who were administered oral or intravenous albuterol. The precipitating factor may be hypokalemia, or sensitization of the heart by sympathomimetics to digoxin-induced cardiac arrhythmias. Finally, the hypokalemic effects of thiazide diuretics may be potentiated by concomitant use of albuterol.[76]

Beta-Agonist Disease Incompatibility Profile (DIP 3-13). Controlled and moderate intake of sympathomimetic agents is generally safe. However, when use of these agents is chronic and excessive, a number of adverse clinical effects may be observed, especially in patients with underlying central nervous system disorders, cardiovascular disease, asthma, and endocrine disorders.[77] Consequently, a number of yellow warning designations appear in the drug incompatibility profile for albuterol, metaproterenol, and isoetharine. Because beta sympathomimetics are potent central nervous system stimulants and can cause stimulation, restlessness, apprehension, anxiety, and fear, these drugs should be administered with caution to individuals suffering from depression, panic attacks, and anxiety disorders. In addition, beta-agonists are associated with palpitations, changes in blood pressure (elevation and depression), tachycardia, arrhythmias, chest discomfort, PVCs (rare), and other cardiac symptoms. Ephedrine, in particular, can precipitate hypertensive episodes severe enough to cause intracranial hemorrhage, and can induce angina in patients with acute coronary insufficiency.

Accordingly, sympathomimetics should be used with caution in patients with a history of coronary artery disease, congestive heart failure, cardiac arrhythmias, and stroke. Because the elderly are at high risk for having these underlying conditions, a yellow designation is issued for beta-agonist use in this age group. Large doses of intravenous albuterol can aggravate preexisting diabetes mellitus; the role of inhaled albuterol is unknown, but insulin or oral hypoglycemic requirements should be carefully monitored in diabetic patients taking oral sympathomimetics. Most of these agents carry a category C pregnancy classification, and should be avoided in this patient subgroup.

Because beta-agonists can produce heartburn and nausea, their use in patients with peptic ulcer disease should be monitored. Finally, on occasion, inhalants can stimulate bronchospasm and coughing in patients with chronic obstructive pulmonary disease. Accordingly, the possibility of paradoxical deterioration of patients with underlying lung disease should be considered.

Theophyllines

Theophylline compounds (Theo-Dur®, Bronkodyl®, Choledyl®, etc.) are used to provide symptomatic relief and for prevention of reversible bronchospasm associated with chronic bronchitis, asthma, and emphysema. Excessive dosage of the drug can produce serious toxicity, which increases at serum levels > 20 mcg/ml (toxic effects are seen in 75% of patients with serum levels > 25 mcg/ml).[78] Decreased clearance of theophylline is common in the elderly, in patients with liver dysfunction, and in individuals taking medications that inhibit the p-450 hepatic cytochrome oxidase system. Because the therapeutic to toxic ratio is extremely narrow with theophylline, and because the cardiovascular and neurologic side effects of this drug can produce serious clinical consequences,

ANTIDEPRESSANTS

TRICYCLIC ANTIDEPRESSANTS
Elavil®, Sinequan®

DRUG Incompatibility Profile

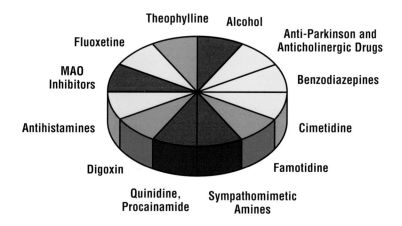

Theophylline · Alcohol · Anti-Parkinson and Anticholinergic Drugs · Fluoxetine · MAO Inhibitors · Benzodiazepines · Antihistamines · Cimetidine · Digoxin · Famotidine · Quinidine, Procainamide · Sympathomimetic Amines

DISEASE Incompatibility Profile

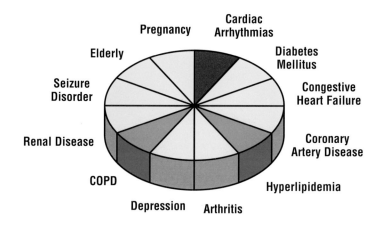

Pregnancy · Cardiac Arrhythmias · Elderly · Diabetes Mellitus · Seizure Disorder · Congestive Heart Failure · Renal Disease · Coronary Artery Disease · COPD · Hyperlipidemia · Depression · Arthritis

ANTIDEPRESSANTS

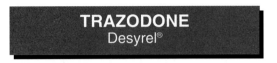

TRAZODONE
Desyrel®

DRUG Incompatibility Profile

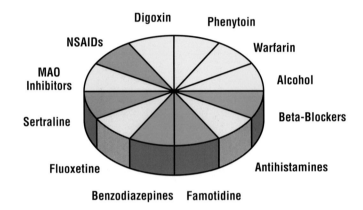

Digoxin   Phenytoin

NSAIDs   Warfarin

MAO Inhibitors   Alcohol

Sertraline   Beta-Blockers

Fluoxetine   Antihistamines

Benzodiazepines   Famotidine

DISEASE Incompatibility Profile

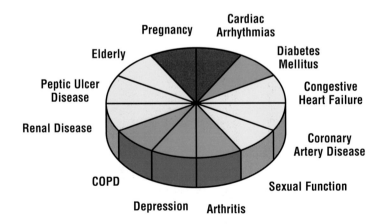

Pregnancy   Cardiac Arrhythmias

Elderly   Diabetes Mellitus

Peptic Ulcer Disease   Congestive Heart Failure

Renal Disease   Coronary Artery Disease

COPD   Sexual Function

Depression   Arthritis

ANTIDEPRESSANTS

FLUOXETINE, PAROXETINE
Prozac®, Paxil®

DRUG Incompatibility Profile

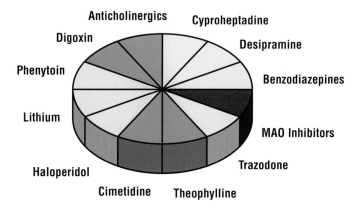

Anticholinergics
Cyproheptadine
Digoxin
Desipramine
Phenytoin
Benzodiazepines
Lithium
MAO Inhibitors
Haloperidol
Trazodone
Cimetidine
Theophylline

DISEASE Incompatibility Profile

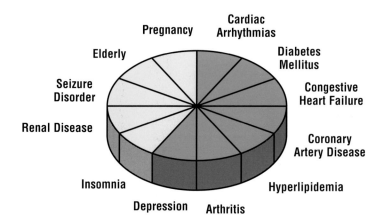

Pregnancy
Cardiac Arrhythmias
Elderly
Diabetes Mellitus
Seizure Disorder
Congestive Heart Failure
Renal Disease
Coronary Artery Disease
Insomnia
Hyperlipidemia
Depression
Arthritis

ANTIDEPRESSANTS

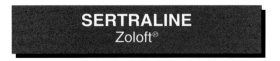

DRUG Incompatibility Profile

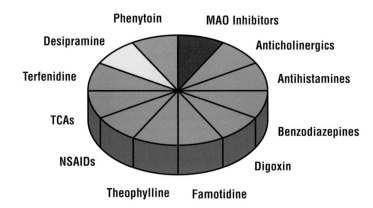

DISEASE Incompatibility Profile

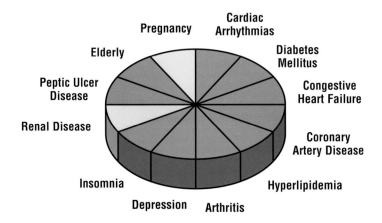

ANTI-INFLAMMATORY AGENTS

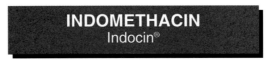

INDOMETHACIN
Indocin®

DRUG Incompatibility Profile

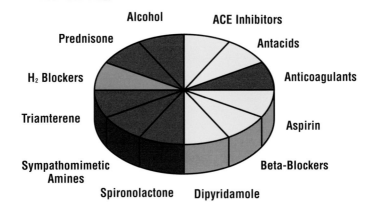

Alcohol
ACE Inhibitors
Prednisone
Antacids
H₂ Blockers
Anticoagulants
Triamterene
Aspirin
Sympathomimetic Amines
Beta-Blockers
Spironolactone
Dipyridamole

DISEASE Incompatibility Profile

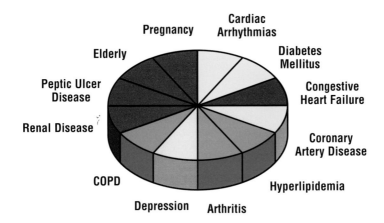

Pregnancy
Cardiac Arrhythmias
Elderly
Diabetes Mellitus
Peptic Ulcer Disease
Congestive Heart Failure
Renal Disease
Coronary Artery Disease
COPD
Hyperlipidemia
Depression
Arthritis

ANTI-INFLAMMATORY AGENTS

NSAIDs
Ibuprofen, Ketorolac, Nabumetone,
Naproxen, Piroxicam

DRUG Incompatibility Profile

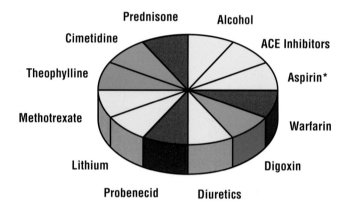

DISEASE Incompatibility Profile

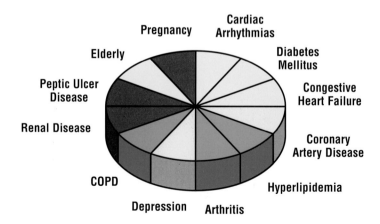

*Aspirin is contraindicated with Ketorolac.

CORTICOSTEROIDS

CORTICOSTEROIDS
Methylprednisolone, Prednisone

DRUG Incompatibility Profile

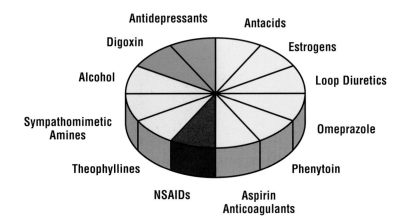

DISEASE Incompatibility Profile

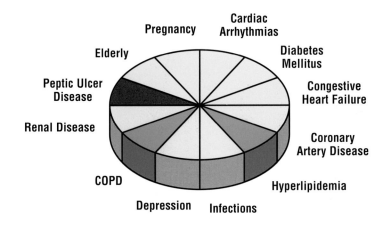

ANTI-PLATELET DRUGS

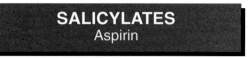

SALICYLATES
Aspirin

DRUG Incompatibility Profile

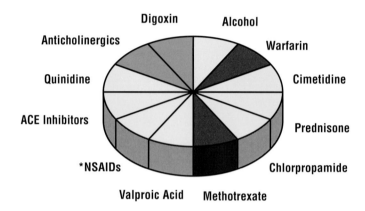

Digoxin   Alcohol
Anticholinergics   Warfarin
Quinidine   Cimetidine
ACE Inhibitors   Prednisone
*NSAIDs   Chlorpropamide
Valproic Acid   Methotrexate

DISEASE Incompatibility Profile

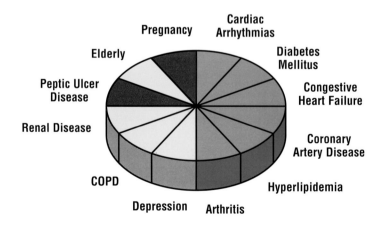

Pregnancy   Cardiac Arrhythmias
Elderly   Diabetes Mellitus
Peptic Ulcer Disease   Congestive Heart Failure
Renal Disease   Coronary Artery Disease
COPD   Hyperlipidemia
Depression   Arthritis

*Except for Ketorolac, which should be red.

H₂-ANTAGONISTS

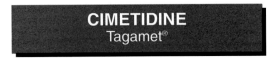

CIMETIDINE
Tagamet®

DRUG Incompatibility Profile

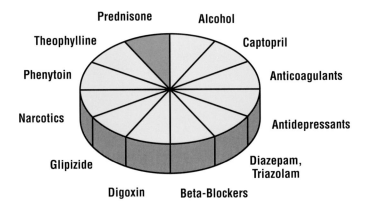

Prednisone Alcohol
Theophylline Captopril
Phenytoin Anticoagulants
Narcotics Antidepressants
Glipizide Diazepam, Triazolam
Digoxin Beta-Blockers

DISEASE Incompatibility Profile

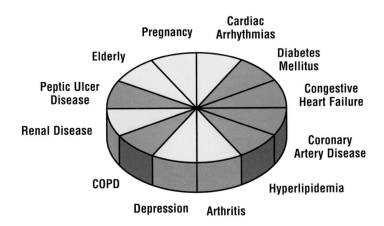

Pregnancy Cardiac Arrhythmias
Elderly Diabetes Mellitus
Peptic Ulcer Disease Congestive Heart Failure
Renal Disease Coronary Artery Disease
COPD Hyperlipidemia
Depression Arthritis

H₂-ANTAGONISTS

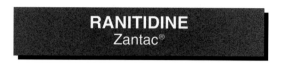

DRUG Incompatibility Profile

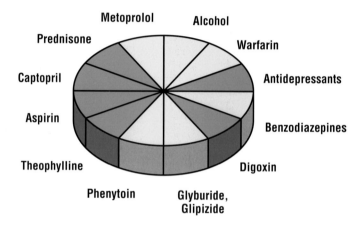

DISEASE Incompatibility Profile

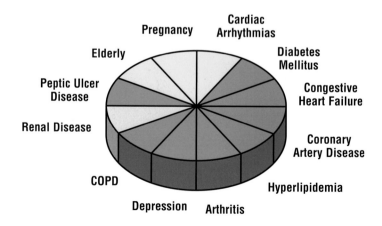

H$_2$-ANTAGONISTS

FAMOTIDINE
Pepcid®

DRUG Incompatibility Profile

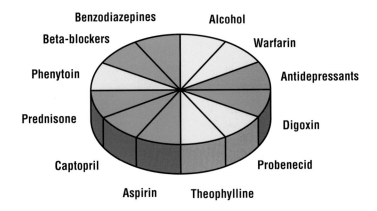

Benzodiazepines Alcohol
Beta-blockers Warfarin
Phenytoin Antidepressants
Prednisone Digoxin
Captopril Probenecid
Aspirin Theophylline

DISEASE Incompatibility Profile

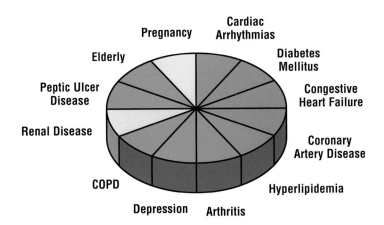

Pregnancy Cardiac Arrhythmias
Elderly Diabetes Mellitus
Peptic Ulcer Disease Congestive Heart Failure
Renal Disease Coronary Artery Disease
COPD Hyperlipidemia
Depression Arthritis

SEDATIVES/ANXIOLYTICS

BENZODIASZEPINES

DRUG Incompatibility Profile

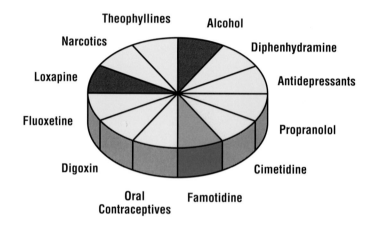

Theophyllines
Alcohol
Narcotics
Diphenhydramine
Loxapine
Antidepressants
Fluoxetine
Propranolol
Digoxin
Cimetidine
Oral Contraceptives
Famotidine

DISEASE Incompatibility Profile

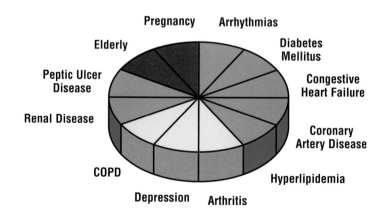

Pregnancy
Arrhythmias
Elderly
Diabetes Mellitus
Peptic Ulcer Disease
Congestive Heart Failure
Renal Disease
Coronary Artery Disease
COPD
Hyperlipidemia
Depression
Arthritis

BRONCHODILATORS

BETA AGONISTS
Albuterol, Metaproterenol, Isoetharine

DRUG Incompatibility Profile

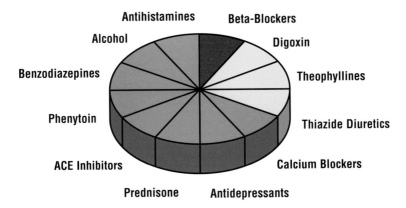

Antihistamines · Beta-Blockers · Alcohol · Digoxin · Benzodiazepines · Theophyllines · Phenytoin · Thiazide Diuretics · ACE Inhibitors · Calcium Blockers · Prednisone · Antidepressants

DISEASE Incompatibility Profile

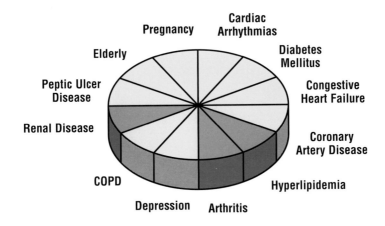

Pregnancy · Cardiac Arrhythmias · Elderly · Diabetes Mellitus · Peptic Ulcer Disease · Congestive Heart Failure · Renal Disease · Coronary Artery Disease · COPD · Hyperlipidemia · Depression · Arthritis

BRONCHODILATORS

THEOPHYLLINES
Bronkodyl®, Choledyl®, Theo-Dur®

DRUG Incompatibility Profile

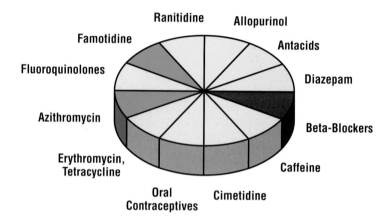

DISEASE Incompatibility Profile

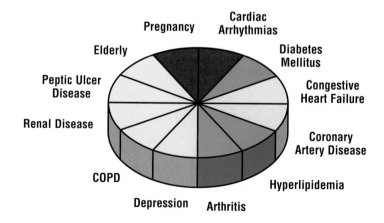

ANTIHISTAMINES

TERFENADINE
Seldane®

DRUG Incompatibility Profile

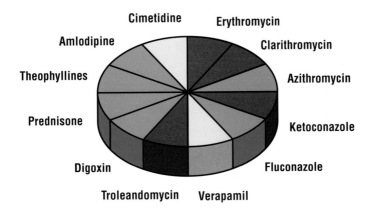

Cimetidine
Erythromycin
Amlodipine
Clarithromycin
Theophyllines
Azithromycin
Prednisone
Ketoconazole
Digoxin
Fluconazole
Troleandomycin
Verapamil

DISEASE Incompatibility Profile

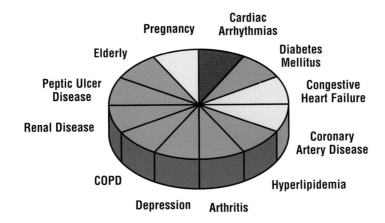

Pregnancy
Cardiac Arrhythmias
Elderly
Diabetes Mellitus
Peptic Ulcer Disease
Congestive Heart Failure
Renal Disease
Coronary Artery Disease
COPD
Hyperlipidemia
Depression
Arthritis

ANTIHISTAMINES

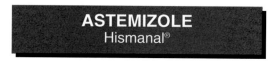

ASTEMIZOLE
Hismanal®

DRUG Incompatibility Profile

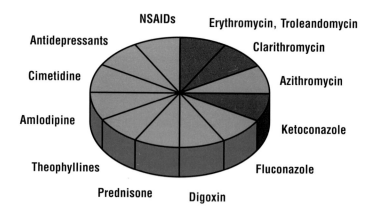

NSAIDs

Erythromycin, Troleandomycin

Antidepressants

Clarithromycin

Cimetidine

Azithromycin

Amlodipine

Ketoconazole

Theophyllines

Fluconazole

Prednisone   Digoxin

DISEASE Incompatibility Profile

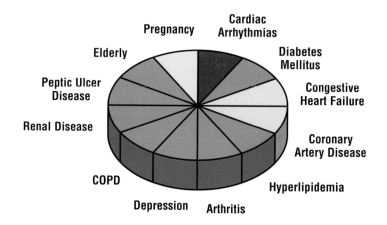

Pregnancy

Cardiac Arrhythmias

Elderly

Diabetes Mellitus

Peptic Ulcer Disease

Congestive Heart Failure

Renal Disease

Coronary Artery Disease

COPD

Hyperlipidemia

Depression   Arthritis

ANTIHISTAMINES

DIPHENHYDRAMINE
Benadryl®

DRUG Incompatibility Profile

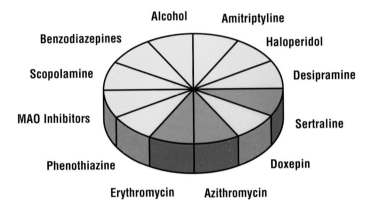

Alcohol
Amitriptyline
Benzodiazepines
Haloperidol
Scopolamine
Desipramine
MAO Inhibitors
Sertraline
Phenothiazine
Doxepin
Erythromycin
Azithromycin

DISEASE Incompatibility Profile

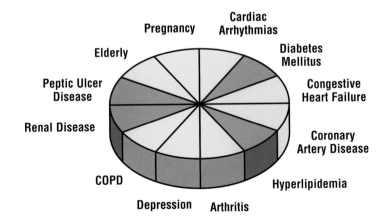

Pregnancy
Cardiac Arrhythmias
Elderly
Diabetes Mellitus
Peptic Ulcer Disease
Congestive Heart Failure
Renal Disease
Coronary Artery Disease
COPD
Hyperlipidemia
Depression
Arthritis

ANTIBIOTICS

FLUOROQUINOLONES

DRUG Incompatibility Profile

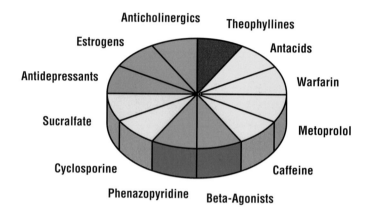

DISEASE Incompatibility Profile

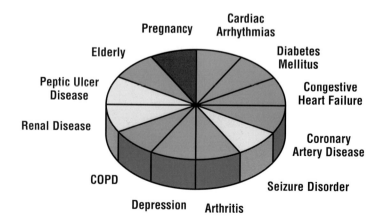

ANTIBIOTICS

ERYTHROMYCIN, CLARITHROMYCIN
Erythrocin®, Biaxin®

DRUG Incompatibility Profile

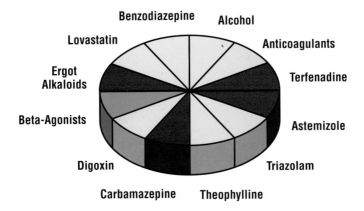

Benzodiazepine Alcohol
Lovastatin
Anticoagulants
Ergot Alkaloids
Terfenadine
Beta-Agonists
Astemizole
Digoxin
Triazolam
Carbamazepine Theophylline

DISEASE Incompatibility Profile

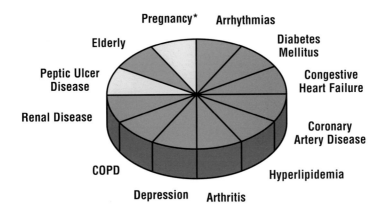

Pregnancy* Arrhythmias
Elderly
Diabetes Mellitus
Peptic Ulcer Disease
Congestive Heart Failure
Renal Disease
Coronary Artery Disease
COPD
Hyperlipidemia
Depression Arthritis

*Clarithromycin should be red and should not be used unless there is no alternative.

ANTIBIOTICS

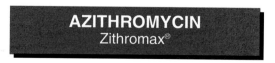

AZITHROMYCIN
Zithromax®

DRUG Incompatibility Profile

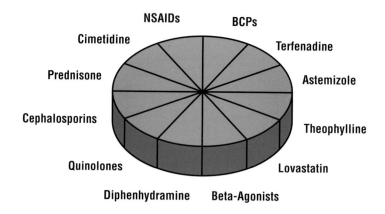

DISEASE Incompatibility Profile

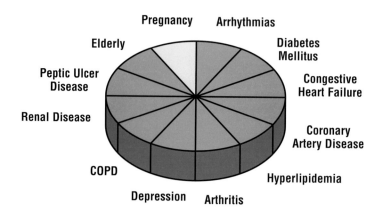

ORAL HYPOGLYCEMICS

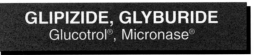

GLIPIZIDE, GLYBURIDE
Glucotrol®, Micronase®

DRUG Incompatibility Profile

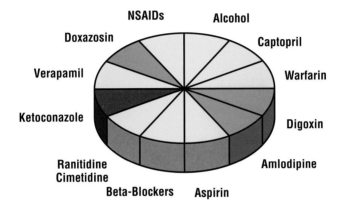

NSAIDs
Alcohol
Doxazosin
Captopril
Verapamil
Warfarin
Ketoconazole
Digoxin
Ranitidine
Cimetidine
Amlodipine
Beta-Blockers
Aspirin

DISEASE Incompatibility Profile

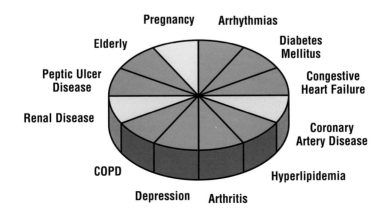

Pregnancy
Arrhythmias
Elderly
Diabetes Mellitus
Peptic Ulcer Disease
Congestive Heart Failure
Renal Disease
Coronary Artery Disease
COPD
Hyperlipidemia
Depression
Arthritis

LIPID - LOWERING DRUGS

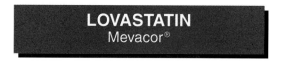

DRUG Incompatibility Profile

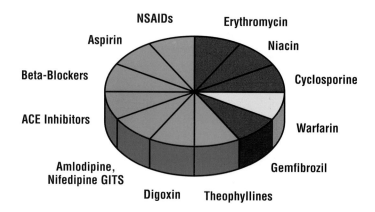

DISEASE Incompatibility Profile

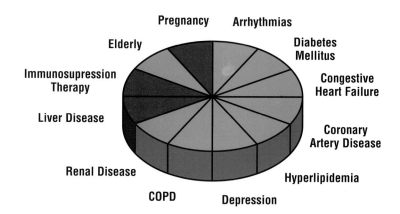

LIPID - LOWERING DRUGS

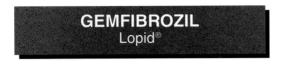

GEMFIBROZIL
Lopid®

DRUG Incompatibility Profile

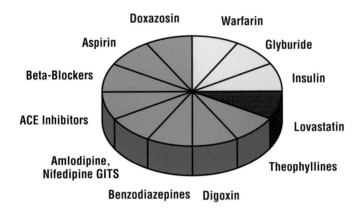

Doxazosin Warfarin
Aspirin Glyburide
Beta-Blockers Insulin
ACE Inhibitors Lovastatin
Amlodipine, Nifedipine GITS Theophyllines
Benzodiazepines Digoxin

DISEASE Incompatibility Profile

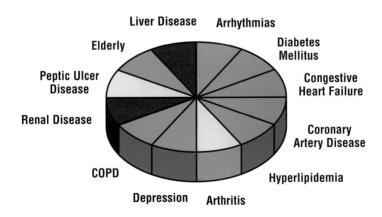

Liver Disease Arrhythmias
Elderly Diabetes Mellitus
Peptic Ulcer Disease Congestive Heart Failure
Renal Disease Coronary Artery Disease
COPD Hyperlipidemia
Depression Arthritis

DIURETICS

THIAZIDE DIURETICS
(Hydrochlorothiazide)

DRUG Incompatibility Profile

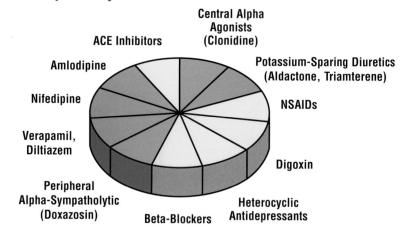

Central Alpha
Agonists
(Clonidine)

ACE Inhibitors

Amlodipine

Potassium-Sparing Diuretics
(Aldactone, Triamterene)

Nifedipine

NSAIDs

Verapamil,
Diltiazem

Digoxin

Peripheral
Alpha-Sympatholytic
(Doxazosin)

Heterocyclic
Antidepressants

Beta-Blockers

DISEASE Incompatibility Profile

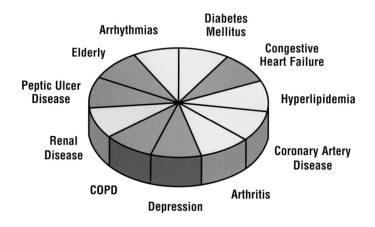

Diabetes
Mellitus

Arrhythmias

Elderly

Congestive
Heart Failure

Peptic Ulcer
Disease

Hyperlipidemia

Renal
Disease

Coronary Artery
Disease

COPD

Arthritis

Depression

BETA-BLOCKERS

BETA-BLOCKERS
(Atenolol, Propranolol, Naldolol)

DRUG Incompatibility Profile

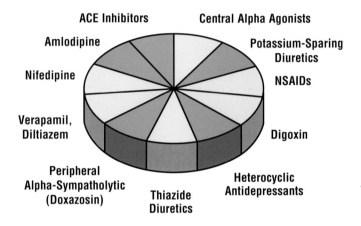

ACE Inhibitors

Central Alpha Agonists

Amlodipine

Potassium-Sparing Diuretics

Nifedipine

NSAIDs

Verapamil, Diltiazem

Digoxin

Peripheral Alpha-Sympatholytic (Doxazosin)

Thiazide Diuretics

Heterocyclic Antidepressants

DISEASE Incompatibility Profile

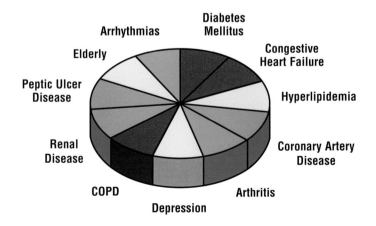

Arrhythmias

Diabetes Mellitus

Elderly

Congestive Heart Failure

Peptic Ulcer Disease

Hyperlipidemia

Renal Disease

Coronary Artery Disease

COPD

Arthritis

Depression

INHIBITORS

ACE INHIBITORS
(Enalapril, Captopril, Lisinopril)

DRUG Incompatibility Profile

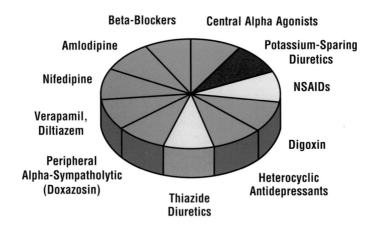

Beta-Blockers Central Alpha Agonists

Amlodipine Potassium-Sparing Diuretics

Nifedipine NSAIDs

Verapamil, Diltiazem

Peripheral Alpha-Sympatholytic (Doxazosin) Digoxin

Thiazide Diuretics Heterocyclic Antidepressants

DISEASE Incompatibility Profile

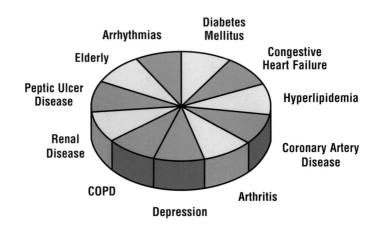

Arrhythmias Diabetes Mellitus

Elderly Congestive Heart Failure

Peptic Ulcer Disease Hyperlipidemia

Renal Disease Coronary Artery Disease

COPD Arthritis

Depression

ALPHA-SYMPATHOLYTIC

PERIPHERAL ALPHA-SYMPATHOLYTIC
(Doxazosin)

DRUG Incompatibility Profile

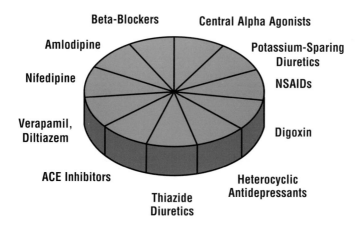

Beta-Blockers
Central Alpha Agonists
Amlodipine
Potassium-Sparing Diuretics
Nifedipine
NSAIDs
Verapamil, Diltiazem
Digoxin
ACE Inhibitors
Heterocyclic Antidepressants
Thiazide Diuretics

DISEASE Incompatibility Profile

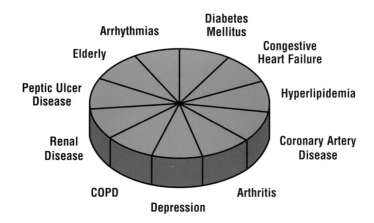

Diabetes Mellitus
Arrhythmias
Congestive Heart Failure
Elderly
Peptic Ulcer Disease
Hyperlipidemia
Renal Disease
Coronary Artery Disease
COPD
Arthritis
Depression

BLOCKERS

CALCIUM CHANNEL BLOCKERS
(Diltiazem, Verapamil)

DRUG Incompatibility Profile

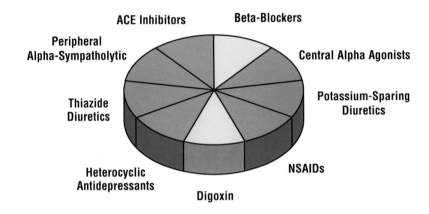

ACE Inhibitors

Beta-Blockers

Peripheral
Alpha-Sympatholytic

Central Alpha Agonists

Thiazide
Diuretics

Potassium-Sparing
Diuretics

Heterocyclic
Antidepressants

NSAIDs

Digoxin

DISEASE Incompatibility Profile

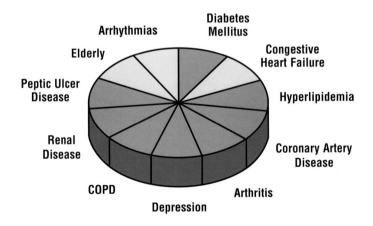

Arrhythmias

Diabetes
Mellitus

Elderly

Congestive
Heart Failure

Peptic Ulcer
Disease

Hyperlipidemia

Renal
Disease

Coronary Artery
Disease

COPD

Arthritis

Depression

BLOCKERS

CALCIUM CHANNEL BLOCKERS
(Nifedipine, Isradipine)

DRUG Incompatibility Profile

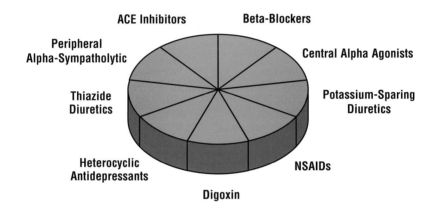

ACE Inhibitors • Beta-Blockers • Peripheral Alpha-Sympatholytic • Central Alpha Agonists • Thiazide Diuretics • Potassium-Sparing Diuretics • Heterocyclic Antidepressants • NSAIDs • Digoxin

DISEASE Incompatibility Profile

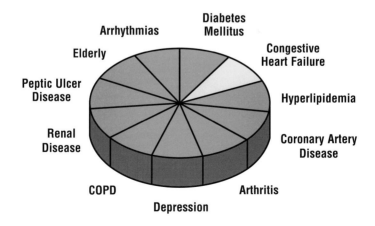

Arrhythmias • Diabetes Mellitus • Elderly • Congestive Heart Failure • Peptic Ulcer Disease • Hyperlipidemia • Renal Disease • Coronary Artery Disease • COPD • Arthritis • Depression

BLOCKER

CALCIUM CHANNEL BLOCKER
(Amlodipine, Norvasc®)

DRUG Incompatibility Profile

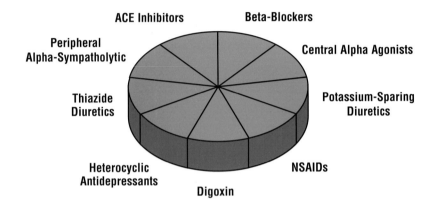

ACE Inhibitors
Beta-Blockers
Peripheral Alpha-Sympatholytic
Central Alpha Agonists
Thiazide Diuretics
Potassium-Sparing Diuretics
Heterocyclic Antidepressants
NSAIDs
Digoxin

DISEASE Incompatibility Profile

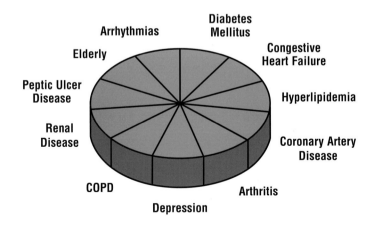

Arrhythmias
Diabetes Mellitus
Elderly
Congestive Heart Failure
Peptic Ulcer Disease
Hyperlipidemia
Renal Disease
Coronary Artery Disease
COPD
Arthritis
Depression

CENTRALLY ACTING AGONISTS

CENTRALLY ACTING AGONISTS (CAA)
(Clonidine, Alpha-Methyl Dopa, Guanfacine)

DRUG Incompatibility Profile

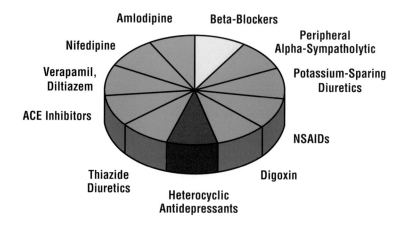

DISEASE Incompatibility Profile

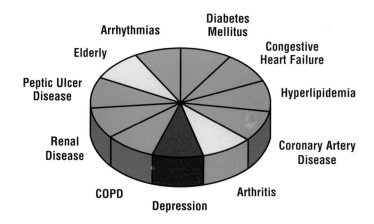

INOTROPIC AGENTS

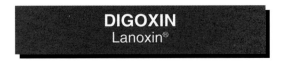

DRUG Incompatibility Profile

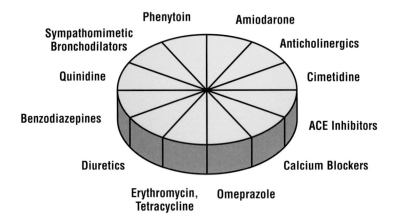

DISEASE Incompatibility Profile

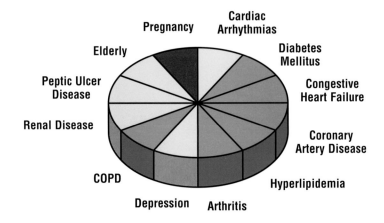

careful monitoring is recommended in a number of patient subgroups, especially in individuals on long-term drug therapy. These concerns are reflected in the drug and disease incompatibility profiles for these agents.[1,6,7,32]

Theophylline Drug Incompatibility Profile (DIP 3-14). A red warning is issued for the combined use of beta-blockers and theophylline,[79] first because beta-blockers should be avoided in asthmatics, and second, because propranolol can decrease theophylline metabolism, thereby producing toxic effects.

Caution is advised when combining theophylline with antacids, as absorption of the bronchodilator may be increased. Allopurinol can produce theophylline toxicity through decreased metabolism. Because cimetidine is a potent inhibitor of the p-450 cytochrome oxidase system, concurrent use of this antiulcer agent can elevate theophylline levels, especially in the elderly and in patients with impaired hepatic function. Ranitidine is a weak binder to the P-450 system and also carries a yellow warning designation, although the risk of inducing theophylline toxicity is extremely rare with this H2-blocker. Famotidine carries a green designation because it has no clinically significant p-450 binding. Theophylline concentrations should be monitored in patients taking cimetidine and ranitidine, as well as in individuals taking oral contraceptives, erythromycin, tetracycline, and flouroquinolones.[80-83] Azithromycin does not appear to affect theophylline levels and is given a green designation. Finally, some of the stimulatory effects of theophylline can be exacerbated by caffeine.

Theophylline Disease Incompatibility Profile (DIP 3-14). Theophylline use is not recommended in pregnancy (category C classification) or in patients with severe coronary artery disease associated with cardiac arrhythmias. Theophylline can cause dysrhythmias or worsen preexisting arrhythmias. Consequently, any change in rhythm or significant change in heart rate warrants determination of theophylline serum levels.

Because the drug can produce serious cardiac arrhythmias, it should be used with caution in patients with congestive heart failure, a condition that may prolong theophylline half-life and is associated with arrhythmogenesis. Theophylline can produce local gastric irritation and abdominal pain, symptoms that dictate cautious use in patients with peptic ulcer disease. Patients with depression should be warned that theophylline can cause central nervous system disturbances, especially irritability, headache, insomnia, and depression. Patients with chronic obstructive pulmonary disease should be advised that theophylline may cause tachypnea and can increase respiratory rate. The elderly, in general, are more susceptible to theophylline toxicity and show decreased metabolism of the drug.[78]

Antihistamines

Generally speaking, antihistamines are remarkably safe considering their widespread use. The principal concern with these agents involves the arrhythmogenic properties of terfenadine and astemizole when used in combination with drugs (e.g., erythromycin, clarithromycin, troleandomycin) that impair metabolism of these antihistaminic agents. In contrast, diphenhydramine drug and disease incompatibilities reflect this agent's anticholinergic and sedating side effects. These concerns are highlighted in the drug and disease incompatibility profiles discussed below.

Terfenadine (Seldane®) Drug Incompatibility Profile (DIP 3-15). As mentioned, the principal concern with terfenadine is the possibility of producing potentially life-threatening cardiac arrhythmias. The clinical consequences of decreased metabolism of terfenadine with concurrent use of such drugs as erythromycin, clarithromycin, and troleandomycin must be recognized.[84-87] As a result, concurrent use of these antibiotics and terfenadine should be avoided. Ketoconazole, an antifungal agent, also should not be used in patients taking this antihistamine because serious cardiac conduction disturbances are reported with combined use. A yellow cautionary designation is issued for verapamil, whose cardiac effects may be potentiated by concomitant use of terfenadine.

Terfenadine Disease Incompatibility Profile (DIP 3-15). Red warning designations accompany the drug-disease pie slices, indicating risk of using terfenadine in patients with cardiac arrhythmias.[85,86] Yellow designations are used for associated cardiac conditions such as congestive heart failure and coronary artery disease. Use in pregnancy is not recommended.

Astemizole Drug Incompatibility Profile (DIP 3-16). Many of the same warnings issued for cardiac arrhythmias resulting from combined use of terfenadine with various antibiotics and antifungal agents also apply to astemizole. The principal concern with astemizole is the possibility of producing life-threatening cardiac arrhythmias. The potential clinical consequences of decreasing metabolism of astemizole with concurrent use of such drugs as erythromycin, clarithromycin, and ketoconazole must be recognized. As a result, concurrent use of these medications with astemizole should be avoided in all situations. There are no reported adverse reactions from the combination of fluconazole and astemizole.

Astemizole Disease Incompatibility Profile (DIP 3-16). Red warning designations accompany the drug-disease pie slices indicating risk of using astemizole in patients with cardiac arrhythmias. Yellow designations are used for associated cardiac conditions such as congestive heart failure and coronary artery disease. Use of astemizole in pregnancy is not recommended.

Diphenhydramine Drug Incompatibility Profile (DIP 3-17). Diphenhydramine can produce clinically significant anticholinergic side effects, central nervous system sedation, impairment of motor function, and urinary retention. Cautious use is advised, especially in the elderly, who may be taking other drugs producing similar side effects. These effects can be exacerbated when this antihistamine is combined with other anticholinergic medications including desipramine, anti-Parkinson drugs, haloperidol, amitriptyline, scopolamine, and phenothiazines. Hallucinations can occur from the combined use of MAOIs and cyproheptadine, although the mechanism is not clear. Caution is recommended for concurrent use of diphenhydramine and central nervous system depressants including alcohol, benzodiazepines, narcotics, antianxiety agents, and barbiturates.[86,88,89]

Diphenhydramine Disease Incompatibility Profile (DIP 3-17).
The central nervous system sedating effects of diphenhydramine can be clinically significant, especially in elderly patients and in individuals consuming other anticholinergic drugs. Accordingly, dosage reduction is the prudent approach in patients over the age of 65, especially men with documented prostatic hypertrophy or symptoms suggestive of prostatism. Use of diphenhydramine in depression is recommended with extreme caution only because lassitude, confusion, insomnia, irritability, and nervousness can occur. The sedative effects of diphenhydramine may be undesirable in patients with arthritis, who should be encouraged to walk and maintain normal physical activity if possible. Because diphenhydramine can produce a number of adverse cardiovascular effects, from tachycardia and palpitations to electrocardiographic changes (widening QRS complex) and hypotension, caution is advised when this antihistamine is used in patients with cardiac arrhythmias, coronary artery disease, and congestive heart failure. When the sedating properties of diphenhydramine are likely to present problems, use of a low-sedating agent such as loratidine or cetirizine is recommended.

Antibiotics

Fluoroquinolones (ciprofloxacin, norfloxacin) Drug Incompatibility Profile (DIP 3-18). Fluoroquinolones are widely used for outpatient management of such common infections as pyelonephritis, prostatitis, and skin infections. Despite their routine use, a number of drug incompatibilities are worth bearing in mind. Theophylline toxicity may be seen with ciprofloxacin and norfloxacin, and this interaction may be potentiated by the concomitant use of cimetidine. At present, there is some data to suggest that ofloxacin and mefloxacin may not produce this theophylline interaction. Nevertheless, a red DIP® warning designation is used to alert pharmacists and physicians of this possible drug interaction. Interestingly, caffeine toxicity may be observed with concurrent enoxacin and ciprofloxacin administration, a finding that suggests large caffeine intake should be avoided in patients taking this class of antibiotics.

Antacids should not be used with fluoroquinolones because decreased antibiotic effects occur with concurrent use of aluminum, magnesium, and calcium-containing antacids. If the patient must take antacids, they should be taken 2 hours after or 6 hours before administration of a fluoroquinolone antibiotic. A yellow warning is used for anticoagulants[90,91] because increased warfarin effects has been reported from the concurrent use of ciprofloxacin and norfloxacin. The possibility of metoprolol toxicity should be monitored in patients taking ciprofloxacin. Renal status should be monitored in patients taking cyclosporine in conjunction with either ciprofloxacin or norfloxacin. Dosage reduction may be required to avoid nephrotoxicity. Concomitant administration of sucralfate may result in reduced ciprofloxacin or norfloxacin effect.

Fluoroquinolones Disease Incompatibility Profile (DIP 3-18).

These agents carry a category C pregnancy rating and should not be used in pregnant women. Alteration of drug dosage may be required in patients with renal impairment. Central nervous system stimulation may occur with ciprofloxacin, which may lead to tremor, restlessness, confusion, and on very rare occasions, to hallucinations and grand mal seizures. Because of these possible side effects, fluoroquinolones should be used with caution in patients with preexisting central nervous system disorders, including severe cerebrovascular disease and epilepsy. A yellow warning designation is issued for fluoroquinolone use in patients with peptic ulcer disease because the drug can cause abdominal pain and nausea. In addition, many patients with peptic ulcer disease may be taking antacids, which are known to interfere with the absorption of this antibiotic.

Erythromycin and Clarithromycin Drug Incompatibility Profile (DIP 3-19).

The most important drug interactions associated with erythromycin include avoidance of concurrent use with terfenadine, astemizole, carbamazepine, and ergot alkaloids. The potentiation of terfenadine- and astemizole-induced cardiac arrhythmias were discussed in a previous section. Carbamazepine toxicity can be precipitated by concurrent erythromycin therapy, which causes a decrease in carbamazepine metabolism. Ergot alkaloid toxicity can be potentiated by erythromycin, and concurrent use is not recommended.

Yellow warning designations are used for the combined use of erythromycin and benzodiazepines (i.e., triazolam and midazolam) because increased toxicity is observed as a result of decreased metabolism. The risk of erythromycin-induced elevations of serum theophylline concentration was emphasized in a previous section. Alcohol use should be discouraged during erythromycin therapy, because erythromycin absorption may be reduced. A single report of lovastatin-induced rhabdomyolysis was reported in a patient taking erythromycin. Finally, increased bleeding times are observed in patients who take this antibiotic and oral anticoagulants in combination.

Many of the drug interactions cited for erythromycin also apply to clarithromycin.

Erythromycin Disease Incompatibility Profile (DIP 3-19).

Erythromycin can be administered with relative safety in most patients. Because of its propensity to cause gastric distress and abdominal cramping, it should be used with caution in patients with gastrointestinal disorders. It carries a category B rating for pregnancy. It may be used in these patients if no other alternatives are available.[1,6,12,32,92]

Azithromycin Drug Incompatibility Profile (DIP 3-20).

Azithromycin has an excellent drug incompatibility profile, and, unlike erythromycin and clarithromycin, this antibiotic can be used in conjunction with terfenadine, astemizole, and theophylline. A cautionary yellow designation is issued for use in patients taking oral contraceptives; absorption of oral contraceptives may be decreased by concurrrent administration of azithromycin.[1,6,92]

Azithromycin Disease Incompatibility Profile (DIP 3-20).

Azithromycin can be used without the risk of adversely affecting the symptoms of most commonly encountered medical disorders. Although it carries a category B pregnancy rating, this antibiotic is the drug of choice for pregnant women with chlamydia cervicitis.

Oral Hypoglycemic Agents (Sulfonylureas: glipizide, glyburide)

The risk of producing hypoglycemia must always be considered in patients taking chronic oral sulfonyurea therapy. Many other drugs can interact with these agents and produce clinically significant adverse effects. These are highlighted in the drug and disease incompatibility profiles discussed below.

Oral Hypoglycemic Drug Incompatibility Profile (glipizide, glyburide) (DIP 3-21). Through an unknown mechanism, miconazole can produce severe hypoglycemia, so a red warning designation against concurrent use appears in the profile.

A yellow warning designation is used for concurrent use of alcohol and sulfonylureas. Patients taking these drugs should be counseled to avoid consumption of large amounts of alcohol, which can potentiate or prolong the hypoglycemic effects of both glipizide and glyburide. On very rare occasions, the increase in insulin sensitivity produced by captopril therapy may cause blood glucose reductions when used in combination with high doses of oral hypoglycemic agents. Both blood sugar levels and prothrombin time should be closely monitored in patients taking warfarin and oral hypoglycemic agents concurrently; increased hypoglycemic effects and increased dicumarol effects may be seen from combined use of these agents.

Beta-blockers should be used with extreme caution in diabetic patients taking oral hypoglycemic agents because (1) beta-blocker receptor blockade can mask the tachycardia and tremor caused by hypoglycemia; and (2) beta-blockers may cause a decreased hypoglycemic effect, possibly as a result of decreased insulin release. NSAIDs can displace first-generation (chlorpropamide) hypoglycemics from their binding sites, causing hypoglycemia, but this is not a problem with second generation agents such as glipizide and glyburide. Finally, verapamil may produce an increased hypoglycemic effect in conjunction with these agents and blood sugar should be monitored.[93]

Oral Hypoglycemic Disease Incompatibility Profile (glipizide, glyburide) (DIP 3-21). Because insulin requirements frequently diminish in patients with progressive renal parenchymal destruction, individuals with renal impairment are at higher risk for developing spontaneous hypoglycemia, especially when taking oral hypoglycemic agents. Careful monitoring of blood glucose concentrations is warranted in this patient population.

Lipid-Lowering Drugs

Lovastatin Drug Incompatibility Profile (DIP 3-22). Lovastatin is a cholesterol-lowering agent that inhibits HMG-CoA reductase, the enzyme which catalyzes the conversion of HMG-CoA to mevalonate, an early step in the biosynthetic pathway for cholesterol. The most worrisome drug-related side effects concern the development of myalgia, transient mild elevations in creatine phosphokinase levels, and in rare cases, rhabdomyolysis with its serious nephrotoxic sequelae. This life-threatening complication is observed most often in cardiac transplant patients taking immunosuppressive therapy with cyclosporine. Other drugs associated with lovastatin-mediated myopathy include gemfibrozil, nicotinic acid, and erythromycin, all of which carry DIP warning designations. In general, these agents should not be used concurrently with lovastatin. Finally, bleeding and prolonged prothrombin times are reported as a result of combined lovastatin and anticoagulant therapy.

Lovastatin Disease Incompatibility Profile (DIP 3-22). Lovastatin is contraindicated in pregnancy. Extreme caution is required when used in patients with liver disease and in those undergoing immunosuppression therapy.

Gemfibrozil Drug Incompatibility Profile (DIP 3-23). As mentioned in the previous section, avoid concurrent use of gemfibrozil and lovastatin therapy. In unusual cases, warfarin effects can be potentiated by the concurrent use of gemfibrozil. Hypoglycemia is observed in patients taking gemfibrozil and glyburide concurrently. In diabetic patients managed with insulin, hypoglycemic effects may be attenuated by concomitant use of gemfibrozil.

Gemfibrozil Disease Incompatibility Profile (DIP 3-23). Gemfibrozil carries a category B pregnancy classification. It is associated with a high incidence of dyspepsia, making its use in patients with gastrointestinal disorders, including ulcer disease, potentially problematic. This drug can also produce myopathy, arthralgias, painful extremities, and other arthritic symptoms. Accordingly, arthritic patients should be observed for possible deterioration of musculoskeletal symptoms after initiation of gemfibrozil therapy.

The DIP™ System In Cardiovascular Drug Prescribing

The use of the DIP system for cardiovascular disease and hypertension must be considered against the backdrop of many drug interactions and comorbid conditions that characterize the clinical spectrum of heart disease. Over the past decade, the pharmacotherapeutic landscape for the treatment of hypertension has witnessed major tectonic shifts. With more than 40 million Americans currently suffering from elevated blood pressure, and an additional 8 million persons inflicted with either congestive heart failure or chronic angina pectoris, selection of antihypertensive and cardioprotective agents is a major clinical priority for primary care practitioners. However, choosing among specific agents from myriad drug classes—some of which correct one clinical parameter (e.g., blood pressure, chest pain) while deleteriously altering another (e.g., lipid levels, heart rate)—is an increasingly problematic and challenging aspect of pharmacotherapy for cardiovascular disorders.

To a great extent, difficulties in drug prescribing arise because agents with varying pharmacologic effects are frequently added to a preexisting drug regimen, a maneuver which may produce one or more drug interactions. The resulting interactions may be helpful or harmful to the patient, depending on clinical circumstances. Patients taking cardiovascular drug therapy may have other diseases, such as lipid disorders, diabetes, and arthritis, which can be adversely affected by the addition of a new drug to the pharmacologic landscape. Finally, for patients with hypertension, congestive heart failure, or coronary artery disease, it should be stressed that optimal intervention not only requires amelioration of the primary clinical derangement, but careful attention to prevention-oriented pharmacotherapy.

Selection of Cardiovascular Drugs: DIP™ Considerations

A wide variety of agents are available to treat cardiovascular disorders, creating new challenges for practitioners. Optimal pharmacotherapeutic management is becoming less a matter of treating abnormal test results or disabling symptoms and now includes treating a spectrum of coexisting conditions and reducing the patient's overall coronary heart disease risk profile.

An approach aimed at optimizing as many clinical variables as possible requires that: (1) drug interactions are minimized; (2) newly introduced agents do not compromise therapy of associated underlying conditions; (3) drug therapy that successfully treats one abnormality (e.g., hypertension) also will positively affect, or has a neutral affect on, other cardiovascular risk factors; and (4) the newly introduced drug does not impair a patient's functional status, but rather, improves quality of life.

Given the multiple considerations that come into play for an individual patient, pharmacologic intervention for cardiovascular disease can be a formidable task. A drug selection system based on drug and disease incompatibility profiles can guide practitioners through a labyrinthine pharmacologic landscape that, for hypertension and coexistent conditions, has become increasingly complex. In recent years, for example, physicians have been deluged by newly approved pharmaceuticals for the primary treatment of hypertension. With the wide spectrum and proven efficacy of so many agents, optimal antihypertensive therapy requires more than merely selecting a drug that will adequately control diastolic and systolic blood pressure. Ideally, an agent or regimen should be selected that is associated with: (1) high patient compliance; (2) a low incidence of adverse drug reactions and interactions; (3) positive effects on modifiable cardiac risk factors; and (4) preservation or enhancement of quality of life, including cognitive and sexual function.

Aside from DIP considerations, much of the controversy concerning optimal initial antihypertensive therapy revolved around the issue of whether old standbys such as thiazide diuretics and beta-blockers should be replaced with newer drugs such as once-a-day calcium blockers, peripheral alpha-1 blockers, and ACE inhibitors. The issue has fueled fierce debate. In 1989, hydrochlorothiazide was the most frequently dispensed pharmaceutical drug in America, with over 70 million prescriptions filled. The efficacy of hydrochlorothiazide and its acceptable cost to most patients has made this drug a favorite for treatment of essential hypertension. However, recent studies report that up to 70% of patients with elevated blood pressure have elevated serum lipids, prompting experts to raise questions about the wisdom of using diuretics as initial agents of choice for the management of patients with essential hypertension.[94]

One disturbing observation is that although thiazide-based pharmacotherapy for hypertension decreases the incidence of stroke, congestive heart failure, and onset of hypertension-induced nephropathy, no controlled clinical trials have convincingly demonstrated a significant reduction in the rate of myocardial infarction in middle-aged men and women. To explain this apparent paradox (i.e., the lack of effect of antihypertensive therapy on myocardial infarction) some have suggested that the adverse metabolic effects of thiazide diuretics counteract the potential end-organ salvage promoted by blood pressure reduction. Based on what is known about risk factors and coronary artery disease, it can be argued that the impaired glucose tolerance, hyperinsulinemia, lipid abnormalities, hypokalemia, and hyperuricemia induced by thiazide diuretics might contribute significantly to the progression of atherosclerosis or might place *selected* individuals at increased risk for arrhythmias, especially hypertensive patients with underlying coronary artery disease or left ventricular hypertrophy.

Although the precise impact of these metabolic factors is still a matter of speculation, thiazide diuretics have had their image tarnished by numerous investigations painting them as metabolic spoilers.[94-97] Although it is not yet time to abandon thiazide diuretics, the effects that antihypertensive drugs have on blood lipid profiles, platelet aggregation, endothelial vasoreactivity, and insulin sensitivity (i.e., metabolic and hematological parameters that are of paramount importance for cardiopreventive drug therapy) are increasingly important factors in choosing specific therapeutic agents for patients at high risk for coronary artery disease.

In an attempt to clarify some of these issues, investigators participating in the "Treatment of Mild Hypertension Study (TOMHS),"[98,99] the most important and comprehensive recent trial of its kind, have reported on the association between blood lipids and a wide range of commonly used antihypertensive drug classes. In this randomized, placebo-controlled, double-blind clinical trial that followed several hundred patients for 24 months, blood lipid changes associated with five active drugs and a placebo were evaluated. The active drug classes included a selective beta-1 blocker with intrinsic sympathomimetic activity (acebutolol), a calcium channel blocker (amlodipine), a diuretic (chlorthalidone), an alpha-1 blocker (doxazosin) and an ACE inhibitor (enalapril).

The variable effects of these agents on cardiac risk factors and quality of life were analyzed over the study period. Chlorthalidone raised total serum cholesterol level 3 mg% at 12 months from baseline in the study group and 9% more than the placebo group, which had a reduction of almost 6 mg/dl. Other agents had reductions similar to or slightly greater than the placebo, with the peripheral alpha-blocker doxazosin producing the greatest drop (12.9 mg/dl) in total serum cholesterol among the active treatment groups.

With respect to serum triglyceride levels, acebutolol, chlorthalidone and enalapril produced reductions less than the placebo group, whereas doxazosin produced the most dramatic reductions (37.7 mg/dl) as well as the highest HDL/Total Cholesterol ratio after 24 months of therapy. In this study, as in others, the calcium channel blocker had a neutral effect on blood lipids. Based on these results, investigators calculated coronary heart disease (CHD) risk. Although such estimates are not based on actual experience with the drugs, careful calculations based on the Framingham equation estimated an increased annual CHD risk of 8% with the diuretic chlorthalidone and a reduced annual risk of cardiovascular disease of 14% with the alpha-1 blocker doxazosin as compared with the placebo.

Newer trials in progress increasingly focus on generating data that will help practitioners to select cardiovascular agents according to CHD risk, inter-drug compatibility and quality of life measurements. The DIP system discussed below organizes findings from recent clinical studies into a drug prescribing scheme that takes into account both CHD and pharmacologic risk factors as they influence drug use in the contemporary outpatient environment.

DIP™ Profiles For Specific Cardiovascular Agents

With respect to the complex group of cardiovascular drugs, the DIP system incorporates those classes of antihypertensive, antianginal, CHF-ameliorating, and cardioprotective agents which are in widest use (beta-blockers, diuretics, peripheral alpha blockers, ACE inhibitors, calcium blockers, and centrally acting agonists) and then evaluates their suitability based on drug and disease compatibilities. Frequently, drugs within a given class have unique properties, some of which suggest windows of opportunity or, conversely, windows of vulnerability as far as clinical outcomes are concerned. One of the purposes of the DIP system is to clarify such distinctions in order to optimize drug selection within and between pharmacologic classes.

To enhance its usefulness, the DIP system also evaluates pharmacologic suitability against the backdrop of those diseases most commonly encountered in middle-aged and older Americans (e.g., coronary artery disease, lipid disorders, arthritis, diabetes, congestive heart failure, depression) as well as against the pharmacologic landscape of agents most likely to be encountered in this patient population. This strategy for optimizing drug selection represents a comprehensive distillation of information gleaned from clinical trials reported in the current medical literature. It also reflects opinions published in expert consensus reports in which the desirability of using different classes of antihypertensives and cardiovascular agents for patients on certain drug regimens or with specific disease risks are carefully analyzed.[6,76,100-104]

Thiazide Diuretics Drug Incompatibility Profile (DIP 3-24). Hydrochlorothiazide is an antihypertensive agent that is also effective in the treatment of congestive heart failure. However, caution is required when it is used in combination with digoxin, NSAIDs, and ACE inhibitors. Thiazide diuretics can cause hypokalemia, an electrolyte disturbance that can potentiate digoxin-induced arrhythmias.[105] Monitoring and maintenance of potassium levels is imperative in patients taking thiazide diuretics and concomitant digoxin therapy; many experts now recommend *empiric* potassium supplementation in all patients taking thiazides in combination with digoxin. NSAIDs can precipitate renal dysfunction, especially in the elderly and other individuals with diminished renal perfusion or a reduced glomerular filtration rate. The combined use of an NSAID and thiazide diuretics can place such patients at greater risk for a drug-related adverse patient event. In susceptible patients (e.g., the elderly, those with preexisting renal disease, individuals with diabetes mellitus) the renal complications associated with ACE inhibitors, as well as hypotensive effects, are potentiated by the simultaneous use of a thiazide diuretic.

Thiazide Diuretics Disease Incompatibility Profile (DIP 3-24). With respect to disease incompatibility profiles, thiazide diuretics are associated with a number of potential incompatibilities that may affect their desirability in specific patient subgroups.[95,96,106] These agents are known to impair glucose tolerance, elevate blood insulin levels (due to impairment of insulin-mediated glucose disposal), and increase total serum cholesterol and triglyceride levels. As a result, patients with either insulin or non-insulin dependent diabetes mellitus (NIDDM), individuals with hyperlipoproteinemias, and patients with two or more risk factors for coronary artery disease (CAD), may be suboptimal candidates for thiazide therapy when other options are available.[97]

Beta-Blocker Drug Incompatibility Profile (DIP 3-25). Beta-blockers were once considered flagship drugs for the monotherapy of elevated blood pressure, despite such well-documented side effects as depression, impotence, and sleep disturbances reported with their long-term use.[107,108] Because of the rapid evolution of antihypertensive drugs that have fewer side effects and which are better suited for CHD risk factor reduction, the use of beta-blockers as monotherapy for lowering blood pressure has waned in relative importance compared to other drug classes. As a result of their capacity to cause drug and disease interactions, they have been recast primarily as agents of choice for the secondary prevention of myocardial infarction and as cotherapeutic agents (i.e., in combination with nitrates and/or calcium blockers) for the medical management of angina.

Beta-blockers can reduce both resting and exercise-mediated increases in heart rate. Attenuation of exercise capacity may be undesirable in individuals who wish to pursue nonpharmacologic therapy (exercise, weight reduction, etc.) for blood pressure reduction. The negative chronotropic effects also can be problematic in older patients taking other sinoatrial node suppressing agents such as verapamil or diltiazem. Consequently, caution is always recommended when combining these two drug classes, especially in the elderly, in patients with underlying conduction disease, and in those with marginal left ventricular function. Moreover, hepatic metabolism of the lipophilic beta-blockers propranolol and metoprolol may be affected by coadministration of verapamil and diltiazem. Although in most patients the clinical significance of this effect is minimal, clinicians should be aware of the potential for increased cardiodepressant activity when combining beta-blockers with either verapamil or diltiazem.

Fortunately, beta-blockers are almost always compatible with nifedipine and amlodipine, once-daily calcium channel blockers with both antianginal and antihypertensive properties. Consequently, optimal calcium blocker therapy of patients with angina and hypertension who already are on a beta-blocker, usually consists of therapy with amlodipine, a drug that will not suppress sinus node rates.[109]

Patients who are on digoxin therapy for inotropic enhancement of left ventricular function may undergo clinical deterioration with the addition of myocardial suppressant agents such as beta-blockers. Beta-blockers usually are contraindicated in patients with overt heart failure. Even the presence of digoxin in the patient's drug regimen should suggest caution regarding addition of drugs from the beta-blocker class, inasmuch as these patients may have been taking digoxin for improvement of left ventricular function. Finally, reports show that such CNS-penetrating, lipophilic beta-blockers as propranolol can cause depression. Consequently, patients already taking antidepressants for management of psychiatric disorders may respond more favorably to other antihypertensives.

Beta-Blocker Disease Incompatibility Profile (DIP 3-25). With respect to its drug-disease incompatibility profile, beta-blockers are generally contraindicated in individuals with clinically apparent congestive heart failure and in patients with bronchospastic chronic obstructive pulmonary disease. Because perception of the peripheral manifestations of hypoglycemia is blunted in diabetic patients on beta-blockers, this class of drugs is generally not recommended for this subgroup. Finally, for reasons discussed earlier, beta-blockers may exacerbate clinical depression and hyperlipoproteinemias, thus necessitating caution when used in these patient populations.

ACE Inhibitors Drug Incompatibility Profile (DIP 3-26). For the most part, ACE inhibitors have acceptable clinical profiles as far as drug interactions and compatibility with underlying diseases. However, this class can cause some problematic drug and disease interactions. Because ACE inhibitors inhibit production of angiotensin II, and thereby decrease aldosterone synthesis, they can cause potassium retention. On occasion, the resulting electrolyte disturbance can be clinically significant. Consequently, the combination of an ACE inhibitor with a potassium-sparing diuretic or potassium-containing salt substitutes (e.g., triamterene, amiloride) is generally not recommended without careful monitoring of the patient.[110]

NSAIDs inhibit cyclooxygenase production, which decreases synthesis of prostaglandins, alters intrarenal hemodynamics, and indirectly leads to suppression of aldosterone secretion. This increases the potential for potassium retention, especially in hyperreninemic patients. As a result, the combination of an ACE inhibitor plus an NSAID is potentially problematic in elderly patients, in diabetics, and in others with diminished renal function. Moreover, because both agents independently have the capacity for causing renal dysfunction, clinicians should avoid, or exercise caution with these two drug classes in combination, especially if other effective agents (e.g., calcium blockers, peripheral alpha-1 blockers) are clinically acceptable.

ACE Inhibitors Disease Incompatibility Profile (DIP 3-26). With respect to drug-disease interactions, a number of clinically important profiles recently surfaced that deserve attention. Although ACE inhibitors are not contraindicated in patients with chronic obstructive pulmonary disease, in smokers, or in others with chronic cardiopulmonary conditions, a recent study analyzing 209 outpatients provides convincing evidence that the incidence of cough associated with enalapril is significantly underestimated and that as many as 10% of patients actually stop the drug within the first several weeks due to the severity of tussive symptoms. Moreover, an additional 15% of patients experience enalapril-mediated cough that is clinically apparent but not severe enough to warrant drug cessation. In light of these findings, clinicians should be aware of the potential difficulties in distinguishing ACE inhibitor-induced cough from symptoms associated with underlying cardiopulmonary disease. When cough is a recurrent symptom in a given patient, to avoid possible confusion with drug-mediated side effects, selection of another blood pressure-lowering drug may be the prudent therapeutic course.

ACE inhibitors can reduce proteinuria associated with diabetic glomerulosclerosis by decreasing efferent, postglomerular arteriolar resistance. This potential advantage may be offset by the fact that diabetics who already have renal impairment are probably at higher risk for developing increased renal dysfunction with ACE inhibitors than with alpha-blockers or calcium channel blockers. Preliminary results from some small studies suggest that ACE inhibitors also elevate serum triglyceride levels, suggesting this drug class is not appropriate for patients with this form of dyslipoproteinemia. Finally, because patients with chronic arthritic disorders frequently require therapy with anti-inflammatory drugs that are known to affect renal hemodynamics, ACE inhibitors should be used with caution in this vulnerable subgroup.

Peripheral Alpha-Blockers Drug and Disease Incompatibility Profiles (DIP 3-27). In an attempt to identify a blood pressure lowering agent that does not impair exercise performance, is associated with minimal interdrug toxicity, and that produces appreciable improvements in coronary heart disease risk, there has been a resurgence of interest in peripheral alpha sympatholytic agents, of which doxazosin is an example. In particular, this peripheral alpha-1-blocker offers a unique window of opportunity for the management of hypertension because: (1) there are no clinically significant drug incompatibilities, which means peripheral alpha-1-blockers can be safely used in conjunction with a wide variety of agents commonly encountered in patients with coronary heart disease risk factors (calcium blockers, beta-blockers, oral hypoglycemics, etc.); (2) at present, there are no known drug-disease incompatibilities, (i.e., peripheral alpha-blockers such as doxazosin do not compromise therapy of or adversely affect the natural history of diseases that frequently co-exist with atherosclerosis, diabetes, or hypertension); and (3) its documented capacity for reducing total serum cholesterol, LDL, and triglycerides (while simultaneously increasing HDL levels) in patients with essential hypertension provides a comprehensive, multifactorial approach to overall coronary heart disease risk reduction, especially in diabetics and those with lipid abnormalities.

Recent studies indicate that doxazosin may play a special role in patients with diabetes, who frequently have concomitant hypertension. In this subgroup, effective management of both conditions is imperative because each is a significant risk factor for the development of atherosclerotic heart disease. Whereas management of the hypertensive diabetic, who is prone to hyperlipidemia, with such drugs as thiazides or beta-blockers is potentially problematic, the peripheral alpha-blockers are free of adverse metabolic sequelae. Their well-documented lipid-lowering effects prompt many experts to advocate their use for the diabetic hypertensive who requires long-term cholesterol and triglyceride control.

Calcium Channel Blockers

Any analysis of calcium channel blockers must begin with the following caveat: *Calcium channel blockers are not created equally.* And neither, for that matter, are most drugs within a so-called "drug class." But the differences among calcium blockers are so significant, that prudent selection of these agents requires a detailed understanding of their specific pharmacokinetic features and, in particular, their effects on cardiac function. In this regard, it should be stressed that, although effective for the treatment of hypertension, the calcium blockers verapamil (Calan® SR) and diltiazem (Cardizem® CD) both have the potential for producing a negative inotropic effects (i.e., impairment of myocardial pump function and, in vulnerable patients, congestive heart failure), sinoatrial node slowing (bradycardia), and conduction disturbances (AV node conduction block).

Moreover, both verapamil and diltiazem are known to produce unfavorable outcomes when used acutely in selected patients (i.e., those with congestive heart failure) with myocardial infarction and poor left ventricular function. Available as once-daily preparations—which are preferred because of enhanced medication compliance—both of these calcium blockers are effective for management of supraventricular tachyarrhythmias. Nevertheless, because of their negative inotropic effects, propensity for producing or exacerbating conduction disturbances, and the risk of producing bradycardia (especially when used concurrently in patients taking cardioprotective beta-blockers, in the elderly, and in those with known brady-tachy syndrome), most experts agree that verapamil and diltiazem now represent "second-line" calcium channel blockers. This second tier status within the calcium blocker group is justified, *except* in patients who have *both* high blood pressure *and* supraventricular tachycardia (SVT), a subgroup in which these agents can play an important (i.e., dual) therapeutic role. With respect to non-cardiac side effects, verapamil is associated with constipation in up to 20% of patients. No calcium blocker has been shown to have cardioprotective properties.

From a practical clinical perspective, the overwhelming majority of patients with hypertension do not require therapy for SVT, and therefore, are better served (from both a safety and therapeutic perspective) with once-daily calcium channel blockers that do not suppress myocardial contractility, that do *not* adversely effect conduction system, and that do *not* slow heart rate. These "first-line" calcium blockers are members of the dihydropyridine class and include such agents as amlodipine (Norvasc®), isradipine (Dynacirc®), felodipine (Plendil®), and nifedipine GITS (Procardia XL®).

Even among the dihydropyridines, however, there are significant differences suggesting some agents within this group are preferrable to others. For example, because isradipine is given on a twice-daily basis, it does not stand up to the improved medication compliance observed with the once-daily dihydropyridines such as amlodipine or nifedipine GITS. With respect to side effects, felodipine is associated with peripheral edema in about 10% to 30% of patients and is more likely to produce irritative side effects such as flushing and headache. Nifedipine GITS is associated with peripheral edema in about 9% to 12% of patients on the 60 mg/d dose; although it has minimal negative inotropic effects, it produces a small increase in cardiac output. Because it is the most potent peripheral vasodilator among the dihydropyridines, nifedipine GITS is the preferred calcium blocker in patients with *severe* hypertension (i.e., patients with diastolic BP > 120 mm Hg).

Amlodipine, which like nifedipine GITS, is approved for treatment of both high blood pressure and angina, has a unique cardio-friendliness profile. It produces no impairment of myocardial pump function, no adverse effect on conduction system (including the SA and AV node), does not decrease heart rate, can be used safely in combination with beta-blockers, and, like ACE inhibitors, this calcium blocker does not increase serum norepinephrine levels. Moreover, because amlodipine has been shown *not* to adversely affect clinical outcomes in patients with congestive heart failure (NYHA functional classes II-IV, PRAISE Trial), has no known clinically significant drug-drug or drug-disease interactions, and produces peripheral edema in only 3% to 5% of patients taking the 5 mg dose, this agent has emerged as the calcium blocker of choice in patients with mild-to-moderate hypertension.

Finally, although selection of a calcium channel blocker will depend upon specific patient needs, comorbid conditions (diabetes, congestive heart failure, supraventricular tachycardia, etc.), the fact is, treatment of hypertension almost always is a long-term affair. Consequently, anti-hypertensive drugs must be evaluated not only according to their capacity for achieving short-term results in clinical trials but according to their capacity for "standing the test of time" as *monotherapy* over the long haul—i.e., many years after onset of therapy—in a real world environment. This feature, called regimen durability, has been assessed in the case of at least one calcium blocker in the "Treatment of Mild Hypertension Study (TOMHS, JAMA, August 1993)."

One of the most rigorous investigations of its kind since Framingham, TOMHS demonstrated that 84% of patients started on the calcium blocker amlodipine will achieve blood pressure-lowering goals on *monotherapy* (i.e., using only this agent) *four years down the road,* whereas *only 67%* of patients started on the ACE inhibitor enalapril, and only 64% of patients on the diuretic chlorthalidone were still taking only a *single* agent four years later. This *regimen durability* advantage associated with amlodipine has important clinical and cost implications, because it suggests that, although the initial cost of calcium blockers is greater than beta-blockers or diuretics, expenditures associated with having to introduce pharmacologic reinforcements—i.e., "add-on" drugs—into the anti-hypertensive regimen can be prevented with drugs that have regimen durability (i.e., amlodipine).

Regardless of the agent, blood pressure control is central to the prevention of cardiovascular disease and stroke. A long-term NIH study (ALLHAT) enrolling 40,000 patients using several different classes of antihypertensive medications is presently under way in order to help refine antihypertensive drug choices according to clinical outcomes.

Rapid Access Guidelines: Calcium Channel Blockers

The following guidelines are recommended as a prudent and sensible approach to the use of calcium blockers in the contemporary clinical setting: (1) Primary care practitioners should continue to use calcium blockers for approved indications, paying special attention to avoid hypotension as a side effect. (2) Physicians should avoid using calcium channel blockers for non-approved indications. (3) Physicians should avoid short-acting calcium blockers. (4) As a drug class, calcium channel blockers are *not* indicated, and therefore, should not presently be used in the setting of *acute* coronary ischemia, unstable angina, or for secondary prevention of myocardial infarction. Initiation of calcium channel blocker therapy in the peri- or early post-infarction period should be avoided whenever possible. (5) Short-acting *nifedipine capsules* and diltiazem preparations have few, if any, clinical indications for which other, better-tolerated drugs are not available. Hence, their use should be avoided whenever possible. (6) Patients with or without ischemic heart disease who are taking *short-acting* nifedipine capsules for the treatment of hypertension or chronic stable angina should be switched to the slow release, long half-life calcium blocker, amlodipine, for reasons cited above ("Calcium Blockers"). (7) Patients who are taking and tolerating well a *long-acting,* nifedipine GITS preparation should remain on their medication. (8) Patients with or without ischemic heart disease who are taking a long-acting nifedipine GITS preparation but experiencing even mild, drug-related side effects such as peripheral edema should be switched to the slow release, long half-life calcium blocker, amlodipine, for reasons cited above ("Calcium Blockers"). (9) Patients with known or suspected congestive heart failure, or mild-to-moderate degrees of left ventricular dysfunction, who are taking long- or short-acting preparations of verapamil or diltiazem for *hypertension,* and who do *not* have a history of suprventricular tachycardia, should be switched to the slow release, long half-life calcium blocker amlodipine for reasons cited above. (10) Patients with new onset hypertension who do not require verapamil or diltiazem for atrial or ventricular rate control and who are appropriate candidates for calcium blocker therapy should be started on the slow release, long half-life calcium blocker amlodipine for reasons cited above. (11) Patients who are taking and tolerating long-acting calcium blockers verapamil or diltiazem for the treatment supraventricular tachycardia should remain on their medications. (12) Generally speaking, patients who are currently taking and tolerating well once-daily, long-acting, calcium blockers should remain on their medications, except for exceptions cited in #(6) and (7) above. (13) Patients on long-acting calcium blockers who present to their primary care physician with concerns about their therapy should be *reassured* that recently published studies have focused almost exclusively on short-acting agents that are no longer widely used for the treatment of hypertension. (14) Except when heart rate control is an issue, the overall trend in calcium blocker prescribing should be *away* from long-

or short-acting agents that produce either myocardial suppression (verapamil and diltiazem) or precipitous vasodilatation (nifedipine capsules) and toward once-daily agents (amlodipine) with a gradual onset of action that also have been shown *not* to suppress myocardial pump function, adversely affect cardiac conduction, or cause precipitous changes in heart rate or blood pressure.

Verapamil and Diltiazem Drug Incompatibility Profile (DIP 3-28). Although lacking cardioprotective properties, the calcium blockers verapamil and diltiazem are effective antihypertensive and antianginal agents. Unlike amlodipine, isradipine, and nifedipine—which, in most cases, spare the sinoatrial node and conduction system—these two calcium blockers must be used with caution in combination with beta-blockers.[102,109,111] In this regard, symptomatic bradyarrhythmias, AV node conduction disturbances, and clinically significant cardiosuppression are more likely to occur when these calcium blockers are used together in the frail elderly, in patients with impaired left ventricular function, and in those with bradytachycardia. Moreover, verapamil and diltiazem should be titrated carefully in patients who are taking digoxin for control of symptoms precipitated by congestive heart failure. In such patients, the cardio-suppressive effects of calcium blockers must be monitored, as well as serum digoxin levels, which studies show can be elevated by up to 33% and 70% with coadministration of verapamil and diltiazem, respectively.

Verapamil and Diltiazem Disease Incompatibility Profile (DIP 3-28). With respect to drug-disease incompatibility profiles, the calcium blockers are relatively free of contraindications. Congestive heart failure is a relative contraindication for the use of verapamil, while use of diltiazem is not desirable in patients with significant AV node conduction disease in combination with left ventricular failure. With respect to the cardioprotective effects of diltiazem, a randomized investigation of 2,466 patients from 38 North American hospitals demonstrated that in myocardial infarction patients with radiographic or clinical findings of congestive heart failure or an ejection fraction less than 35%, long-term diltiazem therapy (average dose, 180 mg/d) was associated with a significantly increased number of adverse cardiac events (hazard ratio, 1:41), including reinfarction and mortality from other cardiac causes. These findings are supported by a recent study that shows calcium channel blockers, in general, are unlikely to reduce the rate of initial or recurrent infarction, limit infarct size, or reduce overall mortality rates.[112]

Nifedipine Drug and Disease Incompatibility Profiles (DIP 3-29). Nifedipine GITS is a once-daily calcium channel blocker that can be safely coadministered with the majority of pharmacologic agents used to treat cardiovascular diseases in the elderly. It is also safe for diabetic patients and those with lipid abnormalities. Moreover, a number of important nuisance side effects previously associated with nifedipine capsules (e.g., flushing, headache, palpitations) are virtually eliminated by the GITS (Gastro Intestinal Therapeutic System) delivery system, which facilitates gradual gastrointestinal absorption of nifedipine, yielding fairly consistent plasma blood levels over time. Consequently, the precipitous peak and trough blood levels associated with rapid gastrointestinal absorption of nifedipine capsules are substantially reduced with nifedipine. The result is a smooth acting, well-tolerated preparation, which is primarily for severe hypertension as well as angina, and which is compatible with most of the important diseases encountered in patients with cardiovascular disorders. Because of its negative inotropic effect, however, it should be used with caution in patients with severe congestive heart failure.

Amlodipine Drug and Disease Incompatibility Profiles (Calcium Channel Blocker) (DIP 3-30). Amlodipine is a once-daily calcium blocker that is effective for the treatment of hypertension as well as angina pectoris. It has no clinically significant effects on the SA or AV node and, therefore, can be used safely in combination with beta-blockers. The absence of known clinically significant drug interactions makes the agent especially useful in individuals whose drug houses are comprised of many different pharmacologic building blocks. Of special importance is the finding that amlodipine does not adversely affect clinical outcome in patients with New York Heart Association stage II, III, or stage III functional class congestive heart failure. Consequently, within the class of calcium blockers, amlodipine offers a unique window of opportunity for management of patients with impaired cardiac function who also require concurrent therapy for treatment of hypertension or angina.

Centrally Acting Agonists Drug and Disease Incompatibility Profiles (DIP 3-31). This class of agents produces a favorable blood pressure lowering response in a wide variety of patients. Problems include a propensity to cause central nervous system sedation, sexual dysfunction, and fatigue. These properties make these centrally acting drugs less than ideal in patients with clinical depression or arthritis, two conditions in which physical activity and mood elevation are essential for maintaining quality of life. Moreover, cyclic antidepressants and centrally acting agonists mutually compete for binding sites at central alpha-II binding sites, making combination therapy with these two drugs a difficult proposition. Finally, because some beta blockers also have central depressing effects, the addition of a centrally acting antihypertensive to this class is not recommended.

Digoxin Drug Incompatibility Profile (DIP 3-32). Digoxin is characterized by a narrow toxic-to-therapeutic ratio, and consequently digoxin levels should be closely monitored in all patients. Special vigilance is required when patients are concurrently taking medications that affect cardiac conduction, electrolyte levels, arrhythmogensis threshold, drug metabolism, and renal function. Consequently, yellow warning designations appear for such drugs as amiodarone, cimetidine, ACE inhibitors, calcium blockers, diuretics, quinidine, bronchodilators, and phenytoin. Caution is also advised for anticholinergic drugs (possible increased digoxin absorption), antibiotics (possible decreased gut metabolism with erthromycin), benzodiazepines (decreased renal excretion), and omperazole (possible increased absorption). Although the precise clinical significance of all these interactions is not fully understood, cautious administration and monitoring of digoxin effects and side-effects is warranted, especially in patients with coronary heart disease and a history of cardiac arrhythmias or conduction disturbances.

Digoxin Disease Incompatibility Profile (DIP 3-32). Digoxin can safely be used in a wide range of patients, including those with hyperlipidemia, arthritis, coronary artery disease, diabetes, and COPD. It should not be used in pregnant women. Cautionary use is warranted in elderly patients, in patients with gastrointestinal disorders, renal disease, and depression. Because manifestations of digoxin toxicity may include gastric distress and CNS changes, use of this medication should be more carefully monitored in patients with these symptoms.

Pharmatectural Implications of DIP™ System for Heart Disease

At present, comprehensive management of patients with hypertension, diabetes, lipid disorders, or coronary artery disease requires a systematic analysis of drug and disease compatability profiles. When such an analysis is combined with efforts to reduce cardiovascular risk factors, drug prescribing strategies emerge that suggest practical, prevention-oriented approaches for optimizing selection of specific agents. Recent investigations suggest maximal coronary heart disease risk reduction is likely to be achieved with peripheral alpha-1 agonists, calcium blockers and ACE inhibitors. Based on expert consensus reports and current trials reported in the medical literature, "The Drug and Disease Incompatibility Profile (DIP)" system represents an attempt to clarify these drug prescribing issues as they relate to more than 50 million Americans with cardiovascular disorders.

[1]Abernathy DR, Andrawis NS. Critical drug interactions: A guide to important examples. Drug Therapy 1993: Cot 15-27.

[2]Alderman J. Drug interactions: the death pen. [Letter] JAMA 1993 Sept 15; 270(11):1316.

[3]FDA Drug Experience Monthly Bulletin: Reports of Suspected Incidents of Adverse Reactions to Drugs. Rockville, Md. US Food and Drug Administration, Bureau of Medicine 1987:87.

[4]Beers MH, Storrie M, Lee G. Potential adverse drug interactions in the emergency room. An issue in the quality of care. Ann Intern Med 1990 Jan 1; 112(1):61-64.

[5]Lamy PP. The elderly and drug interactions. J Am Geriatr Soc 1986;34:586-592.

[6]Mehta M, ed. PDR Guide to Drug Interactions, Side Effects, Indications. Medical Economics Company, 1994.

[7]Rizack MA, Hillman CDM. The Medical Letter Handbook of Adverse Drug Reactions, 1994.

[8]Biglin KE, Faraon MS, Constance TD, Lieh-Lai M. Drug-induced torsades de pointes: a possible interaction of terfenadine and erythromycin [Letter]. Ann Pharmacother 1994 Feb;28(2):282.

[9]Herings RM, Stricker BH, Leufkens HG, Bakker A, Sturmans F, Urquhart J. Public health problems and the rapid estimation of the size of the population at risk. Torsades de pointes and the use of terfenadine and astemizole in The Netherlands. Pharm World Sci 1993 Oct 15;15(5):212-8.

[10]Melmon KL, Morrelli HF, Hoffman BB, et al. eds. Clinical pharmacology: basic principles in therapeutics. 3rd ed. McGraw-Hill 1992:1073-83.

[11]Amodio-Groton M, Currier J. HIV drug interactions. AIDS Clin Care 1991 April;4(4):25-29.

[12]Brodie MJ, Feely J. Adverse drug reactions. BMJ 1988;296:845-9.

[13]Girgis L, Brooks P. Nonsteroidal anti-inflammatory drugs. Differential use in older patients [Review]. Drugs Aging 1994 Feb;4(2):101-12.

[14]Goff DC, Baldessarini RJ. Drug interactions with antipsychotic agents [Review]. J Clin Psychopharmacol 1993 Feb;13(1):57-67.

[15]Gosney M, Tallis RL. Prescription of contraindicated and interacting drugs in elderly patients admitted to hospital. Lancet 1984;2:564-7.

[16]Hamilton RA, Gordon T. Incidence and cost of hospital admissions secondary to drug interactions involving theophylline. Ann Pharmacother 1992 Dec;26(12):1507-11.

[17]Hodsman GP, Johnston CI. Angiotensin converting enzyme inhibitors: drug interactions. Hypertension 1987;5:1-6.

[18]Houston MC. Nonsteroidal anti-inflammatory drugs and antihypertensives [Review]. Am J Med 1991 May 17;90(5A):425-79.

[19]Jue SG, Vestal RE. Adverse drug reactions in the elderly: a critical review. Medicine in Old Age-Clinical Pharmacology and Drug Therapy London, 1985.

[20]Kramer MS, et al. An algorithm for the operational assessment of adverse drug reactions. I. Background, description, and instructions for use. II Demonstration of reproducibility and validity. JAMA 1979;242(7):623-33.

[21]Larson EB, Kukull WA, Buchner D, et al. Adverse drug reactions associated with global cognitive impairment in elderly persons. Ann Intern Med 1987;107:169-73.

[22]Hansten PD. Drug Interactions 1985; ed 5.

[23]Buchan IE, Bird HA. Drug interactions in arthritic patients. Ann Rheum Dis 1991 Oct; 50(10):680-1.

[24]Johnson AG, Seideman P, Day RO. Adverse drug interactions with nonsteroidal anti-inflammatory drugs (NSAIDs). Recognition, management and avoidance [Review]. Drug Saf 1993 Feb;8(2):99-127.

[25]Nolan L, O Malley K. Adverse effects of antidepressants in the elderly [Review]. Drugs Aging 1992 Sept-Oct;2(5):450-8.

[26]Cannon-Babb ML, Schwartz AB. Drug-induced hyperkalemia. Hosp Pract 1986;21(9A):99-107, 111, 114-27.

[27]Hawkins MM, Seelig CB. A case of acute renal failure induced by the co-administration of NSAIDs and captopril. N C Med J 1990 June;51(6):291-2.

[28]Seeling CB, Maloley PA, Campbell JR. Nephrotoxicity associated with concomitant ACE inhibitor and NSAID therapy. South Med J 1990 Oct;83(10):1144-8.

[29]Alegro S, Fenster PE, Marcus FI. Digitalis therapy in the elderly. Geriatrics 1983;38:98.

[30]Dall JLC. Maintenance digoxin in elderly patients. BJM 1970;2:702.

[31]Blazer DG, Federspiel CF, Ray WA, et al. The risk of anticholinergic toxicity in the elderly: a study of prescribing practices in two populations. J Gerontol 1983;38:31-35.

[32]Callahan AM, Fava M, Rosenbaum JF. Drug interactions in psychopharmacology [Review]. Psychiatr Clin North Am 1993 Sept;16(3):647-71.

[33]Garner EM, Kelly MW, Thompson DF. Tricyclic antidepressant withdrawal syndrome [Review]. Ann Pharmacother 1993 Sept;27(9):1068-72.

[34]May FE, Stewart RB, Cluff LE. Drug interactions and multiple drug administration. Clin Pharmacol Ther 1977;22:322-8.

[35]Wright JM. Drug interactions. Clinical Pharmacology: Basic Principles in Therapeutics. 3rd ed 1992;1012-21.

[36]Jenike MA. Cimetidine in elderly patients; review of uses and risks. J Am Geriatr Soc 1987;30(3):170.

[37]Segal R, Russell WL, Oh T, Ben-Joseph R. Use of I.V. cimetidine, ranitidine, and famotidine in 40 hospitals. Am J Hosp Pharm 1993 Oct; 50(10):2077-81.

[38]Shinn AF. Clinical relevance of cimetidine drug interactions [Review]. Drug Saf 1992 Jul-Aug;7(4):245-67.

[39]Peabody CA, Whiteford HA, Hollister LW. Antidepressants with elderly. J Am Geriatr Soc 1986;34:869-74.

[40]Glassman AH, Roose SP. Risks of antidepressants in the elderly: tricyclic antidepressants and arrhythmia-revising risks. [Review] Gerontology 1994; 40 Supp 1:15-20.

[41]Chan CH, Ruskiewicz RJ. Anticholinergic side effects of trazodone combined with another pharmacologic agent [Letter]. Am J Psychiatry 1990 April;147(4):533.

[42]Beasley CM Jr, Masica DN, Heiligenstein JH, Wheadon DE, Zerbe RL. Possible monoamine oxidase inhibitor-serotonin uptake inhibitor interaction: fluoxetine clinical data and preclinical findings [Review]. J Clin Psychopharmcol 1993 Oct;13(5):312-20.

[43]Ciraulo DA, Shader RI. Fluoxetine drug-drug interactions. II [Review]. J Clin Psychopharmacol 1990 June;10(3):213-7.

[44]Ciraulo DA, Shader RI. Fluoxetine drug-drug interactions: I. Antidepressants and antipsychotics [Review]. J Clin Psychopharmacol 1990 Feb;10(1):48-50.

[45]Levinson ML, Lipsy RJ, Fuller DK. Adverse effects and drug interactions associated with fluoxetine therapy [see comments] [Review]. DICP 1991 June;25(6):657-61.

[46]Messiha FS. Fluoxetine: adverse effects and drug-drug interactions [Review]. J Toxicol Clin Toxicol 1993;31(4):603-30.

[47]Suchowersky O, deVries J. Possible interactions between deprenyl and prozac [letter]. Can J Neurol Sci 1990 Aug;17(3):352-3.

[48]Walley T, Pirmohamed M, Proudlove C, Maxwell D. Interaction of metoprolol and fluoxetine [Letter]. Lancet 1993 Apr 10;341(8850):967-8.

[49]Coplan JD, Gorman JM. Detectable levels of fluoxetine metabolites after discontinuation; an unexpected serotonin syndrome [Letter]. Am J Psychiatry 1993 May;150(5):837.

[50]Bauer LA, Black D, Gensler A. Procainamide-cimetidine drug interaction in elderly male patients. J Am Geriatr Soc 1990 April;38(4):467-9.

[51]Klein WA, Krevsky B, Klepper L, Ljubich P, Niewiarowski TJ, Rothstein KO, Dabezies MA, Fisher RS. Nonsteroidal anti-inflammatory drugs and upper gastrointestinal hemorrhage in an urban hospital. Dig Dis Sci 1993 Nov;38(11):2049-55.

[52]Karsh J. Adverse reactions and interactions with aspirin. Considerations in the treatment of the elderly patient [Review]. Drug Saf 1990 Sept-Oct;5(5):317-27.

[53]Laine L. NSAID-induced gastroduodenal injury: what's the score? Gastroenterology 1991 Aug;101(2):555-7.

[54]Lamy PP. A consideration of NSAID use in the elderly. Geriatr Med Today 1988;7(4):30.

[55]Lamy PP. Renal effects of nonsteroidal anti-inflammatory drugs. Heightened risk to the elderly? J Am Geriatr Soc 1986;34:361-7.

[56]Sager DS, Bennett RM. Individualizing the risk/benefit ratio of NSAIDs in older patients [Review]. Geriatrics 1992 Aug;47(8):24-31.

[57]Shorr RI, Ray WA, Daugherty JR, Griffin MR. Concurrent use of nonsteroidal anti-inflammatory drugs and oral anticoagulants places elderly persons at high risk for hemorrhagic peptic ulcer disease. Arch Intern Med 1993 July 26;153(14):1665-70.

[58]Baxter JD. Minimizing the side effects of glucocorticoid therapy [Review]. Adv Intern Med 1990; 35:173-93.

[59]Piper JM, Ray WA, Daugherty JR, Griffin MR. Corticosteroid use and peptic ulcer disease: role of nonsteroidal anti-inflammatory drugs. Ann Intern Med 1991 May 1;114(9):735-40.

[60]Fraser IM, Buttoo KM, Walker SE, Stewart JH, Babul N. Effects of cimetidine and ranitidine on the pharmacokinetics of a chronotherapeutically formulated once-daily theophylline preparation (Uniphyl). Clin Ther 1993 Mar-Apr;15(2):383-93.

[61]Hansten PD. Overview of the safety profile of the H2-receptor antagonists. DICP 1990 Nov; 24(11 Suppl):S38-41.

[62]Tse CS, Iagmin P. Phenytoin and ranitidine interaction [Letter]. Ann Intern Med 1994 May 15;120(10):892-3.

[63]Wormsley KG. Safety profile of ranitidine. A review. Drugs 1993 Dec;46(6):976-85.

[64]Anonymous. Drugs for treatment of peptic ulcers. Med Lett Drugs Ther 1991 Nov 29;33(858):111-4.

[65]Stocky A. Ranitidine and depression [Review]. Aust N Z J Psychiatry 1991 Sept;25(3):415-8.

[66]Ben-Joseph R, Segal R, Russell WL. Risk for adverse events among patients receiving intravenous histamine2-receptor antagonist. Ann Pharmacother 1993 Dec;27(12):1532-7.

[67]Tollefson GD. Adverse drug reaction/interactions in maintenance therapy [Review]. J Clin Psychiatry 1993 Aug;54 Suppl:48-58; discussion 59-60.

[68]Evans RL, Nelson MV, Melethil S, Townsend R, Hornstra RK, Smith RB. Evaluation of the interaction of lithium and alprazolam. J Clin Psychopharmacol 1990 Oct;10(5):355-9.

[69]Sullivan JT, Sellers EM. Detoxification for triazolam physical dependence. J Clin Psychopharmacol 1992 Apr;12(2):124-7.

[70]Closser MH. Benzodiazepines and the elderly. A review of potential problems [Review]. J Subst Abuse Treat 1991;8(1-2):35-41.

[71]Dilsaver SC. Withdrawal phenomena associated with antidepressant and antipsychotic agents [Review]. Drug Saf 1994 Feb;10(2):103-14.

[72]File SE, Andrew N. Benzodiazepine withdrawal: behavioral pharmacology and neurochemical changes [Review]. Biochem Soc Symp 1993;59:97-106.

[73]Greenblatt DJ, Miller LG, Shader RI. Benzodiazepine discontinuation syndromes [Review]. J Psychiatr Res 1990;24 Suppl 2:73-9.

[74]Wysowski DK, Baum C. Outpatient use of prescription sedative-hypnotic drugs in the United States, 1970 through 1989. Arch Intern Med 1991 Sept;151(9):1779-83.

[75]Longe RL. Triazolam dose in older patients [Letter]. J Am Geriatr Soc 1992 Jan; 40(1):103-4.

[76]Lipworth BJ, McDevitt DG, Struthers AD. Hypokalemic and ECG sequelae of combined beta-agonist/diuretic therapy. Protection by conventional doses of spironolactone but not triamterene. Chest 1990 Oct;98(4):811-5.

[77]Ernst P, Habbick B, Suissa S, Hemmelgarn B, Cockcroft D, Buist AS, Horwitz RI, McNutt M, Spitzer WO. Is the association between inhaled beta-agonist use and life-threatening asthma because of confounding by severity? Am Rev Respir Dis 1993 July;1489(1):75-9.

[78]Sessler CN. Theophylline toxicity: clinical features of 116 cases. Am J Med 1990;88:567-76.

[79]Jankel CA, McMillan JA, Martin BC. Effect of drug interactions on outcomes of patients receiving warfarin or theophylline. Am J Hosp Pharm 1994 Mar 1;51(5):661-6.

[80]Grasela TH Jr., Dreis MW. An evaluation of the quinolone-theophylline interaction using the Food and Drug Administration spontaneous reporting system. Arch Intern Med 1992 Mar;152(3):617-21.

[81]Richardson JP. Theophylline toxicity associated with the administration of ciprofloxacin in a nursing home patient. J Am Geriat Soc 1990 Mar;38(3):236-8.

[82]Rockwood RP, Embardo LS. Theophylline ciprofloxacin, erythromycin: a potentially harmful regimen [Letter]. Ann Pharmacother 1993 May;27(5):651-2.

[83]Spivey JM, Laughlin PH, Goss TF, Nix DE. Theophylline toxicity secondary to ciprofloxacin administration. Ann Emerg Med 1991 Oct;20(10):1131-4.

[84]Crane JK, Shih HT. Syncope and cardiac arrhythmia due to an interaction between itraconazole and terfenadine. Am J Med 1993 Oct;95(4):445-6.

[85]Hirschfeld S, Jarosinski P. Drug interaction of terfenadine and carbamazepine [Letter]. Ann Intern Med 1993 June 1;118(11):907-8.

[86]Rice VJ, Snyder HL. The effects of Benadryl and Hismanal on mood, physiological measures, antihistamine detection, and subjective symptoms. Aviat Space Environ Med 1993 Aug;64(8):717-25.

[87]Swims MP. Potential terfenadine-fluoxetine interaction [Letter]. Ann Pharmacother 1993 Nov; 27(11):1404-5.

[88]Kranzelok EP, Anderson GM, Mirik M. Massive diphenhydramine overdose resulting in death. Ann Emerg Med 1982;11(4):212.

[89]Marquardt D. Antihistamines and the heart. West J Med 1993 June;158(6):613-4.

[90]Kamada AK. Possible interaction between ciprofloxacin and warfarin. DICP 1990 Jan;24(1):27-8.

[91]Renzi R, Finkbeiner S. Ciprofloxacin interaction with sodium warfarin: a potentially dangerous side effect. Am J Emerg Med 1991 Nov;9(6):551-2.

[92]Michocki RJ, Lamy PP. A "risk" approach to adverse drug reactions J Am Geriatr Soc 1988; 36:79-81.

[93]Sugarman JR. Hypoglycemia associated hospitalizations in a population with a high prevalence of non-insulin-dependent diabetes mellitus. Diabetes Res Clin Pract 1991 Nov;14(2):139-47.

[94]McVeigh G, Galloway D, Johnston D. The case for low dose diuretics in hypertension: comparison of low and conventional doses of cyclopenthiazide. BMJ 1988;297:95-98.

[95]Kaplan NM. How bad are diuretic-induced hypokalemia and hypercholesterolemia? Arch Intern Med 1989 Dec;149:2649.

[96]Freis ED. Critique of the clinical importance of diuretic-induced hypokalemia and elevated cholesterol level. Arch Intern Med 1989 Dec;149:264-2647.

[97]Warram JH, Laffel LMB, et al. Excess mortality associated with diuretic therapy in diabetes mellitus. Arch Intern Med 1991;151:1350-6.

[98]Anonymous. The effects of nonpharmacologic interventions on blood pressure of persons with high normal levels. Results of the Trials of Hypertension Prevention, Phase I [published erratum appears in JAMA May 6, 1992 267(17):2330] [see comment]. JAMA 1992 Mar 4; 267(9):1213-20.

[99]Whitcroft IA, Thomas JM, Rawsthrone A, Wilkinson N, Thompson H. Effects of alpha and beta adrenoceptor blocking drugs and ACE inhibitors on long term glucose and lipid control in hypertensive non-insulin dependent diabetics. Horm Metab Res Suppl 1990; 22:42-6.

[100]Perks D, Fisher GC. Esmolol and clonidine—a possible interaction [Letter]. Anaesthesia 1992 June;47(6):533-4.

[101]Sagie A, Strasberg B, Kusnieck J, Sclarovsky S. Symptomatic bradycardia induced by the combination of oral diltiazem and beta blockers [see comments]. Clin Cardiol 1991 Apr; 14(4):314-6.

[102]Fisher ML, Lamey PP. Special considerations in the use of antihypertensive agents in the elderly patient with coexisting disease. Geriatr Med Today 1987;6(11):47.

[103]Amery A, et al. Mortality and morbidity results from the European working party on high blood pressure in the elderly. Lancet 1985;1:1349-1354.

[104]Amir M, Cristal N, Bar-On D, Loidl A. Does the combination of ACE inhibitor and calcium antagonist control hypertension and improve quality of life? The LOMIR-MCT-IL study experience. Blood Press 1994;Suppl 1:40-2.

[105]Levy DW, Lye M. Diuretics and potassium in the elderly. J R Coll Physicians Lond 1987;21(2):148.

[106]Hollifield JW, Slaton PE. Thiazide diuretics, hypokalemia, and cardiac arrhythmias. Acta Med Scand 1981;647(suppl):67.

[107]LaPalio L, Schork A, Glasser S, Tifft C. Safety and efficacy of metoprolol in the treatment of hypertension in the elderly. J Am Geriatr Soc 1992 Apr;40(4):354-8.

[108]Wassertheil-Smoller S, Blaufox DM, et al. Effect of antihypertensives on sexual function and quality of life: The TAIM study. Ann Intern Med 1991;114:613-20.

[109]Ben-Ishay D, Leibel B, Stessman J. Calcium channel blockers in the management of hypertension in the elderly. Am J Med 1986;81 (Suppl 6a):30-4.

[110]Lee HC, Pettinger WA. Diuretics potentiate the angiotensin converting-enzyme inhibitor-associated acute renal dysfunction [Letter]. Clin Nephrol 1992 Oct;38(4):236-7.

[111]Arstall MA, Beltrame JF, Mohan P, Wuttke RD, Esterman AJ, Horowitz JD. Incidence of adverse events during treatment with verapamil for suspected acute myocardial infarction. Am J Cardiol 1992 Dec 15;70(20):1611-2.

[112]Held PH, Yusuf S, Furberg CD. Calcium channel blockers in acute myocardial infarction and unstable angina: an overview. Br Med J 1989;299:1187-92.

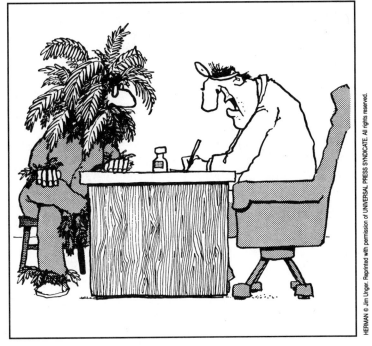

"We'll take you off the vitamins for a couple of days."

Drug House Demolition: Pearls and Pitfalls

The problems associated with inappropriate,[1,2] suboptimal,[3-5] and excessive drug prescribing[6] in middle aged and older Americans are more than everyday clinical issues. They have become a public health problem.[7-11] In fact, nearly every physician and pharmacist is challenged by the need to recognize and react to the pitfalls of polypharmacy.

For example, consider the following 72-year-old female patient who is taking a number of different medications: theophylline, albuterol, beclomethasone inhaler, lorazepam, amitriptyline, cimetidine, furosemide, potassium, digoxin, diltiazem, and a bisacodyl rectal suppository. Clearly, this is a veritable pharmacopoeia of drugs, and it may not even include any over-the-counter medications the patient is taking without physician knowledge or approval.

Several questions immediately come to mind. Is this 72-year-old woman really taking all of these medications? Is she able to keep them all straight? How does she find the time to do anything other than take her medications? How many physicians are prescribing these drugs? Are any of these agents causing or contributing to her present symptoms and clinical deterioration? What drug interactions might explain her chief symptoms of fatigue and lightheadedness? Are some of these medications inappropriate for an elderly patient? Have any of these drugs been used beyond their accepted duration limits? Should these assorted agents be taken together? Why is she taking so many different drugs? Can any of these medications be discontinued without adversely affecting her clinical status?

Polypharmacy is a common problem, and, perhaps, nowhere are its manifestations more visible—and potentially more life-threatening—than in the elderly.[11,14,15] In particular, the risk of polypharmacy increases with the patient's age, the number of diseases with which an individual is afflicted, and the number of different physicians simultaneously providing care for the patient. Although it is hard to lay the blame for polypharmacy on any single factor, the fact is, two-thirds of all physician visits result in a prescription,[6,8] many of which may be unnecessary.

The pressures producing this epidemic of excessive drug prescribing in middle-aged and older Americans are well known. First, there is a perception that modern medicine ought to provide a cure for every symptom or complaint. Patients often expect a drug for everything that ails them, and physicians or pharmacists are often guilty of fostering this expectation. After all, it is much easier and less time consuming to write a prescription than to educate and reassure patients that all they need is a little "tincture of time."

Polypharmacy is not only a risk factor for medication noncompliance, but it increases the risk of drug reactions and interactions, which can range in severity from minimal to life-threatening. With these clinical and pharmacologic concerns in mind, the purpose of this chapter is to discuss and characterize the multiple factors contributing to polypharmacy. This section also reviews and outlines strategies for identifying drug-related adverse patient events (DRAPEs) and for responding to the pitfalls associated with the so-called "Brown Bag Syndrome," a reference to a patient's collection of prescription drugs brought to the physician or pharmacist in a brown paper bag.

DECIPHERING THE BROWN BAG

When a patient who is taking multiple medications presents to the physician or pharmacist with a new sign, symptom, complaint, or deterioration of a previously stable chronic condition, complications associated with polypharmacy must be considered. Fortunately, a meticulous medication history can frequently uncover problems associated with complex medication regimens. These include medication noncompliance-mediated therapeutic failures,[16-21] recent addition of drugs known to produce side effects,[22] drug interactions,[23,24] self-medication with a potentially toxic agent,[25] precipitous withdrawal of drugs resulting in an exacerbation of symptoms[26-28] or clinical deterioration.[29-31] The goal of the physician or pharmacist is to recognize these pitfalls of polypharmacy,[28,32] document them, notify the patient's primary physician of potential problems, and, if a new drug must be added as a part of management, to select an agent that will reduce the patient's risk of future drug interactions.

The danger signs of polypharmacy are obvious to the experienced practitioner and pharmacist: too many drugs, too many pills, dosages that are too high, too many prescribers, and too many high-risk medications (i.e., medications with a narrow therapeutic index, agents with steep dose-response relationships, and drugs known to inhibit or induce hepatic enzymes). In addition, four types of patients warrant special attention because of their increased risk of incurring DRAPEs. At particular risk are the critically ill, the elderly, patients with AIDS, and substance abusers. There is some controversy as to whether AIDS is an independent risk factor for drug interactions. In the elderly, the case is quite clear. A number of studies suggest the incidence of drug interactions and inappropriate prescribing practices is increased in the geriatric population.[1,3,7] A landmark study recently demonstrated that about 25% of all Americans over 65 years of age were taking at least one medication deemed to be inappropriate by a panel of national experts.[11]

Patients with AIDS have a higher incidence of toxic reactions to medications than other subgroups treated with similar drugs.[33] These individuals frequently consume five to six different medications daily, including antiretroviral drugs, as well as a number of antibiotic or antifungal agents that are used for prophylaxis against opportunistic infections. AIDS patients with advanced disease are especially susceptible to the toxic effects of their complicated drug houses. Although the precise reasons for this increased sensitivity to drug-related side effects are not fully understood, it may be that HIV-infected individuals tend to take multiple medications for long periods and also have multiorgan system compromise.[33] Finally, such commonly abused drugs as alcohol and stimulants contribute to clinically significant drug interactions, and therefore, substance abuse patients should be screened carefully for the consumption of prescription drugs that are known to potentiate adverse effects.

CLEANING UP THE BROWN BAG

Streamlining drug regimens, deleting problematic agents, and performing clinically advantageous drug substitutions or deletions in the patient's drug regimen ideally should fall within the province of a *single* physician. Nevertheless, all practitioners and pharmacists involved in the patient's care can help in recognizing and rectifying clinical problems and complications associated with polypharmacy. The job begins with a meticulous documentation of all drugs, including prescription, OTC, and recreational drugs being taken by the patient. In addition, an attempt should be made to confirm that the dose and frequency of each medication. Correlating clinical deterioration with medication noncompliance or potential drug toxicity is an integral part of this screening process. Special attention should be paid to the recent addition, deletion, or substitution of medications, since such alterations may explain changes in the patient's clinical status. The physician may be able to pinpoint a pharmacologic basis for the patient's clinical deterioration, but more often than not, an association between medication intake and clinical status will be difficult to establish.[15]

Even when a direct link cannot be found between drug intake and patient symptoms, the physician or pharmacist can still perform an extremely valuable function by screening the drugs assembled in the "brown bag" for possible toxicity or inappropriate use.[34] In particular, the medication list should always be thoroughly evaluated for the following pitfalls: (1) possible inclusion of unnecessary prescription drugs;[6,35] (2) inclusion of medications that have been prescribed at doses much higher than usually required to achieve clinical results;[36] (3) inclusion of drugs that are considered unsuitable or that should be avoided in the elderly;[7,11,24] either because their side effect profile is problematic[2,37] or because other agents with equal therapeutic efficacy, but less toxicity, are available;[3,38] (4) drugs that may be suitable for elimination because of inappropriate or questionable initial indications for their clinical use;[39-42] (5) drugs that may be unnecessary because usage exceeds usual duration limits;[32,43] and (6) drugs that should be avoided because of their propensity to cause drug interactions.

Although the pharmacist or physician may not be able to act on his or her findings during the first patient encounter, clinical impressions regarding polypharmacy should be documented in the patient's chart and communicated to the primary care physician or appropriate specialist. Finally, judicious screening and consultation with authoritative sources before prescribing additional medications will help minimize the adverse consequences of polypharmacy.

BROWN BAG VICTIMS

The pitfalls associated with inappropriate prescribing in middle aged and older adults can be life-threatening. Consider the following case: An 83-year-old white female was brought to the emergency department complaining of bilateral leg cramps, shortness of breath, generalized weakness, and inability to walk for the past 12 hours. The patient had heart disease, high blood pressure, and osteoarthritis, but no history of intrinsic renal disease. On physical examination, the patient was weak and short of breath. She was alert and oriented and able to move all of her extremities. Her cardiovascular examination revealed an irregular rhythm with an S3 gallop. Pulmonary examination revealed bilateral inspiratory rales. Her abdominal examination was normal, and her EKG showed a new, diffusely widened QRS complex. The laboratory examination revealed a BUN concentration of 48, the potassium level was 7.3, and blood glucose was 132 mg. The remainder of the electrolytes were within normal limits. The chest x-ray showed mild congestive heart failure.

The patient's medication list included the following:

(1) insulin, 20 units NPH, 8 regular subq q.a.m.,

(2) amitriptyline, 50 mg PO q.h.s.,

(3) quinidine, 300 mg PO q.i.d.,

(4) isosorbide dinitrate, 20 mg PO t.i.d.,

(5) captopril, 12.5 mg PO b.i.d.,

(6) furosemide, 40 mg PO q.daily,

(7) digoxin, 0.125 mg PO q.daily,

(8) thyroid, two grain q.daily PO,

(9) dipyridamole, 50 mg PO b.i.d.,

(10) aspirin, 325 mg PO q.daily,

(11) calcium, 250 mg PO b.i.d. and

(12) ibuprofen, 400 mg PO t.i.d.

Of special note is that the ibuprofen was started *four days prior to admission.*

This case study illustrates the potential clinical deterioration that can result from drug interactions and polypharmacy. This patient had a number of drug-related adverse reactions, some of which were life-threatening. The newly widened QRS complex, which indicates a serious conduction system abnormality, can result from toxicity associated with three of the medications she was taking. These possibilities include: quinidine, digoxin, and amitriptyline. Hyperkalemia can also be a contributing factor. The most likely precipitating factor that led to this cascade of drug-drug and drug-disease interactions, however, was the introduction of ibuprofen, a nonsteroidal anti-inflammatory drug (NSAID), which precipitated this patient's acute renal deterioration and led to accumulation of quinidine, digoxin, and hyperkalemia.

Most physicians and pharmacists are aware that you cannot take an 83-year-old woman who has 30% reduction in renal function because of her age alone, renal hypoperfusion secondary to congestive cardiomyopathy, diabetic renal disease, is taking multiple drugs affecting kidney function, and then add an NSAID without incurring significant drug/drug or drug/disease interactions. In fact, it is well known that the risk of inducing renal dysfunction with NSAIDs is increased in the elderly, in patients with coronary artery disease, in diabetics, and in patients who are taking diuretics.

What about the patient's acute hyperkalemia? There are a number of possible causes, including: (1) ACE inhibitor-induced inhibition of renin angiotensin and resulting potassium retention; (2) NSAID-mediated inhibition of aldosterone secretion, resulting in hyperkalemia caused by decreased potassium excretion; and (3) possible insulin deficiency. Complicating this patient's renal deterioration and acute hyperkalemia is furosemide-induced prerenal azotemia, which is exacerbated by renal hypoperfusion associated with low cardiac output. In addition, it is important to emphasize that this patient had a high likelihood of having digoxin toxicity. Not only is digoxin excreted through the kidneys, but the patient also was taking quinidine, which is known to inhibit renal excretion of digoxin. In addition, the ibuprofen-induced renal failure contributed to elevated serum digoxin and quinidine levels.

This case is a dramatic illustration of the risks for incurring drug interactions with commonly used medications, such as NSAIDs, ACE inhibitors, digoxin, and antidepressants. The impaired cardiac conduction, renal deterioration, and hyperkalemia—as well as the possible quinidine, digoxin, and amitriptyline toxicities—reflect a life-threatening cascade of interactions and reactions caused by the addition of a single agent to a patient's drug regimen. Pharmacologic management of this patient required a number of steps to both decrease the effects of potentially toxic agents and to correct metabolic abnormalities. Clearly, all of the involved medications should be stopped. The hyperkalemia is best treated by an insulin-glucose infusion and administration of sodium bicarbonate to lower serum potassium level and mitigate the toxic effects of quinidine and amitripty-line. Although use of calcium gluconate is possible for the treatment of hyperka-lemia, this patient's likelihood of digoxin toxicity precludes the use of calcium, unless absolutely necessary.

All of these strategies were employed, and within 12 hours of treatment, the patient's QRS complex returned to normal, and renal function improved dramatically.

In addition to the acute, life-threatening drug interaction resulting from the NSAID, it also is important to note that many other agents in this drug house may have been inappropriate for patients in this age group or had questionable indications at best. For example, this elderly patient was taking amitriptyline, which can produce potent anticholinergic side effects, including urinary retention, blurry vision, dry mouth, sedation, confusion, and orthostatic hypotension. A careful examination of the indications for amitriptyline suggested that the patient would be more appropriately treated with a selective serotonin reuptake inhibitor (SSRI). Reevaluation of quinidine therapy also is mandatory. Patients with atrial fibrillation and congestive heart failure who take quinidine for cardioversion have a mortality rate that is twice that observed in patients who are treated with digoxin solely for the purpose of ventricular rate control and continue in atrial fibrillation. In other words, although quinidine may successfully cardiovert the patient and maintain normal sinus rhythm, the patient is also more likely to die on quinidine, presumably because of its proarrhythmogenic properties. Therefore, the use of quinidine in this patient requires careful reexamination. Captopril, which is prescribed three times per day, also requires review. Dipyridamole (Persantine®) is probably unnecessary in this patient because aspirin alone will provide ade-quate anti-platelet effects.

EVALUATION OF MEDICATION COMPLIANCE

Strategies for drug reduction, elimination, simplification, and consolidation, (The DRESC   Program, Chapter 5) are designed to prevent violation of pharmatectural safety codes that can lead to life-threatening drug interactions. From a pharmatectural perspective, drug house deconstruction and reconstruction should not proceed before verifying the patient's pattern of medication compli-ance.[20,45,46,47] Poor medication compliance is a multifaceted problem that can: (1) prevent effective treatment of a clinical condition; (2) compromise the natural history of a disease; (3) cause additional unnecessary prescriptions to be added in order to compensate for subtherapeutic drug levels and inadequate clinical effects; (4) induce patients to self-medicate with OTC drugs or make alterations in their drug regimens; and (5) precipitate drug-induced side effects.

Defining the relationship between compliance and daily dose frequency is complicated because most published studies use the pill count method for verifying compliance.[21] Results of studies using this methodology must be interpreted with caution because subjects may provide false information about drug intake or little information is provided about the day or time of dose interval. Consequently, the need for clinical trials elucidating factors that enhance or compromise medication compliance has never been greater. Medication compliance is frequently imperfect, and partial compliance with prescribed regimens is difficult to diagnose.[48] Suboptimal medication intake can lead to additional hospitalizations caused by therapeutic failure. In short, major gaps in taking cardiovascular drugs can predispose patients to fluctuating drug concentrations and to withdrawal phenomena.

The Science of Compliance

To evaluate the precise relationship between daily dose frequency and medication compliance, a team of investigators from Washington University School of Medicine and St. Louis University School of Medicine undertook a study[49] designed to investigate the relationship between prescribed daily dose frequency for antihypertensive medications and patient compliance by analyzing the compliance data obtained from unique pill containers that electronically record the date and time of medication removal. When medication compliance was calculated as a simple ratio (number of pill doses removed/number of doses prescribed) times 100, mean patient compliance was higher in the once-daily (96%) and twice-daily (93%) dose regimens than in the three-times daily regimen with which compliance was only 83.8%. More detailed insight into compliance, however, was obtained by examining drug-intake behavior according to a definition in which compliance was measured by the number of days during which the patients took the correct number of prescribed doses within a 24-hour period. Using this more refined index of medication compliance, investigators found that for patients on a once, twice, or thrice daily antihypertensive medication dose regimen, the prescribed number of doses was taken on 83.6%, 74.9%, and 59% of days, respectively.

Based on this study's design, it is clear that if dose frequency decreases from three times to once daily, medication compliance improves by about 42%. Dramatic improvements in drug intake can be made simply by decreasing the daily dose frequency. The clinical implications of these findings are clear. For the purposes of long-term therapy, medication compliance is best assured when patients are prescribed once-daily medications, and any program designed to simplify the drug regimen should take this factor into account.[50,51]

Despite considerable data to the contrary,[21,49] many physicians and pharmacists believe that they can successfully recognize and interpret deviations in medication consumption. However, few practitioners are able to recognize gaps in medication taking. An important study performed at Stanford University[52,53] attempted to identify major gaps in medication-taking behavior and factors that predispose patients to cardiovascular morbidity and mortality because of inadequate medication consumption. In this study, which enrolled 33 patients with cardiovascular conditions, medication intake was evaluated for drug regimens consisting of fewer than six prescription medications. Using electronic surveillance of pill bottle access, these investigators determined that medication-taking gaps of greater than two times the prescribed dosing interval occurred in about 48% of patients. In addition, patient's dosing patterns often produced uncovered intervals ranging from 3 to 25 days with doubtful pharmacologic effectiveness. These lapses in drug intake were underestimated by the patients and not recognized by their treating physicians. Major treatment gaps occurred frequently, even in carefully selected ambulatory populations, and generally escaped detection. These compliance patterns and gaps may contribute to reported excesses of cardiovascular morbidity and mortality in patients who require cardiovascular drug intake to maintain clinical stability.

The degree to which patients, even those with serious cardiovascular diseases, deviated markedly from the prescription was dramatic. The largest single group in this study consisted of near-optimal compliers, which accounted for about 50% to 60% of the total population. These patients were convinced about the value of treatment and are effective in maintaining dose frequency within acceptable limits. The second group, totalling 30% to 40% of ambulatory patients, could be considered partial compliers. These individuals accepted the principle of treatment but failed to adhere with sufficient consistency to avoid clinical problems. Their most common deviation from adequate medication intake was dose omission. Prolonged dosing gaps clearly carry risks of suboptimal clinical benefit, withdrawal or rebound phenomena, and unnecessary and inappropriate escalation of the regimen. The final group, comprising up to 10% of patients, were noncompliers. Even if their intentions were excellent, execution remained poor. Some patients may take medications especially well just before seeing their physicians, confounding the clinical assessment. Consequently, any attempt at streamlining and simplifying drug regimens must be made on the assumption that physicians and pharmacists, even when familiar with their patients, are unable to identify major deviations in medication-taking behavior.[52,53] The fact is, dose omissions are particularly difficult to detect.

Generally speaking, satisfactory adherence to a drug regimen should never be assumed, since potentially important gaps may occur in up to 40% of outpatients. Regular inquiries about obstacles to full compliance should take place at each visit in nonconfrontational ways, seeking solutions rather than fault-finding. Whenever reasonable, longer-acting preparations are preferred to blunt the impact of gaps in medication taking. On occasion, electronic monitoring may prove useful for selected patients when therapeutic goals remain elusive despite apparent adherence to medication compliance.

In summary, any attempts at drug reduction, elimination, simplification, or consolidation must be based on an adequate knowledge of the patient's medication intake patterns. If there is evidence to suggest that a patient is noncompliant with a drug regimen, measures should be taken to simplify the drug regimen and establish a pattern of regular medication intake. On the other hand, if the patient is compliant with the regimen, measures aimed primarily at consolidation of drug therapy are more appropriate.

DRUG HOUSE DEMOLITION: THE ART OF DISCONTINUING MEDICATIONS

There is now a substantial body of evidence[54,55] suggesting that many medications can be discontinued without adversely affecting clinical outcomes.[29,36,56-58] Much of this data comes from studies that evaluate the effect of antipsychotic medication withdrawal in elderly nursing home residents.[10,13,32,58] The implementation of the Nursing Home Reform Amendments of 1987[10,59,60] (Omnibus Reconciliation Act-87) sought to narrowly restrict the use of antipsychotic medications in nursing home patients, invigorating the debate concerning appropriate use of medications in long-term care facilities. It is well known that the primary use of antipsychotic medications is for the treatment of behavioral manifestations of dementia (see Table 4-1). Although there is substantial clinical experience that antipsychotic drugs can calm acutely agitated patients, their effectiveness and appropriateness for long-term management of chronic behavior problems are less well defined.[61] After all, the adverse effects of antipsychotic drugs include tardive dyskinesia and other movement disorders, dystonia, peripheral and central anticholinergic toxicity, impaired alertness, postural hypotension, social withdrawal, and an association with an increased risk of falls and hip fractures. In light of these findings, the OBRA-87 regulations attempt to restrict antipsychotic medication use in dementia to those behaviors that are dangerous to the patient or others, that interfere with the provision of adequate care, or impair resident function.[10,59,60]

Nonpharmacologic Measures. These guidelines also require a trial of nonpharmacologic therapy to control behavior problems, as well as a trial of gradual dose reduction in patients who remain stable over a period of time. Although one study[32] found a 36% decrease in prescriptions for neuroleptic drugs without apparent adverse affects, other experts argue that regulations encouraging withdrawal of antipsychotic medications can have inadvertent negative effects.[32] Some of these concerns are reinforced by the effects of an educational program that encouraged reduction of antipsychotic drug use in nursing home residents.[58] When compared with baseline antipsychotic medication users in control nursing homes, those in the homes in which education for medication reduction was provided had an 18% reduction in antipsychotic medication use, but no increase in behavior problems and less deterioration in short-term memory. However, these patients did have increased reports of depressive symptoms, which led to speculation that anti-psychotic drugs might have been inappropriately discontinued. Most recent studies show that antipsychotic medications, such as benzodiazepines, cyclic antidepressants, and nonbenzodiazepine hypnotic/anxiolytic drugs, with careful clinical monitoring, can be reduced or discontinued in many nursing home residents without adverse consequences.[2,32,62-64]

Table 4-1

Antipsychotic Medications

Category and Drug	Sedative Potency	Anticholinergic Potency	Orthostatic Hypotensive Potency	Extrapyramidal Potency	Equivalent Dosage (mg)
Aliphatic					
Chlorpromazine	High	Moderate	High	Low	100
Triflupromazine	High	Moderate	High	Moderate	30
Piperidines					
Mesoridazine	Moderate	Moderate	Moderate	Moderate	50
Thioridazine	High	High	High	Low	95
Piperazines					
Acetophenazine	Low	Low	Low	Moderate	15
Fluphenazine	Moderate	Low	Low	High	2
Perphenazine	Low	Low	Low	High	8
Trifluperazine	Moderate	Low	Low	High	5
Aliphatics					
Chlorprothixene	High	High	High	Low	75
Piperzines					
Thiothixene	Low	Low	Low	High	5

Table 4-1

Antipsychotic Medications — cont'd.					
Category and Drug	Sedative Potency	Anticholinergic Potency	Orthostatic Hypotensive Potency	Extrapyramidal Potency	Equivalent Dosage (mg)
Dibenzodiazepines					
Loxapine	Moderate	Moderate	Moderate	High	10
Clozapine	High	High	High	Very low	100
Butyrophenones					
Droperidol	Low	Low	Low	High	1
Haloperidol	Low	Low	Low	High	2
Indolones					
Molindone	Moderate	Moderate	Low	High	10
Diphenylbutylpiperidines					
Pimozide	Low	Low	Low	High	1

Miscellaneous   Thioxanthenes   Phenothiazines

Neuropsychiatric Medications. One study conducted in 12 community nursing homes that participated in a randomized, controlled trial of an educational program[32] designed to reduce antipsychotic medication use, found that the frequency of behavior problems did not increase in those residents who had their antipsychotic drugs discontinued. In fact, for these residents, psychiatric symptoms *decreased* by 21%. Residents who had their drug discontinued had no deterioration in any of the measures of psychological or behavioral function. Psychiatric and behavioral improvement was most pronounced in those residents who were *not* using other psychotropic drugs. When compared with those nursing home residents remaining on drugs, residents with antipsychotic medications discontinued had no general increase in the frequency of behavior problems; nor was there an increase in specific types of behaviors such as aggression, hostility, and psychotic symptoms, that might be most likely to deteriorate after medication withdrawal. In fact, patients in whom antipsychotic drugs were discontinued had a marked improvement in many psychiatric parameters; moreover, there was no deterioration in any of several other measures of resident functions.[27,28,41]

With careful clinical observation, discontinuation of neuropsychiatric medications can be successfully conducted in both the outpatient setting and in community skilled-care facilities. Numerous studies[3,32,58] suggest that, given the availability of alternative behavioral management techniques, antipsychotics and other psychotropic medications can be successfully discontinued in a large subset of these nursing home patients.[32] These studies provide support to trials of withdrawal in long-term care settings.[64] Nevertheless, it is still difficult to identify those specific patients in whom withdrawal is most likely to succeed. Most educational programs aimed at decreasing antipsychotic drug use *exclude* patients with a history of psychosis or substantial violence. These guidelines are also present in OBRA-87. In general, however, drug withdrawal is more likely to be successful in nursing home residents receiving *lower* antipsychotic drug doses, as well as those not using other psychotropic drugs.

Adverse Drug Withdrawal Events (ADWE's). In addition to benzodiazepines,[30,65] antidepressants, and antipsychotics, other drug classes including antihypertensive medications[66,67] can be withdrawn or have their dosages reduced in a significant percentage of patients without adverse clinical consequences.[36,38,43,55,68] Unfortunately, few studies have systematically evaluated the risk of broad-based drug reduction programs. In part, identifying the hazards of drug discontinuation is limited by the lack of accepted, explicit, standardized criteria that can be applied to determine the probability that an adverse clinical event is related to drug discontinuation. Nevertheless, recent studies[32] performed in a Veteran's Hospital attempted to develop and standardize criteria that might link adverse drug withdrawal events (ADWEs) to drug discontinuation. In this study evaluating 62 patients who had 94 ADWEs, it was found that the majority of such events were probably related to drug discontinuation (62%). Most ADWEs were minor (72%); one was associated with hospitalization for myocardial infarction, and none were associated with death. All ADWEs were recurrences of the condition for which the drug was prescribed. Most ADWEs (80%) were associated with three classes of drugs: cardiovascular, CNS, and gastrointestinal. Of all ADWEs, 32% were cardiovascular in nature, with recurrence of hypertension accounting for 11%, exacerbation of heart failure 9%, recurrence of angina 5%, and myocardial infarction 1%. Eleven percent of ADWEs affected the central nervous system, including seizures (7%), hallucinations (2%), and dyskinesia (2%). Four gastrointestinal hemorrhages occurred, but none required hospitalization.

The frequency with which medications required reinstitution varied widely. For example, ranitidine was reinstituted in 17% of cases, haloperidol in 20% of patients, and theophylline in 25% of patients discontinued from the drug. Phenytoin was reinstituted in 30%, digoxin in 40%, and furosemide in 72%. Overall, 60% of all discontinued drugs were not reinstituted. These findings lend support to the idea that drug reduction programs may be successful and have acceptable risks. In this regard, digoxin, furosemide, and ranitidine were those agents most commonly associated with an ADWE of major severity; and, therefore, if discontinued, these patients require careful monitoring.[69,70] It also should be stressed that careful clinical protocols should be followed when withdrawing drugs such as benzodiazepines, theophylline, antidepressants, beta-adrenergic blockers, and many other agents, since discontinuation can be followed by serious physiologic withdrawal symptoms.[26,29-31,42,71]

MEDICATION WITHDRAWAL AND DOSE REDUCTION: WINDOWS OF OPPORTUNITY AND VULNERABILITY.

Antihypertensive Medications

There are as many as 50 million Americans with elevated blood pressure (systolic blood pressure of 160 mm Hg or greater and/or diastolic blood pressure of 90 mm Hg or greater) who are taking antihypertensive medication.[66] Although the majority of these individuals need pharmacologic intervention for their elevated blood pressure, a significant percentage of patients can probably be treated with nonpharmacologic means.[66,68,72,73] The goal of treating hypertensive patients is to prevent morbidity, target organ disease, and mortality associated with high blood pressure, and to control the patient's blood pressure by the least intrusive means possible. Lifestyle modifications, such as weight reduction, increased physical activity, and moderation of dietary sodium and alcohol intake, are used as definitive or adjunctive therapies for the treatment of hypertension. Accordingly, physicians and pharmacists should vigorously encourage their patients to adopt these lifestyle modifications in the hope that medication usage can either be eliminated or reduced.

Nonpharmacologic methods also offer some hope for disease prevention, and they also can modify other risk factors for premature cardiovascular disease. It should be emphasized that the capacity of lifestyle modifications to reduce morbidity or mortality in patients with hypertension is not conclusively documented. However, because of their ability to improve the overall cardiovascular risk profile, lifestyle modification interventions, when properly used, offer multiple benefits at little cost and with minimal risk. Even when these changes are not adequate in themselves to control high blood pressure, they may help reduce the number and dosage requirements of medications needed to manage hypertension. Lifestyle modifications are especially helpful in the large percentage of hypertensive patients who have additional risk factors for premature cardiovascular disease, such as hyperlipidemia or diabetes.[67]

Lifestyle modifications that can improve hypertension control include weight loss, limitation of alcohol intake, aerobic exercise, and reduction of sodium intake. Cessation of cigarette smoking, although not directly associated with a reduction in blood pressure, is strongly advocated in the hypertensive smoker since, along with hypertension and hyperlipidemia, it represents one of the major risk factors for coronary artery disease.

Weight Reduction. Weight reduction alone will reduce blood pressure in a large proportion of hypertensive individuals who are more than 10% above ideal weight. A reduction in blood pressure usually occurs early during a weight loss program, often with a weight loss as little as ten pounds. Moreover, weight reduction in overweight, hypertensive patients enhances the blood pressure-lowering effect of concurrent antihypertensive agents and can significantly reduce concomitant cardiovascular risk factors. Therefore, all hypertensive patients who are above their ideal weight should initially be placed on an individualized weight reduction program involving caloric restriction and regular physical activity.

Alcohol Intake. Excessive alcohol intake, also, can raise blood pressure and cause resistance to antihypertensive therapy. Therefore, a detailed history of current alcohol consumption should be elicited in all patients in whom pharmacologic therapy is being contemplated. In general, hypertensive patients who drink alcoholic beverages should be counseled to limit their daily intake to one ounce of ethanol (two ounces of 100-proof whiskey, eight ounces of wine, or 24 ounces of beer a day). Significant hypertension may develop during withdrawal from heavy alcohol consumption, but the pressor effect of alcohol withdrawal reverses a few days after alcohol consumption is reduced. Minimal to moderate alcohol consumption may reduce the risk of coronary heart disease.

Physical Activity. Regular aerobic physical activity, adequate to achieve at least a moderate level of physical fitness, may be beneficial for both prevention and treatment of hypertension. Physical activity can also enhance weight loss and functional health status, and reduce the risk of cardiovascular disease and overall mortality. Sedentary and unfit normotensive individuals have a 20% to 50% increased risk of developing hypertension when compared with their more active and physically fit peers.

Regular aerobic physical activity can reduce *systolic* blood pressure in hypertensive patients by approximately 10 mm Hg. Effective lowering of blood pressure can be achieved with only moderately intense physical activity. Therefore, physical activity need not be complicated or expensive; for most sedentary patients, such moderate activity as 30 to 45 minutes of brisk walking three to five times weekly is beneficial. When such a program is adopted by the patient, it may be possible to reduce dosages of antihypertensive medications.

Diet. Epidemiologic observations and clinical trials also support an association between dietary sodium intake and blood pressure. A number of therapeutic trials[67] have documented a reduction of blood pressure in response to reduced sodium intake. African-Americans, older people, and patients with hypertension are generally more sensitive to changes in dietary sodium chloride. Because the average consumption of sodium is in excess of 150 mmol/day, moderate dietary sodium chloride reduction to a level of < 100 mmol/day (approximately < 6 grams of sodium chloride or < 2.3 grams of sodium per day) is recommended. With appropriate counseling, this is an achievable diet. In fact, blood pressure may be completely controlled by this degree of sodium chloride restriction in patients with borderline or mild hypertension; in those patients who still need drug therapy, the medication requirements may be decreased.

A high dietary potassium intake also may protect against developing hypertension, and potassium deficiency may increase blood pressure and induce ventricular ectopy. Therefore, normal plasma concentrations of potassium should be maintained, preferably through food sources. If hypokalemia occurs during diuretic therapy, additional potassium may be needed from potassium-containing salt substitutes, potassium supplements, or use of a potassium-sparing diuretic. In many, but not all epidemiologic studies, there is an inverse association between dietary calcium and blood pressure. Calcium deficiency is associated with an increased prevalence of hypertension, and a low calcium intake may amplify the effects of a high sodium intake on blood pressure. An increase in dietary calcium intake may lower blood pressure in some patients with hypertension, but the overall effect is minimal, and there is no way to predict which patients will benefit. Therefore, there is currently no rationale for recommending calcium supplements in excess of the recommended daily allowance.[74-77]

Step-Down Therapy. In patients with *mild* hypertension, these lifestyle modifications should be attempted *prior* to initiation of pharmacologic therapy. However, if an inadequate response is observed *after* an attempt to implement these lifestyle modifications, pharmacologic therapy is indicated. Sound patient treatment includes attempts to decrease the dosage or number of antihypertensive drugs while maintaining lifestyle modifications.[74] In general, complete cessation of an antihypertensive treatment program is usually not indicated. However, after blood pressure is effectively controlled for 1 year and at least four doctor visits, it may be possible to reduce antihypertensive drug therapy in a deliberate, slow, and progressive manner.[75,76] Step-down therapy is especially successful in patients who are also following lifestyle modifications, and a higher percentage of these patients maintain normal blood pressure levels with less, or no medication. Patients whose drugs are discontinued should have regular follow-up, because blood pressure usually rises again to hypertensive levels. In these patients, hypertension can recur, sometimes months or years after discontinuation, especially in the absence of sustained improvements in lifestyle activities known to facilitate nonpharmacologic management.[77]

Digoxin

A number of clinical studies suggest that digoxin is an over-used medication.[39,70] Although it is clear that many individuals are started on digoxin therapy without adequate clinical indications it is inappropriate to discontinue digoxin in patients who require this medication for maintenance of their cardiovascular status.[78] Based on recent studies, specific criteria for digoxin discontinuation are now available.[70,79] Most patients who are on digoxin therapy, who are in normal sinus rhythm, and who have echocardiographic evidence of *normal* systemic ventricular function, probably can have digoxin safely discontinued from their regimen. It should be stressed that discontinuation should be incremental, gradual, and carefully monitored. Patients who have normal systolic ventricular function, but who are taking digoxin for ventricular rate control in the setting of chronic atrial fibrillation, *should not* have digoxin discontinued. The usefulness and effectiveness of digoxin for maintaining ventricular rate control in patients with supraventricular tachyarrhythmias such as chronic atrial fibrillation are well established. Its role in preventing recurrent episodes of paroxysmal supraventricular tachycardia, however, is less certain.

Digoxin should *not* be discontinued in patients who have documented congestive heart failure.[79] For patients who have congestive heart failure, normal sinus rhythm, systolic dysfunction, and an ejection fraction < 35%, digoxin is an important component of the medical regimen. In addition, patients responding favorably to a program of digoxin, diuretics, and ACE inhibitors should not have their digoxin withdrawn, because there is significant risk of cardiovascular deterioration. There are insufficient data at present comparing the relative benefits and adverse effects of digoxin and ACE inhibitors in chronic congestive heart failure to determine which drug to use first—an important clinical decision. However, digoxin is effective in patients with chronic, stable mild-to-moderate heart failure and most studies documenting a beneficial effect of ACE inhibitors on survival in patients with heart failure used ACE inhibitors in conjunction with a stable regimen of digoxin and diuretics. There is strong evidence of the clinical efficacy of digoxin in patients with normal sinus rhythm and this degree of congestive heart failure. Specifically, withdrawal of digoxin in patients with mild congestive heart failure results in a significant worsening of exercise performance and an increased incidence of, and a decreased time to, treatment failure.

Consequently, digoxin discontinuation is recommended only in patients who have normal sinus rhythm and echocardiographic confirmation of normal systolic ventricular function. When these two variables coexist, gradual and incremental discontinuation of digoxin is indicated but only with careful clinical observation.

Antiarrhythmic Medications

Although mortality from cardiovascular disease decreased over the last 10 years, sudden cardiac death remains a medical problem of epidemic proportion. It is presently estimated that over 250,000 persons die suddenly each year in the United States, and most of these deaths are believed to be a consequence of ventricular tachyarrhythmias.[80,81] The majority of patients who experience sudden death have coronary artery disease, often with prior myocardial infarction. Attempts to reduce sudden cardiovascular mortality have focused on the use of antiarrhythmic agents designed to suppress potentially lethal arrhythmias.[82] In particular, the Cardiac Arrhythmia Suppression Trial (CAST) was designed as a multicenter, randomized, placebo-controlled trial to test the hypothesis that in patients with prior myocardial infarction, the suppression of ventricular premature depolarization improves survival.[80,81] Because ventricular ectopy is an important risk factor for cardiac arrest in patients with a history of myocardial infarction, it was believed by many that drugs that suppress ventricular ectopy would prevent ventricular tachyarrhythmia-based cardiac arrest.[83]

Historically, the oral drugs most frequently used to suppress ventricular ectopy were the type IA antiarrhythmics such as quinidine, procainamide, and disopyramide. The trial was designed to determine whether these type IA agents or the newer agents encainide, flecainide, and moricizine could reduce the risk of sudden cardiac death in patients at high risk because of previous myocardial infarction and the presence of ventricular ectopy. Patients whose arrhythmia was suppressed by encainide, flecainide, or moricizine were randomly assigned to placebo or active drug treatment. The study demonstrated that patients randomly assigned to active treatment with antiarrhythmic agent experienced a 2.5-fold increase in mortality (encainide and flecainide), or no survival benefit (moricizine), compared with those randomly assigned to placebo.[81,82,84] These results show association between the ability of the type I antiarrhythmic agents to suppress ventricular ectopy and their ability to produce sudden cardiac death after acute myocardial infarction.[85] The study also showed the inadequacy of ventricular ectopy suppression as a marker for prevention of sudden cardiac death. Based on the CAST trial, drugs such as encainide, flecainide, and moricizine should not be used for non life-threatening ventricular tachyarrhythmias.[39,80-82,86-88]

The recently completed conventional-versus-amiodarone drug evaluation study (CASCADE Study) suggests that the CAST results may not be generalizable to other antiarrhythmic drugs.[82] In this secondary prevention trial, patients with out-of-hospital ventricular fibrillation not occurring during an acute Q-wave myocardial infarction were studied. Patients were randomly assigned to empiric treatment with amiodarone or to treatment with other antiarrhythmic drugs (including flecainide and moricizine, which were used in the CAST trial, and eight other antiarrhythmic agents). Ventricular fibrillation, syncope-associated defibrillated discharge, and cardiac death occurred less frequently in the amiodarone-treated group. Based on this study, patients with previously documented out-of-hospital ventricular fibrillation may have improved survival rates with the use of amiodarone.[89]

Guidelines for Drug Therapy in Patients With Ventricular Arrhythmias

Few clinical decisions in outpatients with heart disease require as much thought and critical analysis. Stated simply, the indications for and approach to drug therapy for patients with ventricular arrhythmias is one of the most controversial and misunderstood areas in clinical cardiology. The problem is especially common for primary care practitioners, who encounter many older patients with and without ischemic heart disease who demonstrate ventricular premature complexes (VPCs) or short runs of ventricular tachycardia (VT) on a routine electrocardiogram or during ambulatory Holter monitoring. From a therapeutic perspective, the critical clinical decision is to determine which patient subgroups will benefit from antiarrhythmic therapy, which patients require invasive intervention with automatic implantable cardioverter-defribrillators (AICD), and which patients simply ought to be followed with no pharmacotherapeutic intervention whatsoever.

These are important clinical determinations, given the fact that many studies (CAST) have shown that some pharmacologic interventions (Type IA antiarrhythmic agents) used for management of ventricular arrhythmias are associated with increased mortality, findings that have reframed our approaches to drug therapy for this patient population. The following guidelines-oriented section will review the prognosis and management of ventricular arrhythmias (VA) with and without heart disease.

These recommendations are based on extraction of pertinent articles obtained from a computer-assisted search of the English literature contained in a MEDLINE database, followed by a manual search of the bibliographies of relevant articles. The emphasis is on studies involving older persons and all articles were reviewed and analyzed in depth. These treatment approaches are recommended in specific subgroups, according to the prognosis, risk of treatment, and benefits of therapy.

Patients With No Heart Disease. First, it should be stressed that, in the studies reviewed, in patients with no clinical evidence of heart disease the presence of VPCs, nonsustained ventricular arrhythmias (VA), or complex ventricular arrhythmias (VA) were not associated with an increased incidence of new coronary events at a two-year follow-up. In addition, they were not associated with an increased incidence of primary ventricular fibrillation or sudden cardiac death. Because nonsustained VT or complex VA are not associated with increased mortality in older persons with no clinical evidence of heart disease—defined, for all the analyses in this review as the presence of myocardial ischemia, history of myocardial infarction, or left ventricular hypertrophy (LVH)—this review recommends no antiarrhythmic drug treatment of asymptomatic nonsustained VT, VPCs, or complex VA in older persons without heart disease.

Class I Antiarrhythmic Drugs. Based on the results of The Cardiac Arrhythmia Suppression Trial (CAST) I, encainide or flecainide is not recommended for the treatment of VT or complex VA in older or younger patients, even those with heart disease. Similarly, because investigators in the CAST II trial indicated that the use of the antiarrhythmic morcizine may be not only ineffective or harmful, this agent is not recommended for nonsustained VT, VPCs, or complex VA in older or younger persons without heart disease. Based on a meta-analysis of four randomized trials evaluating quinidine, flecainide, mexilitene, tocainide, and propafenone, there was an increased risk of mortality in patients treated with quinidine as compared to patients treated with the other antiarrhythmic agents. In contrast to findings with the aforementioned drugs, one important study demonstrated a decreased incidence of death and recurrent cardiac arrest in patients treated with beta-blockers versus no antiarrhythmic drug.

Based on cumulative data, the use of any class I antiarrhythmic agent is not recommended for the treatment for VT or complex VA in older or younger patients with heart disease. However, the use of *beta-blockers* is recommended for treatment of patients resuscitated from prehospital cardiac arrest attributable to ventricular fibrillation.

Calcium Channel Blockers. Calcium channel blockers are of no proven value in the management of patients with ventricular arrhythmias and, therefore, are not recommended for this patient population.

Beta-Blockers. In the majority of clinical trials analyzed, beta-blockers were associated with a reduction in cardiac ischemia, mortality, and risk of ventricular fibrillation in patients complex VA and myocardial infarction. Based on these studies, beta-blockers are recommended for treatment of both older and younger patients with VT or complex VA associated with ischemic or nonischemic heart disease and with normal or abnormal LV ejection fraction, provided there are no contraindications to beta-blocker therapy.

Amiodarone. Although amiodarone is very effective in suppressing VT and complex VA, the incidence of adverse effects of amiodarone approaches 90% after 5 years of therapy. In one large trial, the incidence of pulmonary toxicity was 10% at 2 years. Based on available studies, amiodarone use in the setting of complex VA or VT should be reserved for patients with life-threatening ventricular tachyarrhythmias in older or younger patients who cannot tolerate or who do not respond to beta-blockers.

Angiotensin-Converting Enzyme Inhibitors. Although ACE inhibitors do not possess antiarrhythmic properties, per se, these agents have been shown to produce a significant reduction in complex VA in patients with congestive heart failure (CHF). On the basis of limited available data, ACE inhibitors are reasonable adjunctive agents in patients with VT or complex VA associated with congestive heart failure. Combined use with a beta-blocker may produce additional benefits in older or younger patients with asymptomatic LV systolic dysfunction plus ventricular arrhythmias.

Invasive Intervention. Patients who have life-threatening recurrent VT or ventricular fibrillation that is resistant to antiarrhythmic drugs require invasive intervention which may include: coronary artery bypass graft surgery, aneurysmectomy or infarctectomy, and endocardial resection with or without adjunctive cryoblation based on activation mapping in the operating room. Although these procedures have their place in a small subset of individuals, the automatic implantable cardio-defibrillator (ACID) is currently accepted as the most effective treatment for patients with life-threatening VT or ventricular fibrillation (VF). Based on available studies, ACID is recommended in older or younger patients who have medically refractory sustained VT or VF.

Based on a review of more than 70 studies evaluating the prognosis and effectiveness of management options in patients with ventricular arrhythmias, recommendations are offered that maximize outcomes while reducing risk. These therapeutic approaches can be recommended for implementation in the primary care setting, as indicated, and include the following principles: (1) patients without heart disease who have non-lifethreatening VA should not be treated with antiarrhythmic drugs; (2) Class I antiarrhythmic drugs should not be used to treat complex VA in older patients with ischemic or nonischemic heart disease, if there are no contraindications to beta-blocker therapy, which is preferred therapy; (3) amiodarone should be reserved for life-threatening VA in older persons who are not responsive to or who cannot tolerate beta-blocker therapy; (4) ACE inhibitors should be part of an antiarrhythmic regimen for patients with VA that is associated with CHF; and (5) patients who have life-threatening VA (including sustained VT or VF) that is resistant to drug therapy are best managed with automatic implantable cardio-defibrillator (ACID).

Finally, underlying causes of complex VA should always be treated, whenever possible. In this regard, treatment of digitalis, toxicity, electrolyte disturbances, left ventricular dysfunction, myocardial ischemia, or hypoxia may help reduce or abolish ventricular arrhythmias. With respect to lifestyle, non-pharmacologic measures, patients should be counseled to avoid alcohol and cigarette smoking.[142]

In general, indications for the use of all antiarrhythmic agents in patients with known coronary artery disease should be reevaluated.[88] Even patients who are taking quinidine therapy for pharmacologic cardioversion of atrial fibrillation may require reassessment, based on recent studies showing that mortality rates are increased in some patients taking this antiarrhythmic agent.[90] Consultation with a cardiologist is required prior to adjustment of dose or discontinuation of antiarrhythmic therapy.[87,91,92]

Aspirin

Aspirin has become a bulwark of defense for the prevention of coronary artery disease, transient ischemic attacks, and embolic stroke associated with chronic atrial fibrillation (when anticoagulation with warfarin is contraindicated).[93,94] Despite the widespread use of aspirin to prevent both cardiovascular and cerebrovascular conditions, the precise dosage of aspirin required in each condition is still highly controversial.[95,96] In the case of secondary prevention of myocardial infarction, however, 80 mg of aspirin per day, or 160 mg of aspirin every other day, is sufficient for prevention of recurrent myocardial infarction. Generally speaking, patients who are taking aspirin therapy exclusively for the secondary prevention of myocardial infarction should be maintained on no more than 80 mg of aspirin per day. As a rule, higher doses are not required, and patients can be rapidly tapered to a lower dose, which has the advantage of decreased gastrointestinal side effects.

The appropriate dose of aspirin for the prevention of transient ischemic attacks and stroke, however, is still hotly debated.[93-96] Nevertheless, it is clear that when stroke prevention is studied in the setting of chronic, nonrheumatic atrial fibrillation, patients who receive 325 mg per day of aspirin have a 42% reduction in ischemic stroke and systemic embolism, as compared with placebo. However, those patients who receive only 75 mg per day of aspirin have a smaller and *insignificant* (16%) reduction in cerebrovascular events. This study suggests that patients who, for one reason or another, are not appropriate candidates for warfarin therapy (which is the drug of choice for the prevention of embolic infarction in patients with chronic atrial fibrillation), should be treated with at least 325 mg of aspirin a day.[95,96]

Although many investigations in the United Kingdom suggest that as much as 1,200 mg per day of aspirin may be required to prevent transient ischemic attacks or minor stroke, there is also evidence reported by the Swedish Aspirin Low-Dose Trial (SALT) that patients who take only 75 mg of aspirin per day will have a significant reduction in stroke and death compared to the placebo group.[95] Moreover, a Dutch study compared low dose (283 mg per day) and very low dose aspirin therapy (30 mg per day). In this very well-designed trial, there were no significant differences in the primary end points of vascular deaths, stroke, and myocardial infarction when the two dosage regimens were compared.[95,96] This study suggests that in patients with a history of aspirin intolerance, gastric erosions, ulcer disease, or gastrointestinal hemorrhage, and who also require stroke prevention, a 30 mg per day aspirin dose may provide significant clinical benefits, while reducing the risks of aspirin-induced side effects. However, it should be stressed that findings suggesting that aspirin doses of 325 mg or less are successful in preventing stroke are not universal. Further circumstantial evidence concerning low- and high-dose aspirin therapy is available from carotid endarterectomy studies, which demonstrate that doses as high as 1000 to 1500 mg of aspirin per day may be required to reduce stroke incidence and deaths. At present, the precise dose of aspirin required to prevent cerebrovascular events in patients with normal sinus rhythm is not known.[94-96]

Specifically, no study of patients with cerebrovascular disease has established that an aspirin dosage of 325 mg per day or less is better or even comparable with 975 mg or more. It is possible that lower doses are effective but are not as effective as higher doses. Based on this data, reduction of aspirin dose should be limited to those conditions in which lower doses are demonstrated to be efficacious, including patients who require aspirin therapy for prevention of myocardial infarction.

Indications, Dosages, and Clinical Guidelines for Antithrombotic Therapy in The Outpatient Setting

Antithrombotic therapy is the primary bulwark of defense for patients with thromboembolic diseases of the arterial and nervous circulatory systems. With so many clinical trials, reviews, and consensus reports recently published, it has been extremely difficult for practitioners to stay current with recommendations for the more than thirty clinical conditions for which antithrombotic therapy has proven effective. To provide practicing clinicians a universal and standardized approach to drug therapy for patients with thromboembolic diseases, the third American College of Chest Physicians Consensus Conference on Antithrombotic Therapy convened in order to set forth state-of-the-art guidelines for these disorders. Although many of these guidelines address issues related to in-hospital treatment, prophylaxis, and management of thromboembolic disorders, the following guidelines, which are distilled from this landmark report, focus on indications and strategies for use of antithrombotic agents—aspirin, warfarin, ticlodipine, and dipyridamole—in the *outpatient* setting.[143]

Antiplatelet Agents: General Recommendations. Aspirin is indicated for long-term management of patients with stable angina, unstable angina, transient cerebral ischemia, acute myocardial infarction, thrombotic stroke, and peripheral arterial disease. A dose of 160 to 325 mg/d should be used for all indications, except in patients with cerebrovascular disease, in whom a dose of 160 to 325 mg/d is effective, but in whom higher doses (975 mg/d) may prove to be even *more* effective. The advantages versus risks of these higher doses for prevention of stroke remains a controversial point.

In contrast to previous guidelines urging that aspirin prophylaxis primarily directed at prevention of *recurrent* myocardial infarction, current guidelines suggest that aspirin be used as both *primary* and secondary prophylaxis in asymptomatic men and women who are older than 50 years of age in order to prevent myocardial infarction. Aspirin is also indicated in patients with chronic atrial fibrillation in whom warfarin therapy is contraindicated. Although extreme caution is required when aspirin and warfarin are used in combination, studies suggest patients with mechanical heart valves *at high risk* for systemic embolism be treated with a combination of warfarin (maintaining INR between 2.5 and 3.5) and low-dose aspirin. In general, ticlodipine is reserved for use in patients with allergy to aspirin or aspirin intolerance and in patients who develop recurrent thromboembolism despite aspirin therapy.

Venous Thromboembolism. Although treatment is highly individualized, in patients with deep venous thrombosis or pulmonary embolism, long-term anticoagulant therapy should be continued with warfarin for at least 3 months in order to prolong the PT to an INR of 2.0 to 3.0. Patients with recurrent venous thrombosis should be treated indefinitely, as should patients with AT III deficiency. Symptomatic, isolated calf vein thrombosis should be treated with anticoagulation for 3 months.

Atrial Fibrillation. Long-term oral warfarin therapy (INR 2.0 to 3.0) is recommended for patients with atrial fibrillation (AF) who are eligible to receive anticoagulation therapy. Anticoagulation is presently not recommended for patients who are younger than 60 years of age who have no associated cardiovascular disease (i.e., "lone AF"). Patients with AF who are poor candidates for anticoagulation therapy should be treated with aspirin at a dosage of 325 mg/d.

It is strongly recommended that warfarin therapy (INR, 2.0 to 3.0) be given for 3 weeks before elective cardioversion of patients who have been in AF for more than 2 days and be continued until normal sinus rhythm has been maintained for 4 weeks. In contrast, antithrombotic therapy is *not* recommended for cardioversion of atrial flutter or supraventricular tachycardia or for cardioversion of patients who have been in AF for not more than 2 days, unless other risk factors for systemic embolism are present.

Valvular Heart Disease. Patients with a history of rheumatic mitral valve disease who have either a history of systemic embolism or paroxysmal or chronic AF, should be treated with long-term warfarin therapy sufficient to achieve an INR of 2.0 to 3.0. This antithrombotic approach is also recommended for patients with rheumatic mitral valve disease and normal sinus rhythm if the left atrial diameter is in excess of 5.5 cm. If systemic embolism occurs despite adequate warfarin therapy, the addition of 160 mg to 325 mg aspirin/d should be considered. Because of the risks attending concurrent use of aspirin and warfarin, these patients should be carefully monitored. In patients with recurrent embolism who are unable to take aspirin, or who are deemed inappropriate candidates for *concurrent* aspirin and warfarin therapy, an alternative strategy would be to increase the warfarin dose sufficient to prolong the PT to an INR of 2.5 to 3.5.

Long-term antithrombotic therapy is *not* recommended for patients with mitral valve prolapse who have not experienced systemic embolism, unexplained TIAs, or AF. Those who have manifested signs of TIAs should be treated with long-term aspirin therapy at a dose of 325 to 975 mg/d. Those with documented systemic embolism—and paroxysmal or chronic AF—should be treated with long-term warfarin therapy (INR, 2.0 to 3.0).

Prosthetic Heart Valves. All patients with mechanical prosthetic heart valves should receive long-term anticoagulation therapy with warfarin (INR, 2.5-3.5). Aspirin (100 mg/d) offers additional protection when added to warfarin, but with an increased risk of bleeding. Dypyridamole (400 mg/d) may be added to warfarin for additional protection.

Post-Myocardial Infarction. Following acute myocardial infarction, aspirin (80-160 mg/day) is recommended for long-term therapy in preference to warfarin because of aspirin's simplicity, safety, and low-cost. It should be stressed that long-term warfarin therapy is recommended in clinical settings associated with increased embolic risk (duration, 1 to 3 months following acute myocardial infarction complicated by severe left ventricular dysfunction, congestive heart failure, previous emboli, or two-dimensional echo evidence of mural thrombi; duration indefinite in patients with AF). Dipyridamole is *not* recommended for survivors of acute MI.

Chronic Coronary Artery Disease. All patients with clinical or laboratory evidence of chronic coronary artery disease (angina, angiographic confirmation, etc.) should receive oral aspirin therapy (160 to 325 mg/d) indefinitely. The indications for primary prevention of MI have been clarified by the consensus conference and are as follows: all patients older than 50 years of age who are free of contraindications to aspirin should be considered for primary prevention with aspirin doses of 160 to 325 mg/d. The absolute benefits of this strategy increase with advancing age and, most likely, with the presence of diabetes mellitus, systolic or diastolic hypertension, cigarette smoking, and lack of exercise. In contrast, the routine use of aspirin for primary prevention of coronary heart disease is *not* recommended for individuals who are younger than 50 years of age, *unless* they have a history of MI, stroke, or TIA.

Patients With Coronary Bypass Grafts. Aspirin alone is recommended to reduce the incidence of saphenous vein bypass graft closure. The aspirin dose shown to be beneficial in graft patency is 325 mg/d or higher. One study has shown that dypyridamole therapy (225 mg/d) in addition to aspirin is more effective than aspirin (150 mg/day) therapy alone. Although the duration of benefits seen with aspirin therapy is uncertain, one-year of therapy is currently recommended. For patients who are allergic to aspirin, ticlodipine (250 mg twice daily) has been shown to be effective in one study if started 48 hours after surgery, and may be considered an alternative.

Coronary Angioplasty. Long-term aspirin therapy (160-325 mg/d) is recommended in patients following angioplasty, primarily because of its effects on coronary heart disease. Its effect on recurrent stenosis, per se, has not been clarified and is inconsistent.

Peripheral Vascular Disease. Although it is uncertain whether aspirin alone or aspirin with dipyridamole will modify the natural history or clinical course of patients with peripheral vascular disease, because these patients are at high risk for cardiovascular events (stroke and myocardial infarction), they should be given lifelong aspirin therapy (160-325 mg/d) in the absence of contraindications. Long-term anticoagulation with warfarin with or without aspirin should *not* be used routinely after femoropopliteal bypass and other vascular reconstructions.

Cerebrovascular Disease. Following carotid endarterectomy, aspirin (325 to 650 mg twice daily) should be given to prevent continuing TIAs and stroke. Although the optimal approach to patients with symptomatic carotid stenosis is uncertain, all patients with asymptomatic carotid disease should be treated with aspirin whether or not they undergo endarterectomy. This recommendation extends to all patients with asymptomatic bruits as well as individuals with TIAs and a history of minor ischemic strokes, where aspirin has been established to be effective in doses ranging from as low as 30 mg/d (TIAs) to 1300 mg/day. While many experts recommend 325 mg/d of aspirin, other authorities believe that higher doses, i.e., 975 to 1300 mg/d confer greater benefit. Although studies suggest ticlodipine is more effective than aspirin in the setting of cerebrovascular disease, it is also more toxic, and, therefore, ticlodipine is recommended for patients who are intolerant to aspirin and those who experience recurrent ischemic events during aspirin therapy.

Clinical Monitoring. Most clinicians agree that oral anticoagulation for venous thromboembolism or atrial fibrillation should be monitored with the goal of maintaining a prothrombin time (PT) 1.3-1.5 times control; in patients with mechanical heart valves the PT should be maintained at 1.5-2.0 times control. It has become increasingly clear that recommendations such as these are not generalizable and may lead to significant errors in clinical practice, since laboratories throughout North America use different thromboplastin reagents when determining PT valves. The sensitivity of these reagents varies widely and can be measured by the international sensitivity index (ISI). Therefore a PT of 15 at one laboratory might be equivalent to a PT of 24 at another. In order to circumvent this difficulty the INR (International Normalized Ratio) was developed. The INR equals the ratio of patient to control PT taken to the power of the ISI for the particular thromboplastin reagent used. Use of the INR eliminates uncertainty involved in monitoring oral anticoagulation. Unfortunately, most laboratories report only prothrombin times, and clinical decisions based on the PT or ratio of patient to control PT are only accurate when the sensitivity of the thromboplastin reagent is in a narrow range (ISI: 2.2-2.6).[144,145]

In one trial investigators from the University of Texas developed a questionnaire for institutional laboratories to determine the sensitivity index (ISI) of the thromboplastin they use and their method of reporting PT values (in seconds, as PT ratios, or as INRs). The survey was completed by 140 institutions participating in the SPAF study (Stroke Prevention in Atrial Fibrillation). An additional 50 teaching and community hospitals were surveyed by phone or during the winter forum of the American College of Clinical Pharmacy. Finally, three major pharmaceutical firms were contacted and asked to disclose the sensitivity index of the thromboplastin reagents they market.

Of 190 participating institutions, only 28 used reagents with sensitivity indices within the range which allows standard interpretation of PT values (2.2-2.6 times control). Thirty one institutions could not even determine the sensitivity index of the thromboplastin reagent they were currently using, and at the other sites the sensitivity index ranged from 1.4-2.8. Only 21% of the laboratories reported results as an INR; 75% reported only PT values in seconds. The range of ISI values reported by pharmaceutical firms was 1.2-2.8, and none of them were currently marketing a product with a sensitivity index in the desired range (2.2-2.6).

The INR is the most reliable guide in the management of patients receiving warfarin. The therapeutic goal in patients with deep venous thrombosis (DVT), pulmonary embolus (PE), atrial fibrillation, and tissue heart valves is an INR from 2.0-3.0. In patients with mechanical heart valves or a cardiogenic embolus the INR should be maintained in a higher range, i.e., 3.0-4.5. When dealing with referral laboratories that do not report INRs, anticoagulation can be properly managed through knowledge of the international sensitivity index (ISI) of the thromboplastin reagent that particular lab is currently using. If the ISI falls between 2.2 and 2.6, traditional recommendations are valid. If not, the following chart can be referred to. Choose the row corresponding to the ISI that your lab is using, and underline the adjacent therapeutic goals in order to safely and effectively anticoagulate your patients.

ISI	LESS INTENSIVE ANTICOAGULATION (e.g., DVT, PE, atrial fib., tissue heart valve) INR 2.0-3.0		MORE INTENSIVE ANTICOAGULATION (e.g., Cardiogenic embolus, Mechanical heart valve) INR 3.0-4.5	
	Protime (secs)	PT ratio patient/ control	Protime (secs)	PT ratio patient/ control
1.2	21-30	1.8-2.5	30-42	2.5-3.5
1.4-1.6	20-24	1.6-2.0	26-30	2.2-2.6
1.8-2.0	18-21	1.5-1.7	22-25	1.8-2.1
2.2-2.4	16-19	1.4-1.6	20-22.5	1.6-1.9
2.6-2.8	15.5-18	1.3-1.5	18-21	1.5-1.7

Beware the laboratory that cannot provide you with the ISI of the reagents they use. If they are not willing to correct this shortcoming, a laboratory that is more up-to-date would better serve your patients.[144,145]

Dipyridamole

Attempts to maintain patency of carotid vessels in patients who undergo carotid endarterectomy focus on the use of aspirin and dipyridamole (Persantine®), which is widely administered to patients having mechanical vascular procedures in hopes of reducing the risk of subsequent vascular restenosis. Despite the widespread practice of using dipyridamole to prevent stroke and to prevent carotid artery restenosis following surgery, its value and efficacy have never been formally substantiated in these patient populations. Given the significant cost of dipyridamole and the potential gastric toxicity of aspirin, it is important to establish the role of these agents in preventing stroke and restenosis in patients undergoing endarterectomy. The most comprehensive studies evaluating this issue confirm that restenosis after carotid endarterectomy is not prevented by aspirin and dipyridamole therapy.[97] Consequently, patients who undergo carotid endarterectomy should have dipyridamole eliminated from their perioperative and postoperative management.

On the other hand, because long-term aspirin therapy reduces the risk of nonfatal myocardial infarction, stroke, and vascular mortality in patients with symptomatic coronary, peripheral, or cerebral atherosclerotic vascular disease, aspirin should be useful for patients with stenotic carotid vascular disease as well. The ideal dose of aspirin that should be used to prevent carotid restenosis is not determined, but a range of 30 to 325 mg of aspirin per day seems justified. As for the role of dipyridamole therapy in preventing cerebral thrombotic infarction, there are presently no studies that show that this agent plays any significant role in reducing the risk of cerebrovascular disease.[97,98]Therefore, dipyridamole can be eliminated in virtually all patients who are taking the medication exclusively for the secondary prevention of atherothrombotic cerebral infarction. Individuals who are taking dipyridamole in combination with warfarin to prevent thrombus formation associated with cardiac valve replacements should be maintained on this agent pending further studies.[99]

Nitrates

Nitrates are central to the treatment of chronic stable angina pectoris. They are the oldest and, perhaps, most reliable form of antianginal therapy. These agents are effective in all forms of angina (classic, variant, mixed), and are relatively low in cost. Moreover, they are helpful in reducing preload and congestive symptoms, and they are available in a variety of preparations, routes of administration, and dosages. Longer acting oral and transdermal nitrates are widely used to provide angina prophylaxis. However, their ability to deliver long-acting, continuous nitrate therapy is associated with the rapid development of tolerance (defined as a decrease in magnitude and duration of effects despite constant or increased dose and plasma concentration). Because of tolerance, more intermittent dosing of longer acting nitrates (i.e., isosorbide dinitrate orally three times daily in an asymmetrical schedule, or removal of nitrate patches for 12 hours at night time) to provide a nitrate-free interval is standard practice. While this strategy does reduce the development of tolerance, sometimes there is an increase in anginal episodes during periods of low nitrate levels. The relative inconvenience of using nitrate preparations prompted many experts to recommend their discontinuation in favor of using calcium channel blockers or beta adrenergic receptor antagonists to treat anginal episodes. Recent studies, however, suggest that older nitrate preparations can be discontinued in favor of isosorbide-5-mononitrate (e.g., ISMO®, Monoket®), the major active metabolite of isosorbide dinitrate, and is approved for clinical use in the United States in a regimen of 20 mg twice per day, given 7 hours apart.

Recent studies have suggested that isosorbide mononitrate provides long-acting prophylactic antianginal therapy without the development of either nitrate tolerance, increased rebound angina attacks, or reduced efficacy at the end of its duration of action. Furthermore, this preparation is more convenient due to its twice daily dosing.

Nitrates are clearly important agents for the medical therapy of angina. Many nitrate formulations give clinicians the opportunity to use them in several ways to manage angina. All patients with angina should carry a rapidly acting, short duration preparation, such as nitroglycerin tablets for sublingual use, or a nitroglycerin spray, to alleviate acute anginal attacks. They can also be used before specific activities known to induce angina, such as walking uphill and sexual intercourse.

Theophylline

Although the use of theophylline to treat bronchospastic pulmonary disease and asthma decreased significantly over the past several years, studies suggest that theophylline is still an overused medication. Physicians and pharmacists encounter many patients on theophylline therapy in whom the dose can be reduced, or the medication eliminated entirely.[54] It should be stressed that theophylline toxicity can be a serious and life-threatening problem. One study evaluating theophylline overdose in 249 consecutive patients referred to the Massachusetts Poison Control Center attempted to identify risk factors for major toxicity associated with this medication.[100] Major toxicity occurred in 62 patients and caused death in 13. It is important to note that 37% of the patients with theophylline toxicity were inadvertently overmedicated while receiving *long-term* theophylline therapy. Major toxicity was more common in this group than in those with acute (presumably intentional) overdosage. Moreover, the study showed that peak level is the most important risk factor for major toxicity in acute overdosage, and advancing age was the most critical factor in chronic overdosage.[101,102]

This study demonstrates that in an important subset of older patients who are receiving theophylline therapy for management of chronic asthma, toxicity can be both inadvertent and serious. Up to 20% of such patients receiving long-term theophylline therapy may have at least some toxic manifestations.[100] In fact, the longstanding controversy over the appropriateness of theophylline use has centered not only on the question of its effectiveness when compared with other more modern drugs, but also its narrow therapeutic range.

At present, there is no dearth of data indicating that theophylline is a relatively weak bronchodilator when compared with beta-2 agonists and inhaled ipratropium bromide. Even in combination with other bronchodilators, there is much evidence to suggest that the addition of theophylline increases side effects without significantly improving bronchodilation. Taken together, these studies suggest that theophylline is a third- or fourth-line agent for the treatment of asthma.

Currently, it seems clear that theophylline should not be a first-line drug for treatment of mild, intermittent asthma because acute exacerbations of asthmatic reactions are most effectively managed by more powerful and rapidly acting beta-2 agonists. Moreover, chronic suppression of inflammatory mediators of the late asthmatic reaction is best achieved by administration of inhaled steroids. In more severe asthma, however, there is an increasing role for the use of theophylline that is supported by a handful of studies. Particularly in patients with nocturnal complaints, long-term theophylline therapy has a clear role in the alleviation of disease symptoms. Despite the lack of evidence that theophylline provides bronchodilator advantages in the acute setting, there is some evidence that lends credence to the concept that hospitalized patients will benefit from early administration of the drug. Clearly, because advancing age increases the likelihood of toxicity from this agent, theophylline should be used with extreme care in elderly patients and should be accompanied by frequent measurements of blood levels (even in the apparently stable patient).

It seems reasonable to consider discontinuation of theophylline therapy in those asthma patients who have *not* been given an adequate trial of beta-2 agonists or inhaled corticosteroid therapy. If a patient presents on theophylline treatment but has no previous history of taking beta-2 agonists or corticosteroids for treatment of asthma, these therapeutic options should be evaluated before continuation of long-term therapy with theophylline. There are, however, some subgroups which seem to benefit from theophylline therapy, including patients who need diaphragmatic stimulation, patients with sleep apnea, and some patients with nocturnal asthma. For most other patients with asthma, however, theophylline is relegated to relatively low standing, and attempts at discontinuing the medication are justified especially in older patients in whom toxicity is more common.

Corticosteroids

Because of the wide range of potential side effects that result from chronic therapy with corticosteroids, these agents should be used very judiciously in patients with rheumatoid arthritis and other chronic inflammatory disorders. Low-dose ($\leq$ 10 mg per day prednisone) treatment with steroids is widely used in patients with rheumatoid arthritis, often to induce potent anti-inflammatory effects and symptomatic relief until other anti-inflammatory agents have a chance to work. The incidence and severity of side effects of low-dose steroid therapy are controversial, and many clinicians and pharmacists feel that the positive effects of steroids on the inflammatory process outweigh the risks when used on a short-term basis. An area of particular concern is the effect of steroids on bone mass, as it is widely known that chronic steroid therapy is a powerful inducer of osteoporosis.[103,104] Most trials examining these effects are nonrandomized and, therefore, are subject to selection bias and confounding factors because rheumatoid arthritis itself is a risk factor for bone loss. Furthermore, it is known that the negative influences of steroids on bone mass are more pronounced in the first few months of therapy, so that longitudinal studies that look at bone mass in the chronic phase of therapy may underestimate the effects of these agents on bone.

The major conclusion of a recent study suggests that even low-dose, short-term corticosteroid therapy can cause a significant decrease in bone mineral density that is only partially reversible.[103] Accordingly, it is imperative that steroids be used at the lowest possible dosages and for the shortest periods of time possible. A common and reasonable approach is to use steroids until other inflammatory agents have a chance to work. However, these medications may require several months before significant impact is noted—well within the timeframe for significant loss in bone mineral density to be induced by prednisone. Recognizing this, preventive strategies to help minimize the degree of bone loss while patients are on steroids are important. However, there is relatively little evidence that documents exactly what treatments are most effective as preventive interventions in this setting. Until there is such evidence, interventions that are effective in other situations, such as estrogen replacement, calcium supplements, vitamin D, and calcitonin may be considered. Measurement of bone density during and following steroid therapy in patients with rheumatoid arthritis can help guide the degree and intensity of these various therapies.

When using steroids to manage *acute* inflammatory conditions, it is clear that rapid, short-term tapering courses of steroids are as effective as longer dose reduction measures occurring over several weeks. Specifically, with regard to asthma, patients can be tapered over a period of 3 to 7 days following an acute exacerbation. There is no justification for prolonged tapering over a several week period. Finally, in those patients who are taking long-term steroid therapy, every attempt should be made to reduce the dose to less than 10 mg per day, to avoid suppression of the hypothalamic-pituitary adrenal axis.[103]

Antidepressants

The indications and criteria for discontinuing antidepressant drug therapy are controversial.[105-107] First, most depressive disorders extend over a lifetime, and for the majority of patients, the risk for future episodes of depression increases as the number of past episodes increases.[108,109] Moreover, the length of the well interval between episodes becomes progressively shorter with each new episode. Those individuals who are older at the onset of their depression have higher probabilities of relapse during future years if not maintained on treatment. As the number of episodes grows larger and the patient becomes older, severity also often intensifies, treatment response to conventional antidepressants may diminish or even disappear, and the potentially destructive behavioral consequences of the disorder progressively worsen.[5] This destructive lifetime pattern can be modified in many, if not most patients, since antidepressants are effective in preventing most future episodes of depression and preserving quality of life.

In recent years, with the introduction of selective serotonin reuptake inhibitor (SSRIs), patterns of antidepressant use have changed dramatically. More and more, this class of antidepressants is being used to treat panic disorders, premenstrual syndrome, obsessive-compulsive disorders, chronic anxiety, as well as other symptoms associated with the trials of modern life. In addition, it is frequently difficult to determine which patients have a depressive illness that requires long-term maintenance therapy and which patients can be discontinued from their antidepressant medication once their situational crisis resolves. Nevertheless, specific recommendations can be given that shed light on windows of opportunity and vulnerability regarding maintenance versus discontinuation of long-term antidepressant therapy.

Maintenance. Lifetime pharmacologic maintenance *is* indicated for patients who are 50 years of age or older when they experience their first episode of depression. Maintenance therapy also appears to be justified in those patients who are 40 years of age or older with two or more prior episodes of depression and for those with three or more prior episodes, regardless of their age.[108,109] Maintenance dosages need to be comparable to established treatment dosages until it is proven that lower doses are effective. When an antidepressant is selected for long-term treatment, strong consideration should be given to the agent's side effect profile (see Table 4-2), since compliance is essential for success. Rapidly accumulating data indicate that the prevailing treatment philosophy for those with major depression probably should *not* shift toward discontinuation of treatment. However, if medications must be discontinued for those at high risk, dosage should be tapered over a prolonged period, patients should be monitored closely, relapses should be expected, and nonpharmacologic treatments such as psychotherapy and phototherapy should be considered, as indicated.

For patients taking antidepressant medication for a situational crisis or anxiety-related symptoms, medication discontinuation is probably more justifiable. It must be emphasized that the pharmacologic consequences of stopping an antidepressant medication may be equal to or greater than those associated with administering it.[31] Discontinuing a medication that is taken for a prolonged period is not an innocuous action. Nevertheless, despite known risks, clinical or personal reasons sometimes lead to a decision to discontinue antidepressant therapy.

Discontinuation. How should discontinuation be accomplished? Ideally, the schedule for cessation should be gradual. Treatment should be tapered over several weeks, or perhaps a few months. Whenever possible, tapering of the medication should be conducted over a much longer period, preferably one year. Data are not available to firmly substantiate that this more gradual reduction strategy is more effective in preventing relapse for most antidepressant medications, but we do know about risks associated with rapid discontinuation, and we have considerable knowledge about the rate of change for receptors and other neurobiological functions following administration and discontinuation of centrally active agents. These clinical and neurobiologic observations suggest that the brain requires months rather than days or weeks to adjust to the changes associated with stopping a medication. For tricyclic or heterocyclic agents, a simple strategy is to reduce the dosage by 25% *every 3 months*. For drugs with a longer half-life and a standardized dosing regimen, such as fluoxetine, this reduction is accomplished by taking the pill at a reduced frequency every quarter, such as every other day, then every third day, and so on, or by switching to lower dosage forms or liquid products and continuing daily administration, and then reducing the dosage by 25% every 3 months. Patients generally tolerate these reduced regimens. The use of a daily diary helps maintain compliance. To assist patients in remaining on course, a withdrawal calendar should be prepared and given to patients and families with clear instructions. It is also important to continue other treatments that are proven valuable, such as interpersonal therapy, phototherapy, or other modalities.

Table 4-2

		Antidepressant Medications				
Category and Drug	Sedative Potency	Anti-cholinergic Potency	Orthostatic Hypotensive Potency	Cardiac Arrhyth-mogenic Potential	Target Dosage (mg/day)	Dosage Range (mg/day)
Tertiary amines						
Amitriptyline	High	Very high	High	Yes	150-200	75-300
Clomipramine	High	High	High	Yes	150-200	75-250
Doxepin	High	Moderate	Moderate	Yes	150-200	75-300
Imipramine	Moderate	Moderate	High	Yes	150-200	75-300
Trimipramine	High	Moderate	Moderate	Yes	150-200	75-300
Secondary amines						
Desipramine	Low	Low	Moderate	Yes	150-200	75-300
Nortriptyline	Low	Low	Lowest of the tricyclics	Yes	75-100	40-150
Protriptyline	Low	High	Low	Yes	30	15-60
Amoxapine	Low	Low	Moderate	Yes	150-200	75-300
Maprotiline	Moderate	Low	Moderate	Yes	150-200	75-200
Bupropion	Low	Very low	Very low	Low	300	200-450
Fluoxetine	Low	Very low	Very low	Low	20	5-80
Sertraline	Low	Very low	Very low	Low	100-150	50-200
Trazodone	High	Very low	High	Low	400	50-600

Row group labels (left margin): Tricyclics; Related Polycyclics; Atypical Agents

Tricyclic antidepressants with anticholinergic potency require special mention when planning discontinuation of treatment, since receptor regulatory changes occur in patients who are taking medications that block muscarinic receptors for a sustained period. If a tricyclic antidepressant is stopped suddenly, a transient but significant cholinergic supersensitivity will develop in many patients.[28,31] Patients may complain of somatic distress, gastrointestinal symptoms, disturbed sleep patterns that include excessive and vivid dreaming or nightmares, or patients may report frequent awakening and insomnia. Psychomotor disruptions, agitation, anxiety, and activation may also occur. This antidepressant withdrawal syndrome has been described in detail, and many of these anticholinergic withdrawal symptoms are indistinguishable from the symptom profile experienced by patients relapsing into depression. This is another important reason for planning a gradual discontinuation of medications whenever possible, especially when tricyclic antidepressants are being used.

Patients who are taking SSRIs (sertraline, fluoxetine, etc.) also require gradual discontinuation from their medication. It is preferable to be cautious and taper these agents gradually to prevent precipitation of a major depressive episode.

In summary, recurrent episodes of depression across a lifetime are an unfortunate but predictable characteristic of this disorder. The consequences of multiple episodes of depression are almost always debilitating and, on occasion, may even be fatal. Therefore, recurrences should be prevented whenever possible. Maintenance treatment with antidepressant medications is effective in most patients, if dosages are at adequate treatment levels. Individuals with multiple prior episodes of depression, especially if they are elderly and if prior episodes were severe, are at especially high risk for relapse if medications are discontinued. As a result, maintenance regimens at treatment dosage levels probably should be the norm for many or most patients with depressive mood disorders.

Since age at onset and the number of prior episodes both may predict risk of subsequent episodes, a workable formula is that anyone age 50 or more at onset of their first episode, age 40 or more at onset with two or more episodes, or any age with three or more episodes, probably should be considered a candidate for maintenance. If medication discontinuation is absolutely essential, despite known risks, it should be performed gradually, with close monitoring, ongoing use of nonpharmacologic treatments, if possible, and with a strategic plan for prompt intervention if the anticipated relapse occurs.[42,43,48,49]

Benzodiazepines

Benzodiazepine drugs such as alprazolam are widely used for the treatment of panic disorders. There is considerable debate, as well as negative perceptions, shared by health professionals, pharmacists, patients, lay public, and the media regarding the syndrome associated with benzodiazepine discontinuation. Clearly, there is a need to determine the optimal time for discontinuing these medications, the appropriate reasons for doing so, how discontinuation should be accomplished, and expected outcomes.[65] Recent studies suggest that the majority of patients taking benzodiazepines (see Table 4-3), when slowly tapered, are able to discontinue these agents without a great deal of trouble, particularly after *short-term therapy.*[30] Patients treated with long-term therapy at higher therapeutic doses tend to experience greater difficulty with discontinuation.[27,110] However, if patients are appropriately and adequately prepared, and discontinuation efforts follow a slow and gradual tapering schedule, discontinuation symptoms, if they occur, tend to be transient, mild to moderate in severity, and are generally tolerable by the average patient.

Panic Disorder. Definitive evidence is not yet available regarding the optimal length of treatment for panic disorders, although one recent study documented that 8 months of treatment led to greater improvement than 2 months of therapy, which is certainly in keeping with the experience of most physicians. Another study compared short-term versus extended maintenance treatment in panic disorder patients treated with imipramine and demonstrated that the group who received 12 months of maintenance therapy, following 6 months of acute treatment, had significantly less relapse at follow-up than did the group who received only 6 months of acute treatment.[111]

After 6 to 18 months of effective pharmacotherapy of panic disorder, most physicians attempt to taper and discontinue medications.[112,113] Although one might question discontinuing treatment that proved effective and allowed the patient to return to a near-normal level of functioning, the expense and potential side effects associated with these medications will justify an attempt at discontinuation in the majority of cases. Moreover, once the patient has maintained maximal improvement for at least 6 months and has reestablished his or her previous state of functioning and confidence, there are several appropriate reasons for reassessing the need for continued treatment.

The most compelling case for discontinuation is that treatment may no longer be necessary.[114] Also, problematic side effects, the wish to conceive, unexpected pregnancy, or emergence of alcohol or drug abuse are all valid reasons for attempting to discontinue effective treatment. Other, less important but equally understandable reasons include the expense and inconvenience involved in taking benzodiazepines or tricyclic antidepressants several times a day and issues of self-esteem. Consequently, the decision to discontinue benzodiazepines, for whatever the reason, should be a mutual one between patient and physician, and the patient should be reassured that in most cases discontinuation can be accomplished without significant adverse consequences. In this regard, it is critical that the medication be tapered slowly and gradually; this minimizes the severity of withdrawal symptoms that may occur with discontinuation. The patient should also be reassured that he or she may experience some anxiety symptoms, but that for most, these will resolve within 1 to 3 weeks. The patient should also be reassured that if it is determined that pharmacologic treatment is required, the medication can be reinstated.

Table 4-3

		Benzodiazepines	
Drug	**Equivalent Dosage (mg)**	**Rate of Onset after Oral Dose**	**Half-life (hr)***
Alprazolam	0.5	Intermediate	6-20
Chlordiazepoxide	10.0	Intermediate	30-100
Clonazepam	0.25	Intermediate	18-50
Clorazepate	7.5	Rapid	30-100
Diazepam	5.0	Rapid	30-100
Estazolam	2.0	Intermediate	10-24
Flurazepam	30.0	Rapid to intermediate	50-160
Halazepam	20.0	Intermediate to slow	30-100
Lorazepam	1.0	Intermediate	10-20
Midazolam	—	Intermediate	2-3
Oxazepam	15.0	Intermediate to slow	8-12
Prazepam	10.0	Slow	30-100
Quazepam	15.0	Rapid to intermediate	50-160
Temazepam	30.0	Intermediate	8-20
Triazolam	0.25	Intermediate	1.5-5.0

*The elimination half-life represents the total for all active metabolites; the elderly tend to have the longer half-lives in the range reported.

Timing. Timing is also critical when considering discontinuation, which should be initiated at a relatively unstressful time in the patient's life. For example, the physician should not consider discontinuation for a student when exams are scheduled. Similarly, it would be inappropriate to begin tapering medication for the executive when he has an important presentation pending or a critical business trip to make.

A number of different outcomes are observed when benzodiazepines are discontinued. The first and, obviously, most desirable result is that the patient remains asymptomatic following benzodiazepine discontinuation. Realistically, however, many patients experience transient withdrawal symptoms or rebound panic, both of which generally resolve within 1 to 3 weeks after complete discontinuation of the drug. Present studies suggest that the extent of relapse varies widely from patient to patient but that about 30% to 45% of patients with panic attacks remain well after discontinuation of their therapy.[115]

As mentioned earlier, patient education and reassurance are critical to successful discontinuation of these agents. If patients *know* to expect withdrawal symptoms during discontinuation, they are usually able to tolerate the symptoms. Studies show that at least some withdrawal symptoms occur in as many as 35% to 90% of patients discontinued from drugs such as alprazolam.[115,116] Given this outcome, the patient should be reassured that if symptoms occur, they are not life-threatening, are generally mild to moderate, and should resolve within a few days or weeks. Again, the patient should understand and agree that tapering will be accomplished slowly, with gradual decreases in dosage to minimize any return of symptoms.

Tapering. The time frame within which discontinuation of benzodiazepines is completed is probably the most important factor in the success of this process. When alprazolam is discontinued rapidly after 8 weeks of acute treatment, 35% of patients experienced rebound panic and withdrawal symptoms; rebound panic can be especially frightening to the patient, since it often occurs with more intensity than the original panic episode.

Unfortunately, much of the clinical data available on discontinuation of benzodiazepines reflects outcomes and symptoms following relatively rapid discontinuation of the drug.[27,30] However, there are some studies that compare rapid versus gradual discontinuation. In general, when benzodiazepines were discontinued abruptly, patients experienced more symptoms than when the drug was discontinued gradually. In one study, 44% of patients suffered recurrent anxiety after abruptly discontinuing compared to none of those in the gradually tapered group.[115] A preponderance of studies suggests that the incidence and severity of withdrawal symptoms can be greatly reduced by slower tapering schedules.[27] Specifically, most patients can discontinue benzodiazepines with few problems if the medication is tapered slowly over a 2 to 4 month period. Finally, discontinuation of benzodiazepine treatment should be discussed in detail with the patient at the beginning of treatment.[111] The patient should be reassured that severe withdrawal symptoms, or exacerbation of psychological symptoms will be managed as required. If the patient is educated about the potential outcomes associated with discontinuation and has adequate support from physician and pharmacist, withdrawal is accomplished with little problem.[65,110]

ANTICONVULSANTS

No definitive rules can be established regarding the discontinuation of anticonvulsant therapy. While some patients have prolonged or permanent remissions of their seizures, it is difficult to predict who will relapse. There are, however, some useful prognostic indicators in children. Slow withdrawal from medication may be considered in patients with idiopathic seizures who are seizure-free for two or more years. The same factors that predict recurrence after a single seizure suggest that the patient will have a relapse off medication. However, even with an electroencephalogram with elliptical activity, the patient may wish to try stopping treatment, so long as the seizure-free period is at least 2 years.[57,58,69]

Phenytoin: Optimal Use

Phenytoin (Dilantin®) is an anticonvulsant medication widely used in the treatment of generalized seizure disorders as well as other forms of epilepsy. It can be used as either ongoing therapy for patients with well established seizure disorders or as prophylaxis in individuals at risk for seizures following neurosurgery, head trauma, or stroke. When used properly, phenytoin is generally safe and highly efficacious but it has a number of properties that can make clinical use complicated.[145] Phenytoin metabolism is non-linear (not directly related to dose and serum concentration) within the therapeutic range. The enzyme system for phenytoin becomes saturated at relatively low plasma concentrations resulting in a progressive *decrease* in the rate of elimination as the dosage is increased. Therefore, after saturation of the enzyme system, a small increase in dosage leads to a large increase in serum phenytoin concentration. Another factor complicating phenytoin dosing is the large individual variation in the disposition of the drug in patients taking the same dosage, so that there can be as much as a fifty fold difference in plasma concentration among individuals taking the drug. Finally, phenytoin has significant interactions with numerous other commonly used medications and its disposition can be affected by variations in serum albumin levels.

Therapeutic Levels. In patients who suffer frequent, recurrent epileptic seizures, a definite reduction in the number of seizures, or the virtual elimination of convulsions, is a well-defined endpoint by which to measure the therapeutic efficacy of phenytoin. In those individuals who have infrequent seizures or are taking phenytoin on a prophylactic basis, the plasma phenytoin concentration is generally the most sensible surrogate marker for assessing a therapeutic response. Unfortunately, there is some uncertainty regarding the optimal plasma concentration for phenytoin. Longitudinal studies have demonstrated that improved seizure control can be achieved for patients with epilepsy when plasma phenytoin concentration exceeds 40 μmol/l. Most of the subjects in these trials had relatively severe seizure disorders, and other studies have suggested that seizure control may be achieved with lower plasma phenytoin concentrations. The overall consensus, however, is that optimal seizure control can be accomplished without toxicity when phenytoin plasma concentration is in the range of 40-80 μmol/l (10-20 μg/ml; 1 μmol/l = 0.25 μg/ml).

The risk for toxicity increases dramatically above 80 μmol/l and is nearly universal above 100 μmol/l. The earliest sign of phenytoin toxicity is usually nystagmus (often seen at levels of 80-120 μmol/l), followed by ataxia (120-160 μmol/l) and mental status changes (>160 μmol/l). Toxicity can develop very insidiously, however, and signs and symptoms may be difficult to distinguish from other neurological diseases, especially in those with underlying neurological disorders or pre-existing cerebellar dysfunction. There is less correlation between plasma concentration and some potential long-term adverse effects of phenytoin. These effects include gingival hyperplasia, acne, hirsutism, coarsening of facial features, folate deficiency and vitamin D deficiency. These manifestations are probably related to the duration of therapy as well as plasma phenytoin concentration.

All methods used to measure phenytoin plasma concentration reflect total concentration, which includes both protein-bound and unbound phenytoin components. In patients with chronic renal or hepatic disease, those in the last trimester of pregnancy, neonates, and individuals taking drugs such as sodium valproate, plasma protein binding can be reduced so that the total phenytoin concentration may greatly underestimate the concentration of unbound, pharmacologically active medication. It is important to recognize these situations, although it is usually not possible to directly estimate the degree of impairment of binding of phenytoin to plasma proteins. Since about 10% of phenytoin is usually unbound in the plasma and the therapeutic range for phenytoin concentration is considered 40-80 μmol/l, a therapeutic range for free (unbound) phenytoin concentration of 4-9 μmol/l has been suggested.

Drug Interactions. A host of commonly used medications interact with phenytoin and may affect its metabolism. They include: Cimetidine (Tagamet®), amiodarone (Cordarone®), allopurinol (Zyloprim®), chlorpromazine (Thorazine®), imipramine (Tofranil®), isoniazid, metronidazole (Flagyl®), omeprazole (Prilosec®), thioridazine (Mellaril®), and sulfonamides. These medications inhibit phenytoin metabolism and may cause an increase in plasma concentration and heightened risk of toxicity. Sodium valproate inhibits phenytoin metabolism but also displaces phenytoin from protein binding sites. These effects counteract each other, making it difficult to predict and interpret phenytoin concentrations in patients also taking valproate. Acute hepatitis also impairs the liver's ability to metabolize phenytoin, which also can increase the risk for toxicity.

Carbamazepine (Tegretol®) and rifampin stimulate hepatic metabolism of phenytoin, which reduces phenytoin concentration and increases the potential for breakthrough seizures. Folic acid also increases phenytoin clearance by an unknown mechanism, thereby lowering plasma concentration. At the same time, long-term treatment with phenytoin can result in folate deficiency, which when treated with folic acid could lower plasma phenytoin concentration and lead to breakthrough seizures.

Monitoring. Phenytoin is an intergral medication for treatment of seizure disorders and for prophylaxis of seizures in patients following neurosurgery, head trauma, and stroke. Clinicians need to be familiar with its unusual pharmacokinetic properties in order to insure its safe and effective use and to interpret and utilize measurements of plasma concentrations appropriately. Plasma concentration should not be checked unless a steady state of concentration has been reached. Generally speaking, this does not occur until three to four weeks after the initiation of treatment. An exception to this principle is if the plasma concentration is being checked because of suspected toxicity, in which case a steady state concentration is unnecessary. Clinical judgement must always be used in conjunction with plasma concentrations. If seizure control is adequate, dosage adjustment is often not necessary, even if the plasma concentration is below the "therapeutic" range. Similarly, if suspicion of phenytoin toxicity is present, reduction of the dosage is appropriate even if the plasma level is below the "toxic" range.

Once a steady state concentration has been achieved, the timing of blood samples to check plasma concentration is unimportant since phenytoin has a rather long half-life and diurnal variation is small even with once daily dosing. Some general guidelines for phenytoin dosage adjustment to achieve desirable levels are as follows: (1) if the plasma concentration is below 20 μmol/l, increase daily dose by 100 mg; (2) if plasma concentration is 20-60 μmol/l, daily dose should be increased by no more than 50 mg; (3) if plasma concentration is above 60 μmol/l, increase daily dose by 25 mg. Finally, clinicians should recognize that many common medications affect phenytoin metabolism and can alter plasma concentration. Moreover, clinical situations also may affect serum protein levels and, therefore, potentially raise the level of unbound plasma phenytoin.

Seizure Management

Nearly 10% of patients who live to 80 years of age will experience a seizure at some point in their life. Most of these patients can be appropriately managed by primary care physicians. It is essential, therefore, for clinicians to be familiar with current concepts in the classification, diagnosis and treatment of seizure disorders.

Seizures can occur secondary to acute processes such as meningitis or hypoxia, but in many instances, normal individuals have a single seizure for which no cause is found. If these idiopathic seizures recur, the patient is said to have epilepsy. Seizures can be partial (originating from a single focus) or generalized at their onset. Examples of partial seizures include simple partial seizures, in which focal motor activity occurs without loss of consciousness, and complex partial (temporal lobe) seizures, in which the patient may act out automatisms but is actually unconscious. Generalized seizures most often encountered in general practice are tonic-clonic (grand mal) and absence (petit mal) seizures. It can often be difficult to clinically distinguish partial seizures which secondarily generalize from true generalized seizures.

The diagnosis of a seizure disorder is made on clinical grounds. Electroencephalography (EEG) is most useful when it is obtained during an event. The interpretation of an interictal EEG is much more difficult because only 30-50% of seizure patients have an abnormal EEG at any given time. Furthermore, a small percent of healthy individuals have EEG findings consistent with epilepsy yet never experience a seizure. Interictal EEG is more sensitive when it is performed repeatedly, or when the patient is either sleep-deprived or sleeping during the study. Magnetic resonance imaging (MRI) is also useful in the evaluation of a patient with a seizure disorder. MRI is more sensitive than CT in identifying lesions related to epilepsy, especially if coronal views are obtained. Several medications including ciprofloxacin, theophylline and tricyclic antidepressants can cause generalized seizures (especially in overdose). More commonly, seizures occur secondary to withdrawal from alcohol or sedative medications such as benzodiazepines (e.g. alprazolam-Xanax®).

Evaluation of the patient with a first seizure should focus on ruling out acute etiologies including hypoglycemia, hypoxia, electrolyte abnormalities, alcohol or medication withdrawal and liver or kidney dysfunction. In selected patients, a urine drug screen can be useful. Lumbar puncture need not be performed unless there is clinical evidence of meningitis or encephalitis. A CT scan or MRI should be performed in virtually all patients greater than 18 years of age, and in younger patients with partial seizures or other evidence of a focal neurologic process. Radiologic studies need not be obtained immediately unless the patient is obtunded, or has suffered an acute brain injury, such as a stroke or subdural hematoma. Hospitalization is not required after a first seizure if the patient is alert during a period of observation, and there is a friend or family member who can drive the patient home and stay with them for at least 24 hours. Specific plans for follow-up are essential if such an approach is taken. It is not necessary to begin anti-epileptic drug treatment after a first seizure unless recurrent seizures are highly likely (as in patients with acute brain injury, or a strong family history of epilepsy).

Drug Therapy. Treatment after a single seizure is controversial. The 12 month recurrence rate of an untreated seizure is 16-62%, and this rate is increased if the patient has a focal brain injury, a positive interictal EEG, or a family history of epilepsy. The recurrence rate in treated patients is 25-41%, and 30% of patients will experience side effects severe enough to warrant discontinuation of the medication. There is no evidence that early initiation of drug therapy improves the natural history of epilepsy. Monotherapy achieves adequate seizure control with tolerable side effects in roughly 50% of patients. Of those who fail, 60% will respond to another single agent. Only a small minority of patients will experience improved control on combination therapy. Dosage should be based on clinical control of seizures and the occurrence of side effects. Some patients will require drug concentrations above the therapeutic range for control, and others will experience toxic effects when drug concentration is in the "therapeutic range." Drug levels are most useful in confirming compliance, evaluating symptoms that might be drug induced, and managing patients who are pregnant or have liver or renal dysfunction.

In adults, most seizures which clinically appear to be generalized are actually partial seizures with secondary generalization. The presence of an aura or focal event at the onset of a generalized seizure suggests the diagnosis of partial seizure with secondary generalization, but an EEG may be necessary to make this distinction. Carbamazepine (Tegretol®) and phenytoin (Dilantin®) are the agents of first choice for partial seizures, whether or not they become secondarily generalized. Carbamazepine is preferable in young women who will wish to avoid facial coarsening and hirsutism (as well as the teratogenic effects) associated with phenytoin. Valproate (Depakene®) is the most effective agent for true generalized seizures. Starting these medications at low doses and gradually increasing them often minimizes side effects. If the initial agent is not effective, another single agent should be tried since combination therapy is rarely superior to properly chosen monotherapy.

If seizures continue to recur after 3 months of treatment, or if there is an associated, progressive neurologic syndrome, a neurologic consultation is advisable. All patients with refractory seizures should undergo MRI scanning, since some epileptic foci can be surgically resected. Refractory symptoms should also prompt the physician to reconsider the diagnosis, since other disorders including pseudoseizure, migraine, narcolepsy, vasovagal attack, arrhythmia, panic disorder and hyperventilation can mimic seizures.

H₂ Receptor Antagonists

H₂ blockers are the most popular drugs for the treatment of peptic ulcer disease. All four of the currently approved agents—cimetidine, ranitidine, famotidine, and nizatidine—are effective, easily taken, and generally well-tolerated (see Table 4-4). These agents competitively block the histamine H_2 receptor of the acid-producing parietal cells, and thus render the cells less responsive, not only to histamine stimulation but also to the stimulation of acetylcholine and gastrin because of postreceptor interactions. The efficacy of these medications is about equal, and there is little to recommend one H_2 blocker over another, although there are some differences in cost, and cimetidine is more likely to produce drug interactions due to its ability to inhibit the P-450 cytochrome oxidase system.[117,118] All of them can occasionally produce central nervous system symptoms, such as headache and mental confusion. When used long-term and in high doses, as in the treatment of hypersecretory states, cimetidine sometimes causes reversible gynecomastia and impotence. However, omeprazole, rather than an H_2 blocker, is probably the drug of choice today in the treatment of the Zollinger-Ellison syndrome. As mentioned, cimetidine, and to a much lesser extent, ranitidine, bind to hepatic cytochrome P-450 microsomal enzymes and may inhibit the catabolism of many drugs metabolized by this system. This interaction, however, is not usually significant clinically, except in older patients on polypharmacy who are taking drugs that have narrow therapeutic-to-toxic ratios, most notable among them, theophylline, phenytoin, and warfarin. Despite the infrequency of serious adverse drug reactions, levels of theophylline and phenytoin and prothrombin times should be monitored more carefully if cimetidine is used in conjunction with these drugs. On the other hand, another H_2 blocker such as famotidine can be used instead and, therefore, reduce the drug-monitoring costs associated with long-term cimetidine therapy.

Table 4-4

Dosage Schedule for H_2-Receptor Antagonists			
Indication	**Cimetidine**	**Ranitidine***	**Famotidine**
ACUTE OR RECURRENT PEPTIC DISEASE	400 mg po, bid or 800 mg po, hs	150 mg bid or 300 mg po, hs	20 mg po, bid or 40 mg po, hs
SEVERELY ILL PATIENTS	37.5 mg/hr IV (continuous infusion)	6-12 mg/hr IV (continuous infusion)	1.7 mg/hr IV (continuous infusion)
PROPHYLAXIS FOR RECURRENT ULCER	400 mg po, hs	150 mg po, hs	20 mg p.o., hs

*Oral dosage for nizatidine is identical to that for ranitidine; an intravenous preparation of nizatidine is not available.

Lifestyle Modification. A number of general therapeutic measures, including lifestyle modifications, dietary alterations, and psychotherapeutic interventions, are recommended in order to reduce the need for long-term maintenance therapy with H_2 blockers. Patients are encouraged to get adequate rest, relaxation, and sleep. The precise role that emotional factors such as anxiety, anger, frustration, and resentment play in the pathogenesis of peptic ulcer disease is hotly debated. In years past, they were widely thought to play a significant role, especially in duodenal ulcer disease, but in recent years their importance has been questioned. At any rate, anxiety and anger should probably be ameliorated as much as possible by simple means, such as by making patients aware of their feelings, encouraging them to vent their problems, manipulating their environments, encouraging participation in regular physical activity, and, when indicated, administering sedatives and tranquilizers. Ulcerogenic drugs, such as aspirin and NSAIDs, should be avoided or, if absolutely required, at least taken in smaller doses. Smoking and alcohol ingestion should also be minimized or completely eliminated if possible.

The role of diet in the treatment of peptic ulcer disease has been reevaluated in recent years. The traditional, restrictive bland diets, eaten in frequent, small meals, are unnecessary and may even be harmful. Patients should eat three regular meals a day while avoiding any foods noted to cause symptoms. Caffeine-containing beverages such as coffee, tea, and colas may also be restricted, although their effects are probably of little significance. Once recommended, frequent meals, and protein in particular, were meant to buffer the acid in the stomach. Unfortunately, these frequent meals also stimulated acid secretion for several hours, while providing satisfactory buffering of the gastric acid for only the first hour. Moreover, the traditional bedtime snack, which was recommended before the advent of H_2 blockers that could control nocturnal acid secretion, was especially harmful because it stimulated acid secretion for several hours, while the patient was asleep, and was unable to take antacids. The traditional bland diets are not only distasteful to patients, but also contain a lot of the milk sugar lactose, which causes abdominal cramps, gas, and even diarrhea in many patients with some degree of lactose intolerance. Bland diets also tend to be high in calories, and because of their high fat content, are possibly atherogenic.

Maintenance Therapy. Therapy of uncomplicated duodenal ulcer disease requires treatment with H_2 blockers. High-dose therapy for a period of 6 to 8 weeks usually results in ulcer healing. The indications for maintaining suppression of ulcer recurrence with chronic therapy using H_2 blockers remains controversial.[43,55,119] However, the preponderance of clinical trials strongly suggests that continued use of an H_2 receptor blocker (or any other ulcer-healing drug) at approximately *half* of the ulcer-healing dose is usually effective for prevention of ulcer recurrence. The mean recurrence rate for duodenal ulcer during maintenance therapy and placebo therapy is dramatically different. Only about 25% of patients taking continuous H_2 receptor blocker therapy experience ulcer recurrence, in contrast to approximately 75% of those patients receiving placebo. Thus, the overwhelming evidence shows that fewer duodenal ulcers recur during sustained maintenance therapy with an H_2 receptor blocker or with sucralfate than with placebo therapy. All of the H_2 receptor blockers appear equally effective in this regard.

Exactly how *long* maintenance therapy should be continued is uncertain.[55] The results of most studies show a consistently high relapse rate if maintenance drug treatment is withdrawn during the first year. Accordingly, maintenance therapy is approved and recommended for 12 months. However, it is also clear that once such maintenance treatment is discontinued, the same high rate of ulcer relapse is observed. This does *not* mean that therapy with H_2 blockers should be continued indefinitely. However, continuation of treatment beyond 1 year is effective in preventing both ulcer relapse and the development of ulcer complications such as hemorrhage and perforation. Accordingly, there is justification for continuing drug therapy, but only in patients who remain at high risk for ulcer recurrence, and in those with a medical condition that might be compromised by ulcer recurrence or complications. Certainly, patients who experience significant bleeding as a complication of their previous ulcers are at high risk for recurrent bleeding in the future, and, therefore, are reasonable candidates for indefinite maintenance therapy. Emerging evidence suggests that this specific patient group should be considered for prolonged maintenance therapy, even if other risk factors can be corrected.[43,55,119]

Exactly which schedule for maintenance therapy with H_2 blockers is best also remains uncertain. Physicians and pharmacists recognize that after ulcers heal, many patients follow a self-guided approach to care, even without our prescribing it. Many experts conclude that symptomatic self-care is an appropriate ulcer maintenance regimen for patients with healed, uncomplicated duodenal ulcer. However, self-care is not recommended for the following groups: elderly patients in whom ulcer relapse might present great risk; patients with serious concomitant illnesses; those with previous ulcer bleeding, with previous perforation, or frequent ulcer relapses (more than twice yearly); and those with ulcers that take a prolonged time to heal. Clearly, the approach to self-care with H_2 blocker maintenance therapy requires additional evaluation.

Cost Effectiveness. Although drug treatment trials adequately document the effectiveness of maintenance therapy in reducing ulcer recurrence and preventing complications, an important question is whether such treatment is also cost effective, especially in view of the high cost for many of these drugs. In making these determinations, it is important to remember that the overall costs related to ulcer disease include a number of different components. The direct costs that get early attention include medication acquisition costs, charges for physician visits, medical testing, expenses incurred by hospitalization, and treatment of complications associated with ulcer disease. However, in addition, there are also important indirect costs that must be considered. While not a complete list, these would include loss of work productivity, absenteeism from work, and overall quality-of-life issues.

A number of investigations in the last few years have specifically addressed the cost-benefit aspects of maintenance ulcer therapy. One such trial, evaluating short-term treatment with famotidine (6 months) concluded that the estimated direct cost for the care of the average ulcer patient prescribed maintenance therapy with famotidine was approximately 30% less than the cost would be if the patient received no maintenance H_2 antagonist therapy. In this study, most of the cost savings resulted from a reduction in risks for hospitalization and surgery. A number of other trials also support the cost-efficacy of maintenance therapy with H_2 blockers to prevent ulcer recurrence and emphasize that the added cost of the drug itself is more than offset by a reduction in other direct cost items such as repeated laboratory and endoscopic testing, and hospitalizations to treat complications of recurrent ulcer disease. In addition, the more difficult to measure quality-of-life issues are significantly improved with maintenance therapy. Therefore, it is reasonable to provide maintenance therapy for at least 6 to 12 months in all patients with documented peptic ulcer disease.

Guidelines. The goals for treating patients with ulcer disease are to relieve symptoms, heal the acute ulcer, reduce the risk of ulcer recurrence and complications, and decrease the economic impact of this chronic disease while maintaining the patient's quality of life. Assuming that a diagnosis of peptic ulcer is firmly established, an adequate period of drug treatment with H_2 blockers is indicated. If the patient is young and generally healthy, with an uncomplicated ulcer and few risk factors favoring relapse, the patient can be given a prescription for 3 to 6 months of medication, told to take full therapy for any recurrent symptoms, and to continue the treatment until symptoms are relieved. Failure of this treatment to relieve symptoms after 2 to 3 weeks, the onset of alarming symptoms such as intense pain, vomiting, or melena—or possibly, the exhaustion of the 6 month supply of medication with continued symptoms—should lead to reevaluation.

On the other hand, if the patient has had a complicated course of ulcer disease, such as bleeding, or has a significant number of risk factors—smoking, aspirin or NSAID use, etc.—that would make early ulcer relapse highly likely, it is most prudent to institute *continuous* maintenance therapy while working to reduce or eliminate the adverse risk factors. Any relapse of symptomatic ulcer disease during noncontinuous maintenance therapy should indicate the need for a return to a continuous-dosing regimen.

For ulcer disease that relapses during full-dose maintenance therapy, the clinician should consider permanent reduction of acid secretion by surgery or, more appropriately, search for gastric mucosal infection by *Helicobacter pylori*. In light of recent studies that show dramatic reductions in ulcer recurrence following successful eradication of *H. pylori*, it is clinically safe to consider treatment for this organism prior to more invasive procedures.[71] Early empiric treatment directed at *H. pylori* is also appropriate in patients with ulcer disease. While most of these recommendations are applicable primarily to duodenal ulcer disease, management of recurrent gastric ulcer is similar, once malignancy is excluded, in that risk factors for recurrence should be considered and corrected when possible. For gastric ulcer, these factors are use of NSAID and heavy cigarette smoking. Recurrent ulcerations should be treated by full-dose therapy, and then maintenance therapy instituted with continuous full-dose treatment. Duration of maintenance therapy is less well defined for gastric ulcer, but can be effective for years.

Recommendations for chronic maintenance therapy with H_2 blockers apply only to patients who have ulcer disease documented radiographically or endoscopically. Those patients who are taking long-term H_2 blocker therapy for symptomatic relief of gastrointestinal complaints, but who do not have documentation of peptic ulcer disease, can probably have H_2 blockers discontinued from their drug regimen. Unfortunately, encouraging patients to discontinue therapy with H_2 blockers may be difficult because many of these patients depend on this drug for symptomatic relief, either real or perceived. This is especially true when underlying symptoms are caused by gastroesophageal reflux (GERD).

Helicobacter Pylori

Helicobacter pylori is a curved gram-negative bacteria which was isolated and identified approximately a decade ago. It is uniquely adapted to survive in the hostile environment of the human stomach (or any area where gastric epithelium is found including metaplastic tissue in the esophagus, duodenum or Meckel's diverticulum) by invading the mucous layer and neutralizing the surrounding acid with a powerful urease enzyme. The organism was originally called *Campylobacter pylori* but was renamed in 1989 as part of the new genus *Helicobacter*. In retrospect, the organism was detected in animals during the 1800s and in humans in the early part of this century but because of misconceptions and faulty reasoning, it was ignored until interest was resurrected in the early 1980s by an Australian medical resident named Marshall. He proved that *H. pylori* can cause acute gastritis when he deliberately ingested an inoculum and subsequently subjected himself to repeated gastric endoscopies. There now is little dispute over *H. pylori's* role as the cause of chronic active gastritis. It is also integral to the pathogenesis of peptic ulcer disease and is epidemiologically linked to gastric cancer and lymphoma.

Transmission of *H. pylori* appears to occur via human-to-human spread since no environmental reservoir has been identified. Isolation of the organism in the stool implies that fecal-oral transmission is the likely route of infection. The exact mechanisms by which *H. pylori* produces the inflammatory and cellular destructive changes that accompany its infection remain unclear. The prevalence of infection in the United States is linked to lower socioeconomic class. An increased prevalence rate (up to 80%) is also found in family members of an affected patient. It appears that *H. pylori* is the predominant cause of type B antral, or environmental (as opposed to type A, or autoimmune) gastritis. This is based on several lines of evidence including a prevalence of the organism that approaches 100% in patients with type B antral gastritis and a decreased prevalence in those individuals with a specific gastritis precipitated by alcohol or nonsteroidal anti-inflammatory drugs (NSAIDs). Furthermore, the development of active gastritis in patients in volunteer ingestion studies as well as an epidemic of gastritis from accidental inoculation during the course of a study of acid secretory disorders, provide additional evidence. Finally, healing of gastritis upon treatment that eradicates *H. pylori* is the last parameter to fulfill Koch's postulates.

Disease Spectrum. Chronic active gastritis and associated infection with *H. pylori* are common, although infection is not necessarily associated with symptoms. There is conflicting evidence on whether nonulcer dyspepsia is associated with gastritis or *H. pylori* infection, but the balance of information does not support a relationship between the organism and dyspeptic symptoms. However, there has been tremendous interest in the link between *H. pylori* infection and duodenal ulcer. In the past it has been felt that the development of duodenal ulcer results from an imbalance between mucosal defensive factors and aggressive factors that insult the mucosa (acid and pepsin). It is now clear that *H. pylori* should also be considered an aggressive factor based upon several lines of evidence. There is the nearly uniform (>90%) finding of the organism, along with antral gastritis, in patients with duodenal ulcer. There are markedly reduced relapse rates of ulcer in patients in whom the organism is eradicated (0-25% relapse) compared to patients treated with conventional anti-secretory therapy alone (relapse of 70-90%).

One trial involved patients presenting at a Veterans Affairs Medical Center with dyspepsia or gastrointestinal hemorrhage who were endoscopically proven to have duodenal ulcers and were invited to participate in a randomized controlled trial to determine whether antibiotic therapy accelerates ulcer healing. All 105 patients who entered the study received ranitidine (Zantac) 300 mg each evening, with or without 2 weeks of "triple therapy" (a regimen with known activity against *H. pylori*). Healing was more rapid in patients receiving triple therapy and only two patients receiving triple therapy suffered persistent infection, whereas all patients treated with ranitidine alone remained positive for *H. pylori*. Although not as well studied as duodenal ulcer, there also is strong evidence for a causative role for *H. pylori* in gastric ulcer. Nearly 100% of patients with ulcers unrelated to NSAIDs have evidence of infection, and there are lower relapse rates in individuals in whom the organism is eradicated. An association between the organism and gastric malignancies is being actively studied.

Diagnosis. The diagnosis of *H. pylori* infection can be made by a variety of noninvasive and invasive tests some of which make use of the organism possessing a potent urease enzyme. Examples include the carbon 13 and carbon 14 urea breath tests which are simple, inexpensive and have sensitivity and specificity between 90 to 95% but will not be commercially available until sometime in the future. Other means to detect the organism include assaying a specimen obtained by biopsy at endoscopy for urease activity (e.g., Clo® test) or histological examination or culture of a mucosal biopsy specimen. Serologic tests are available but do not differentiate between active versus remote infection.

It is now appropriate to detect and eradicate *H. pylori* in patients with peptic ulcer since the natural history of the disease is then markedly improved. The goal of treatment of *H. pylori* infection should be the eradication of the organism since this has been associated with very low rates of recurrence of ulcer (<10% per year). Although less well documented, sumilar low recurrences are likely with eradication of the organism in patients with gastric ulcer. Patients who undergo upper gastrointestinal endoscopy can be tested for *H. pylori* by submitting a biopsy for culture or for an assay of bacterial urease activity (e.g., the CLO® test). In the near future, simple non-invasive tests for *H. pylori* such as ^{13}C-urea breath testing should become more widely available, allowing clinicians to definitively and easily diagnose *H. pylori* infection and facilitate the use of antibiotic therapy. In patients in whom endoscopy is not performed, empiric antibiotic therapy directed at *H. pylori* is not unreasonable, although to date this has been reserved primarily for patients with recurrent disease. There is no indication to treat patients who have *H. pylori* and nonulcer dyspepsia or gastritis because eradication does not reliably affect their symptoms.

Drug Therapy. When antibiotics are used, they should be added to conventional ulcer therapy directed against acid secretion. The most common antibiotic regimen employed is so called "triple therapy": bismuth subsalicylate, 1-2 tablets at each meal and 2 tablets at bedtime, tetracycline, 500 mg 4 times a day and metronidazole, 250 mg 3 times a day, during the first 2 weeks of therapy. The additional cost incurred by "triple therapy" is modest and in view of its marked reduction of ulcer recurrence, it is actually less expensive in the long run. It may, however, be difficult for some patients to comply with such a complicated regimen, and noncompliance appears to be the most common cause for failure to eradicate infection. Newer, simpler regimens using omeprazole and amoxicillin or clarithromycin are easier to use but eradication rates are somewhat less (60-80%).

Proton-Blockers

Omeprazole. Omeprazole inhibits the gastrin/proton pump, which regulates the final pathway for acid secretion. This drug is especially effective for patients with gastroesophageal reflux disease, who have not responded to traditional high-dose therapy with H_2 receptor antagonists and antacids.[120,121] Omeprazole is considerably more expensive than H_2 blockers; therefore, indications for its appropriate use in patients with gastroesophageal reflux disease need to be clarified. Candidates for omeprazole therapy include patients who have severe daytime symptoms, recurrent strictures requiring frequent dilations, or large esophageal ulcerations despite full-dose H_2 blocker therapy. As might be expected, omeprazole yields excellent results; after 4 weeks of treatment, 80% of patients with severe disease heal, and over 90% of patients are free of disease at 8 to 12 weeks. Cessation of the drug prompts recurrences in over 80% of patients by 6 months, and even 40% of patients relapse after switching to full-dose H_2 antagonist therapy for maintenance.[121]

An acceptable treatment strategy might be to cycle omeprazole treatment for 4 to 8 weeks, followed by an H_2 blocker every 2 to 4 months, while monitoring the serum gastrin level. The safety of long-term omeprazole therapy is not proven, although a recent study suggests that maintenance therapy with this agent does not predispose patients to adverse side effects or to the development of tumors. Further investigations are required to confirm long-term safety of this medication.[121] In general, it is not appropriate to initiate therapy with omeprazole until more conservative therapy with full-dose H_2 blockers is attempted. Patients who are presently taking omeprazole and have not been treated with H_2 blocker maintenance therapy are appropriate candidates for discontinuation of omeprazole and substitution with H_2 blockers. It should be stressed that the relapse rate after healing is high when medication is stopped or if a lower dose of H_2 blocker is tried as maintenance therapy.

When discontinuing omeprazole treatment, a full dose of an H_2 blocker (cimetidine, 800 mg per day; ranitidine, 300 mg per day; famotidine, 40 mg per day) is usually necessary on a continuous basis to control symptoms in most patients with gastroesophageal reflux disease.[122] Medication for primarily nocturnal symptoms can be initiated using the full dose administered only at night, preferably with the evening meal. Those with daytime reflux should have their medication divided into 12-hour portions. Ranitidine and famotidine are claimed by some to be marginally more effective than cimetidine. A higher dose of ranitidine, 300 mg every 12 hours, inhibits acid production almost to the same level as omeprazole, but a comparable healing rate is not proven. In general, the decision to maintain patients on H_2 blockers versus continuation of long-term therapy with omeprazole is based on the patient's clinical response, ability to comply with a more expensive medication, and future studies demonstrating the safety of long-term omeprazole therapy.[122-124]

Nonsteroidal Anti-inflammatory Drugs (NSAIDs)

Nonsteroidal anti-inflammatory drugs (NSAIDs) (see Tables 4-5 and 4-6) are potent precipitants of gastrointestinal upset. These adverse effects can range from minor gastric irritation to frank peptic ulceration and bleeding. The most serious of these effects result from NSAID-mediated inhibition of gastric prostaglandin synthesis, which is necessary for maintenance of gastric mucosal integrity. Although NSAIDs clearly can provide symptomatic relief for patients with chronic, inflammatory osteoarthritic disorders, there is also evidence to suggest that these drugs are over-used,[63] especially in light of their potentially serious, and sometimes life-threatening side effects.

There are many opportunities to discontinue NSAID therapy, and patient selection is of paramount importance.[12,118,125] Each year, more than 60 million prescriptions are written for NSAIDs, and more than 15 million patients are presently receiving long-term therapy. It is estimated that approximately 20% of patients receiving long-term NSAID therapy have some degree of gastric ulceration, with nearly one-half of these individuals having erosions verified by endoscopy. However, most of these upper gastrointestinal lesions remain clinically silent. The Food and Drug Administration estimates that each year, 2% to 4% of patients receiving long-term NSAID therapy are at risk of developing serious gastrointestinal complications.[126,127] These data translate into at least 300,000 to 600,000 cases of complicated ulcer disease annually in the United States occurring secondary to the use of NSAIDs.[128]

Reducing Toxicity. However, there are important guidelines for reducing the gastrointestinal toxicity associated with NSAIDs.[12,125] First, the risk of having a gastrointestinal hemorrhage is greatest during the first *6 months* of therapy. Consequently, physicians and pharmacists with patients taking NSAID therapy should be especially vigilant during the early stages of therapy. Second, the risk of having gastrointestinal complications from NSAIDs is related to the *dose* of the medication. Consequently, it is prudent to begin NSAID therapy at a dose less than that recommended by the package insert, and to titrate the medication according to symptomatic response in the patient. In general, the initial dose should be approximately 50% of the average recommended dose in the package insert. The dose should be increased only if symptomatic improvement is not reported by the patient.

Some experts recommend that NSAIDs be discontinued once gastrointestinal symptoms occur. Unfortunately, most patients with NSAID-induced ulceration do not have symptoms of ulcer disease prior to a catastrophic gastrointestinal event. In many cases, the first evidence of ulceration is manifested by bleeding or perforation. Therefore, waiting for symptoms to occur and then intervening with drug discontinuation will probably not have a significant impact on either complication rates or morbidity.

Table 4-5

| Side Effects of Nonsteroidal Anti-inflammatory Drugs* ||
System	Symptoms or Findings
Gastrointestinal	
	Anorexia, nausea, vomiting, dyspepsia, erosive gastritis, peptic ulcer Constipation Diarrhea† Hepatotoxicity
Hematologic	
	Impaired platelet aggregation and prolonged bleeding time Bleeding, especially in association with anticoagulants or clotting-factor deficiencies
Renal	
	Aggravation of renal failure during circulatory stress (e.g., congestive heart failure, nephrotic syndrome) Precipitation of renal failure in volume depleted, high risk patients Fluid retention and aggravation of congestive heart failure Hyperkalemia
Central nervous system	
	Headaches, dizziness, tinnitus, deafness, drowsiness, confusion, nervousness, profuse sweating Toxic amblyopia
Pulmonary	
	Aggravation of asthma and rhinosinusitis in patients with aspirin hypersensitivity
Obstetric	
	Delayed parturition Postpartum and neonatal bleeding Premature closure of the ductus arteriosus
Dermatologic	
	Allergic skin rashes

*Bone marrow toxicity as well as granulocytosis and aplastic anemia occur rarely. The best established example of bone marrow toxicity is that which occurs with phenylbutazone and oxyphenbutazone. Salicylates other than aspirin lack the gastric and antiplatelet side effects seen with aspirin and other nonsteroidal antiinflammatory drugs.
†Diarrhea is most frequently seen with meclofenamate (approximately 15% of patients).

Table 4-6

Nonsteroidal Anti-inflammatory Drugs Useful in Osteoarthritis and Other Rheumatic Diseases		
Generic Name	**Trade Name**	**Usual Dosage***
Aspirin (plain, buffered, or enteric coated) **Salicylates** (eg, sodium, choline, or salicyl-salicylate	(many)	2.4 to 6.0 g daily in four divided doses†
Diclofenac	Voltaren, Cefaflan	50 mg bid or tid or 75 mg bid
Diflunisal	Dolobid	500 mg bid
Etodolac	Lodine	600-1200 mg in divided doses
Fenoprofen	Nalfon	300-600 mg qid
Flurbiprofen	Ansaid	200-300 mg in divided doses bid, tid, or qid
Ibuprofen	Advil, Motrin, Nuprin, Rufen, others	200-800 mg qid
Indomethacin	Indocin	25 mg tid or qid 75 mg bid (slow-release preparation)
Ketoprofen	Orudis, Oruvail	50 mg qid or 75 mg tid
Meclofenamate	Meclomen	50-100 mg qid
Mefenamic acid	Ponstell	250 mg qid
Naproxen	Naprosyn, Anaprox, Aleve	250-500 mg bid
Nabumetone	Relafen	1000-2000 mg once or twice a day
Oxaprozin	Daypro	1200 mg once a day or 1800 mg in divided doses
Piroxicam	Feldene	10 or 20 mg once daily
Sulindac	Clinoril	150-200 mg bid
Tolmetin	Tolectin	200-400 mg qid

*Dosages recommended are for long-term therapy (longer than one week). Higher dosages of some of these drugs may be used for short-term therapy (e.g., in acute gouty arthritis). Lower dosages should be used in elderly patients or patients with impairment of kidney or liver function.
†Blood salicylate levels of 20-30 mg/dl should be reached for optimal effect.

One of the most important questions that should be addressed is, should physicians be treating patients who have a chronic, painful disease with anti-inflammatory drugs known to have significant gastrointestinal toxicity? In fact, many experts now recommend that such patients be managed with analgesics such as acetaminophen that do not cause gastrointestinal side effects. One investigator studied the use of acetaminophen versus ibuprofen in patients with osteoarthritis. In this short-term trial, the use of acetaminophen alone was as effective as use of both drugs together, as well as lower doses of ibuprofen. Nevertheless, many clinicians who treat patients with osteoarthritis think that treatment with NSAIDs offers superior symptom relief compared with treatment with acetaminophen or narcotics, despite lack of published clinical trials supporting this concept. However, in patients with *noninflammatory* disease and chronic pain, there is no reason to think that NSAIDs have greater efficacy than acetaminophen or codeine in pain relief.

Prophylaxis. The next important issue is whether or not patients who are taking chronic NSAID therapy require prophylaxis with either prostaglandins, omeprazole, or H_2 blockers. All of these agents can either prevent or heal NSAID ulcerations to some degree, although the data on omeprazole are limited, and the data regarding H_2 blockers are contradictory. It should be emphasized, however, that agents such as misoprostol can cause significant diarrhea; they are expensive (nearly $100 a month for H_2 blockers and omeprazole), and none of the agents has been proven to prevent or decrease the catastrophic gastrointestinal complications associated with chronic NSAID use.

Should we treat patients with inflammatory arthritic conditions who are elderly, but who have no previous history of peptic ulcer disease, with H_2 blockers, omeprazole, or misoprostol to prevent complications associated with ulceration?[129,130] The answer is no, and therefore, in most cases these drugs can be discontinued. Until such time that data indicate that this therapy decreases complication rates and is cost effective, prophylactic therapy with an H_2 blocker is not recommended.[130] In patients not responding to these agents, the lowest dose NSAID resulting in symptom control should be given, as gastropathy is dose-related. In contrast, patients with *previous* documented peptic or gastric ulcer disease and who absolutely require continued NSAID use for symptom control, prophylaxis is indicated. Misoprostol remains the agent with the most supportive data indicating a decreased ulceration rate, although it is likely that omeprazole is equally effective. However, the conflicting data with H_2 blockers makes recommending any H_2 blocker difficult in this clinical situation.[130]

Attempts to discontinue nonsteroidal therapy should be given high priority as part of a drug discontinuation program. As a first step, whenever possible, NSAIDs should be used at the lowest dose possible to achieve relief of symptoms. In addition, patients should be closely monitored. In patients with non-inflammatory conditions, a trial with acetaminophen may be warranted. Drugs such as misoprostol may be worth considering but only in high-risk patients (i.e., those with previous peptic ulceration) who might be willing to tolerate the diarrhea associated with full-dose misoprostol use in return for being able to take NSAIDs.[131] However, routinely prescribing misoprostol for ulcer prophylaxis in *all* patients taking NSAIDs chronically does not reduce the chances of serious complications or the frequency of adverse gastrointestinal symptoms.[132,133] In fact, there is a 33% chance that bothersome diarrhea may ensue.[134] Lower doses of misoprostol are less likely to cause diarrhea and may be less effective. The drug is not indicated for routine use in older patients who require NSAID use, unless they have a history of previous peptic ulceration. In summary, *routine* prophylactic use cannot be recommended, and those patients taking misoprostol merely for ulcer prevention deserve a trial of drug discontinuation.

Oral Anticoagulants

Hemorrhage is the most serious complication of oral anticoagulant drugs (see Table 4-7), occurring in up to 30% of patients who receive these agents. Hemorrhagic complications associated with warfarin use range in severity from minor to life-threatening. Although bleeding can occur at virtually any body site, the gastrointestinal system is most often affected.[135,136]

Despite the risks associated with oral anticoagulants, these agents are indicated in several forms of arterial and venous embolic diseases common in the elderly population. Furthermore, recent studies demonstrate the efficacy of oral anticoagulants in reducing the risk of embolic stroke in patients with chronic atrial fibrillation, which occurs in 2% to 9% of patients over 60 years of age.[98] Despite the effectiveness of oral anticoagulants in reducing morbidity and mortality, some physicians are reluctant to use these agents in older patients because the perceived risk of bleeding complications outweighs the perceived benefits these drugs offer. This concern is supported by trials suggesting that even though older persons take lower doses of anticoagulants, age may increase the risk of hemorrhagic complications.[136,137]

Oral anticoagulants produce therapeutic results at much lower doses than previously suspected. At the present time, an International Normalized Ratio (INR) of 2 to 3 is sufficient to provide adequate thromboembolic prophylaxis in most patients.[138] Some studies suggest an INR of 2.0 to 3.0 is optimal for atrial fibrillation. Unfortunately, the opportunities for discontinuing anticoagulant therapy are few. For example, patients who take anticoagulants for prevention of embolic disease associated with chronic atrial fibrillation require lifelong therapy.[139] In addition, patients who are taking these agents for prophylaxis of embolic disease after mechanical cardiac valve replacement or tissue valve in the neutral position also require long-term maintenance therapy, and the opportunities for discontinuation are virtually nil. On the other hand, patients who take oral anticoagulation therapy for the treatment of venous embolic disease or nonlife-threatening pulmonary embolism can frequently have the medication withdrawn after 3 months, assuming risk factors that originally caused venous embolism are corrected. (See section, Indications and Guidelines for Antithrombotic Therapy.)

Of the factors that influence the risk of serious bleeding from oral anticoagulation, drug interactions play an important role (see Table 4-7). Many agents, including some NSAIDs, alter warfarin metabolism or protein binding and may theoretically increase the risk of bleeding. But of the many potential interactions,

NSAIDs are of special interest because they are widely used by the elderly and substantially increase the risk of gastric erosions and ulceration.

Although it is frequently difficult to discontinue anticoagulant use, it is sometimes possible to eliminate medications from the drug regimen that are known to potentiate the risk of gastrointestinal hemorrhage. Combined use of NSAIDs and oral anticoagulants theoretically increases the risk of gastrointestinal hemorrhage in the elderly. Until recently, few studies supported the validity of this association. However, it is now clear that the concurrent use of NSAIDs and oral anticoagulants places elderly persons at extremely high risk of hemorrhagic peptic ulcer disease. Specifically, there is a nearly thirteen-fold increase in the risk of developing hemorrhagic peptic ulcer disease. This suggests that NSAIDs should be prescribed with extreme caution in patients undergoing anticoagulation therapy. Moreover, whenever it is possible to use medications other than NSAIDs to provide symptomatic relief, these agents are preferable to long-term NSAID therapy.[140]

Table 4-7

Warfarin antagonists and potentiators	
Antagonists	**Potentiators**
Barbiturates	Amiodarone
Carbamazepine	Anabolic steroids
Cholestyramine (when	Aspirin
administered with warfarin)	Chloramphenicol
Glutethimide	Cimetidine
Griseofulvin	Ciprofloxacin
Rifampin	Clofibrate
Vitamin K	Dextrothyroxine
	Disulfiram
	Erythromycin
	Fluconazole
	Hepatotoxins
	Metronidazole
	Miconazole
	Nalidixic Acid
	Norfloxacin
	Quinine
	Sulfinpyrazone
	Sulfonamides
	Tamoxifen
	Third-generation cephalosporins

Inhaled Beta Agonists

Numerous reports over the past several years suggested that regular use, and especially overuse, of inhaled beta agonists may lead to increased morbidity and mortality in patients with asthma. In particular, chronic use of inhaled beta agonists was implicated in the rising mortality associated with asthma; several mechanisms were proposed to explain why long-term use of these agents may lead to more severe complications. First, paradoxical bronchoconstriction from beta agonist use is reported, although this is more likely due to the propellant used in the metered dose inhaler than to the medication itself. Beta agonists also stimulate airway secretions, which may cause further narrowing of the airways. By using beta agonists regularly, patients may unwittingly cause greater exposure to asthma precipitants, which can exacerbate the disease. Whatever the mechanism, several well-publicized studies show that patients who use inhaled beta agonists regularly have accelerated decline in ventilatory function and higher asthma-related mortality than those who use the medication only *as needed* for exacerbations. Clearly, cautious use is warranted.

Although the opportunities for complete cessation of beta agonist therapy may be limited, patients should be instructed to use their inhalers primarily for acute symptomatic relief associated with exacerbations of asthma or prophylaxis of exercise-induced asthma. Whenever possible, encouraging patients to discontinue *chronic* maintenance use with these agents is a prudent course, based on recent studies. It is important to emphasize that asthma is fundamentally an inflammatory disease of the airways that can be triggered by numerous stimuli, including inhaled allergens, respiratory infections, exercise, cold, and other physical factors. Beta agonists can help alleviate the bronchospasm that results from airway inflammation, but they do little else. Consequently, routine use of beta agonists may actually allow bronchoconstriction to occur more easily in response to allergens and other stimuli. Accordingly, they should be reserved for episodic, short-term, symptomatic relief. Corticosteroid therapy, preferably via inhalation, is more effective and appropriate as the mainstay of preventive and maintenance therapy in asthma and can help wean patients from beta agonist therapy. Patient education also is important. Many asthmatics overuse beta agonists because of the relatively quick short-term relief they provide, but they fail to consider the long-term sequelae that are associated with chronic use of this medication.

Corticosteroids

Chronic corticosteroid therapy has a number of well-recognized side effects, including glucose intolerance, mental status changes, cataracts, osteoporosis, suppression of the immune system, and myopathy. Suppression of the hypothalamic-pituitary-adrenal (HPA) axis and inadequate intrinsic corticosteroid output by the adrenal gland is another widely known complication of chronic steroid treatment. This was initially recognized about 40 years ago when the first episodes of postoperative cardiovascular collapse and death were noted in association with steroid therapy withdrawal. Patients with insufficient adrenal function and a suppressed HPA axis are unable to increase corticosteroid output in the perioperative and postoperative settings and in response to other forms of stress. HPA axis suppression is related to a number of factors, including the duration of steroid therapy, the cumulative steroid dose, maximum steroid dose, and the current steroid dose just prior to discontinuation. Which of these factors is most important in producing suppression of the HPA axis is controversial. However, attempts should be made to reduce the dose or discontinue steroid therapy in patients who are being managed with this agent for long-term inflammatory conditions.

Naturally, discontinuation of steroid therapy or reduction of drug dosage will be dictated by symptomatic improvement of the patient, clinical stability, and monitoring of other laboratory parameters indicating the severity of the chronic inflammatory condition. When dose tapering is implemented, it is important to consider suppression of the HPA axis. Duration of therapy, dose interval, dose level, cumulative dose, and highest steroid dose are all thought to be contributing factors in HPA suppression. However, uncertainty about their significance has led to prolonged tapering courses of steroids, and frequent, empiric short-term increases in steroid dose to cover the stress of surgery and other medical illnesses. A recent study demonstrated that no patients receiving < 5 mg per day of prednisone had suppressed HPA axis function and that the dose of steroid to which the patient is tapered is more important than the rate of tapering.[103]

Accordingly, it is recommended that patients be weaned from steroid therapy by a stepwise reduction in daily dose as quickly as feasible, based on severity of illness and steroid withdrawal symptoms. Duration of chronic therapy, total cumulative dose, and highest steroid dose are not significant. An alternate-day steroid regimen is also unnecessary. With < 10 mg per day of prednisone, partial recovery of the HPA axis takes place. Provocative stress testing can serve to confirm adequacy of the adrenal gland. Alternatively, patients can receive supplemental stress steroid therapy. Below 7.5 mg of prednisone per day, full recovery is possible but variable, and patients should either have rapid intravenous adrenocorticotropic testing or empiric steroid stress therapy. Below 5 mg per day of prednisone, however, full recovery of the HPA axis is expected, and while provocative testing is probably unnecessary, a broader recommendation not to perform this requires larger confirmatory trials.

Steroid Tapering. Recommendations regarding tapering of short-term steroid courses are well established. The short-term side effects of corticosteroids include hyperglycemia, weight gain, fluid retention, peptic ulcer disease, hypertension, aseptic necrosis of the femoral head, and mood alterations. The corticosteroids of choice for use in the acute-care setting are prednisone or its active form, prednisolone, which is also available in an intravenous form, (methylprednisolone). Prednisone and prednisolone are five and six times more potent than endogenous hydrocortisone, respectively. Clinically significant improvement with these drugs is measurable 3 hours after administration, and peak effectiveness is reached at 6 to 12 hours. There is no question that steroids reduce the rate of relapse following acute treatment of asthma. More recently, there has been mounting evidence that early administration of steroids reduces admission rates for asthma in both adults and children.

In general, intravenous administration of steroids is indicated in patients with asthma who also require hospitalization. Despite routine use of intravenous steroids, there is no evidence that this route is any more effective than oral forms of steroids. In fact, recent studies show that there were no significant differences in peak expiratory flow, and ratio of forced expiratory flows at 25% and 75% of vital capacity between oral and intravenous steroid administration. The incidence of minor side effects was the same in both groups, and no patient had difficulty swallowing the large number of pills required for steroid therapy. Moreover, the number of days of hospitalization was similar in intravenous and oral steroid groups, and further analysis of subgroups revealed no differences between patients receiving 160 mg per day orally and those receiving the intravenous regimen. Based on this investigation, many experts conclude that oral methyl-prednisolone is safe and effective in the treatment of acute asthma.[141]

Inhaled steroids, while invaluable in the chronic management of outpatient asthma, do not have a role in acute exacerbations, and patients already receiving such therapy should be given oral steroids during acute exacerbations of their disease. A fear of corticosteroid-induced adrenal suppression has led many physicians to discharge patients with complicated steroid-tapering schedules. It now appears that this is unnecessary. Adrenal suppression is not usually seen until after at least 2 weeks of corticosteroid therapy, and most asthmatics require much shorter courses of therapy for control of their acute exacerbations. Tapering of steroid therapy is clearly indicated for asthmatic patients who are already taking oral steroids prior to their exacerbation and for those in whom a prolonged course of steroid therapy is anticipated. The majority of asthmatic patients, however, who are discharged on a 3 to 7 day course of steroids will benefit from high-dose "burst" therapy without the need to taper the drug. Such therapy results in clinical improvement that is comparable to longer tapering courses and does not increase the risk of asthma relapse or adrenal insufficiency. In conclusion, when administering oral steroids for a short-term course, short tapering courses over a 3 to 7 day period are sufficient.[141]

SUMMARY: THE CASE FOR DEMOLITION AND RENEWAL

This chapter has reviewed a number of commonly used medications that are amenable to discontinuation under appropriate clinical circumstances. Clearly, the decision to discontinue a medication, or to reduce its dose, depends on specific clinical parameters, which take into account the patient's symptoms and severity of disease. Clearly, however, there are windows of opportunity available for discontinuing medications, thereby reducing toxicity and quality-of-life impairment. For example, in the nursing home setting, studies show that given the availability of alternative behavioral management techniques, antipsychotic medications such as amitriptyline, haloperidol, and benzodiazepines can be discontinued successfully in some geriatric patients. Of special note is the fact that this discontinuation can be accomplished without an increase in behavioral disturbances. It is encouraging to note that up to two thirds of elderly patients placed on an antipsychotic drug withdrawal program successfully completed it. In addition, cardiovascular, gastrointestinal, and central nervous system medications can also be discontinued in a significant percentage of elderly patients receiving polypharmacy. Although almost half of drug discontinuations were followed by an ADWE, these events were generally not serious and rarely required hospitalization. In fact, drugs that were discontinued were not reinstituted in 60% of patients, a finding that lends credence to the idea that drug reduction programs for such medications as digoxin, furosemide, H_2 blockers, and many other medications may be successful and have acceptable risk/benefit profiles. Careful clinical protocols should be followed when withdrawing cardiovascular medications, as well as drugs such as benzodiazepines or beta-adrenergic blockers, inasmuch as cessation of these drugs can cause serious physiologic withdrawal symptoms.

In the case of hypertension, a strong case can be made for nonpharmacologic therapy with lifestyle modifications in a large percentage of patients with early, mild hypertension. Dose requirements for beta blockers and thiazide diuretics often times can be reduced in patients who are obese and who follow a successful weight loss program. Moreover, there are also opportunities for step-down therapy in patients who have adequate blood pressure control for at least one year and who are taking only a single antihypertensive agent. The best candidates are those on multiple drug therapy for hypertension; one or more agents can frequently be discontinued in this subgroup. In the case of cardiovascular disease, additional opportunities for drug cessation exist in patients who are on digoxin therapy and have normal sinus rhythm but do not have left ventricular systolic dysfunction. Studies show that patients who have normal cardiac function and do not require digoxin for rate control can usually be discontinued from the medication without adverse clinical consequences. Furthermore, the use of type I antiarrhythmic agents such as encainide and flecainide does not improve mortality outcomes in patients who are taking them for suppression of ventricular ectopy. Although long-term therapy with aspirin is necessary for the secondary prevention of myocardial infarction, dosages as low as 80 mg of aspirin per day appear to be sufficient to provide cardioprotective effects.

Opportunities exist for discontinuing medications used to treat neuropsychiatric conditions, although these cases require careful scrutiny. Patients who have a history of several depressive episodes may require lifelong therapy with antidepressant medications. However, those patients who have only a single episode of depression at a young age may be suitable candidates for gradual withdrawal of antidepressants. It also should be stressed that many individuals are currently being treated with SSRIs (fluoxetine, sertraline, etc.) for anxiety-related conditions that do not satisfy the strict criteria for major depressive disorder. After clinical stabilization is achieved in these patients, drug discontinuation should be considered. Even patients who are being treated with benzodiazepines such as alprazolam for the management of panic attacks can frequently be discontinued from long-term therapy. Patient selection must be careful, although patients who have *not* had panic episodes for 6 to 12 months are considered suitable for drug tapering and cessation of therapy. Studies show that benzodiazepines should be tapered gradually over a several-month period to improve clinical outcomes and reduce the incidence of undesirable side effects associated with benzodiazepine withdrawal.

In the case of gastrointestinal disorders, there is still considerable controversy concerning the wisdom of maintaining patients on long-term H_2 blocker therapy. However, the general consensus is that many patients are maintained on these agents unnecessarily. Patients with mild ulcer disease, as well as those taking H_2 blockers for dyspeptic symptoms, are ideal candidates for withdrawal of H_2 blockers. On the other hand, those patients at high risk for recurrent complications associated with ulcer disease may require life-long maintenance therapy. Patients with suspected *H. pylori* infection should receive definitive therapy to eradicate the organism. Opportunities for discontinuation of corticosteroids, NSAIDs, and dipyridamole ought to be investigated for all patients on long-term therapy with these medications.

Ultimately, the decision to discontinue a medication depends on a combination of factors that includes patient compliance, severity of the underlying disease, and the response of the individual patient to the therapeutic agent being considered for discontinuation. Careful monitoring during the discontinuation process is always advised, and patients should be encouraged to report exacerbations of symptoms or clinical deterioration to their physician or pharmacist.

[1]Beers MH, Ouslander JG, Fingold SF, Morgenstern H, Reuben DB, Rogers W, Zeffren MJ, Beck JC. Inappropriate medication prescribing in skilled-nursing facilities [see comments]. Ann Intern Med 1992 Oct 15;117(8):684-9.

[2]Closser MH. Benzodiazepines and the elderly. A review of potential problems [Review]. J Subst Abuse Treat 1991;8(1-2):35-41.

[3]Beers MH, Ouslander JG, Rollingeer I, Reuben DB, Brooks J, Beck JC. Explicit criteria for determining inappropriate medication use in nursing home residents [Review]. Arch Intern Med 1991 Sep;151(9):1825-32.

[4]Gurwitz JH, Goldberg RJ, Chen Z, Gore JM, Alpert JS. Beta-blocker therapy in acute myocardial infarction: evidence for underutilization in the elderly. Am J Med 1992 Dec;93(6):605-10.

[5]Heston LL, Garrard J, Makris L, Kane RL, Cooper S, Dunham T, Zelterman D. Inadequate treatment of depressed nursing home elderly. J Am Geriatr Soc 1992 Nov;40(11):1117-22.

[6]Anonymous. Why do GPs overprescribe antibiotics? [news]. Br J Hosp Med 1991 Jul;46(1):59.

[7]Beers MH, Fingold SF, Ouslander JG, Reuben DB, Morgenstern H, Beck JC. Characteristics and quality of prescribing by doctors practicing in nursing homes. J Am Geriatr Soc 1993 Aug;41(8):802-7.

[8]Gilley J. Toward rational prescribing [editorial]. BMJ 1994 Mar 19;308(6931):731-2.

[9]Parrish RH. Understanding physician prescribing behavior [letter]. Am J Hosp Pharm 1991 Mar; 48(3):463.

[10]Rovner BW, Edelman BA, Cox MP, Shmuely Y. The impact of antipsychotic drug regulations on psychotropic prescribing practices in nursing homes. Am J Psychiatry 1992 Oct;149(10):1390-2.

[11]Willcox SM, Himmelstein DU, Woolhander S. Inappropriate drug prescribing for the community-dwelling elderly. JAMA 1994 Jul 27;272(4):292-6.

[12]Jordan LK 3d, Jordan LO. Prudent prescribing. Prescribing suggestions for physicians. N C Med J 1992 Nov;53(11):585-8.

[13]Kroenke K, Pinholt EM. Reducing polypharmacy in the elderly. A controlled trial of physician feedback [see comments]. J Am Geriatr Soc 1990;38(1):31-6.

[14]Colley CA, Lucas LM. Polypharmacy: the cure becomes the disease [Review]. J Gen Intern Med 1993 May;8(5):278-83.

[15]Soumerai SB, McLaughlin TJ, Avorn J. Quality assurance for drug prescribing [Review]. Qual Assur Health Care 1990;2(1):37-58.

[16]Col N, Fanale JE, Kronholm P. The role of medication noncompliance and adverse drug reactions in hospitalizations of the elderly. Arch Intern Med 1990 April;150(4):841-5.

[17]Deyo RA, Inui TS, Sullivan B. Noncompliance with arthritis drugs: magnitude, correlates, and clinical implications. J Rheumatol 1981;8:931-6.

[18]Halpern MT, Irwin DE, Brown RE, Clouse J, Hatziandreu EJ. Patient adherence to prescribed potassium supplement therapy. Clin Ther 1993 Nov-Dec;15(6):1133-45; discussion 1120.

[19]Hood JC, Murphy JE. Patient noncompliance can lead to hospital readmissions. Hospitals 1978; 52:79-82, 84.

[20]Weintraub M. Compliance in the elderly. Clin Geriatr Med 1990;6:445-52.

[21]DuBard MB, Goldenberg RL, Copper RL, Hauth JC. Are pill counts valid measures of compliance in clinical obstetric trials? Am J Obst Gynecol 1993 Nov;169(5):1181-2.

[22]Larson EB, et al. Adverse drug reactions associated with global cognitive impairment in elderly persons. Ann Intern Med 1987;107:169-73.

[23]Colley CA, Lucas LM. Polypharmacy: the cure becomes the disease. J Gen Intern Med 1993 May;8(5):278-83.

[24]Arstall MA, Beltrame JF, Mohan P, Wuttke RD, Esterman AJ, Horowitz JD. Incidence of adverse events during treatment with verapamil for suspected acute myocardial infarction. Am J Cardiol 1992 Dec 15;70(20):1611-2.

[25]Holden MD. Over-the-counter medications: Do you know what your patients are taking? Postgrad Med 1992 June;91(8):191-4, 199-200.

[26]Egstrup K. Transient myocardial ischemia after abrupt withdrawal of antianginal therapy in chronic stable angina. Am J Cardiol 1988;61:1219.

[27]File SE, Andrews N. Benzodiazepine withdrawal: behavioural pharmacology and neurochemical changes [Review]. Biochem Soc Symp 1993;59:97-106.

[28]Garner EM, Kelly MW, Thompson DF. Tricyclic antidepressant withdrawal syndrome [Review]. Ann Pharmacother 1993 Sep;27(9):1068-72.

[29]Ballenger JC, Pecknold J, Rickles K, Sellers EM. Medication discontinuation in panic disorder [Review]. J Clin Psychiatry 1993 Oct;54 Suppl:15-21; discussion 22-4.

[30]Burrows GD, Norman TR, Judd FK, Marriott PF. Short-acting versus long-acting benzodiazepines: discontinuation effects in panic disorders [Review]. J Psychiatr Res 1990;24 Suppl 2:65-72.

[31]Dilsaver SC. Withdrawal phenomena associated with antidepressant and antipsychotic agents [Review]. Drug Saf 1994 Feb;10(2):103-14.

[32]Gerety MB, Cornell JE, Plichta DT, Eimer M. Adverse events related to drugs and drug withdrawal in nursing home residents. J Am Geriatr Soc 1993 Dec;41(12):1326-32.

[33]Greenblatt RM, Hollander H, McMaster JR, Henke CJ. Polypharmacy among patients attending an AIDS clinic: utilization of prescribed, unorthodox, and investigational treatments. J Acquir Immune Defic Syndr 1991;4(2):136-43.

[34]Sadler C. A pill for every ill? Nurs Times 1991 Feb 27-Mar;87(9):21.

[35]Beers MH, Ouslander JG, Fingold SF, Morgenstern H, Ruben DB, Rogers W, Zeffren MJ, Beck JC. Inappropriate medication prescribing in skilled-nursing facilities.

[36]Bowler SD, Mitchell CA, Armstrong JG. Corticosteroids in acute severe asthma: effectiveness of low doses [see comments]. Thorax 1992 Aug;47(8):584-7.

[37]Rothschild AJ. Disinhibition, amnestic reactions, and other adverse reactions secondary to triazolam: a review of the literature [Review]. J Clin Psychiatry 1992 Dec;53 Suppl:69-79.

[38]Fries JF, Williams CA, Ramey DR, Bloch DA. The relative toxicity of alternative therapies for rheumatoid arthritis: implications for the therapeutic progression. Semin Arthritis Rheum 1993 Oct;23(2 Suppl 1):68-73.

[39]Alegro S, Fenster PE, Marcus FI. Digitalis therapy in the elderly. Geriatrics 1983; 38:98.

[40]Anonymous. Misoprostol for co-prescription with NSAID [Review]. Drug Ther Bull 1990 Apr 2; 28(7):25-6.

[41]DeSantis G, Harvey KJ, Howard D, Mashford ML, Moulds RF. Improving the quality of antibiotic prescription patterns in general practice. The role of educational intervention. Med J Aust 1994 Apr 18;160(8):502-5.

[42]Forman DE, Coletta D, Kenny D, Kosowsky BD, Stoukides J, Rohrer M, Pastore JO. Clinical issues related to discontinuing digoxin therapy in elderly nursing home patients. Arch Intern Med 1991 Nov;151(11):2194-8.

[43]Gurwitz JH, Noonan JP, Soumerai SB. Reducing the use of H_2-receptor antagonists in the long-term-care setting [see comments]. J Am Geriatr Soc 1992 Apr;40(4):359-64.

[44]Lamy PP. Renal effects of nonsteroidal anti-inflammatory drugs. Heightened risk to the elderly? J Am Geriatr Soc 1986;34:361-7.

[45]Green LW, Purrell CO, Koop CE, et al. Programs to reduce drug errors in the elderly: direct and indirect evidence from patient education. In: Improving Medication Compliance. Reston, Va: National Pharm Council, 1985.

[46]Lamy PP. Compliance in long-term care. Geriatrika 1985;1(8):32.

[47]Botelho RJ, Dudrak R 2d. Home assessment of adherence to long-term medication in the elderly. J Fam Prac 1992 July;35(1):61-5.

[48]Hamilton RA, Briceland LL. Use of prescription-refill records to assess patient compliance. Am J Hosp Pharm 1992 July;49(7):1691-6.

[49]Eisen SA, Miller DK, Woodward RS, Spitznagel E, Przybeck TR.The effect of prescribed daily dose frequency on patient medication compliance. Arch Intern Med 1990 Sept;150(9):1881-4.

[50]Keen PJ. What is the best dosage schedule for patients? J R Soc Med 1991 Nov;84(11):640-1.

[51]Litchman HM. Medication noncompliance: a significant problem and possible strategies. R I Med 1993 Dec;76(12):608-10.

[52]Kruse W, Weber E. Dynamics of drug regiment compliance—its assessment by microprocessor-based monitoring. Eur J Clin Pharmacol 1990;38:561-5.

[53]Rudd P, Marshall G. Resolving problems of measuring compliance with medication monitors. J Compliance Health Care 1987;2:23-35.

[54]Kirsten DK, Wegner RE, Jorres RA, Magnussen H. Effects of theophylline withdrawal in severe chronic obstructive pulmonary disease [see comments]. Chest 1993 Oct;104(4):1101-7.

[55]McCarthy DM. Maintenance therapy for peptic ulcer—who needs it? [Review]. Gastroenterol Jpn 1993 May;28 Suppl 5:172-7.

[56]Applegate WB, Miller ST, Elam JT, Cushman WC, el Derwi D, Brewer A, Graney MJ. Nonpharmacologic intervention to reduce blood pressure in older patients with mild hypertension. Arch Intern Med 1992 Jun;152(6):1162-6.

[57]Galimberti CA, Manni R, Parietti L, Marchioni E, Tartara A. Drug withdrawal in patients with epilepsy: prognostic value of the EEG. Seizure 1992 Sep;2(3):213-22.

[58]Jenck MA, Reynolds MS. Anticonvulsant drug withdrawal in seizure-free patients [Review]. Clin Pharm 1990 Oct;9(10):781-7.

[59]Semla TP, Palla K, Poddig B, Brauner DJ. Effect of the Omnibus Reconciliation Act 1987 on antipsychotic prescribing in nursing home residents. J Am Geriatr Soc 1994 Jun;42(6):648-52.

[60]Shorr RI, Fought RL, Ray WA. Changes in antipsychotic drug use in nursing homes during implementation of the OBRA-87 regulations [see comments]. JAMA 1994 Feb 2;271(5):358-62.

[61]Suck JA. Psychotropic drug practice in nursing homes. J Am Geriatr Soc 1988;36:409-18.

[62]Daly MP, Lamy PP, Richardson JP. Avoiding polypharmacy and iatrogenesis in the nursing home. Md Med J 1994 Feb;43(2):139-44.

[63]Edouard L, Rawson NS. Cutting costs by targeting prescribing practices [letter]. Can Med Assoc J 1994 July 1;151(1):14-5.

[64]Gilbert A, Owen N, Innes JM, Sansom L. Trial of an intervention to reduce chronic benzodiazepine use among residents of aged-care accommodation. Aust N Z J Med 1993 Aug;23(4):343-7.

[65]Lader M. Long-term anxiolytic therapy: the use of drug withdrawal. J Clin Psychiatry 1987; 48:12-6.

[66]Kaplan NM. Long-term effectiveness of nonpharmacological treatment of hypertension [Review]. Hypertension 1991 Sep;18(3 Suppl):I153-60.

[67]Kaplan NM. The potential benefits of nonpharmacological therapy. Am J Hypertens 1990 May; 3(5 Pt 1):425-7.

[68]Fuchs Z, Viskoper JR, Drexler I, Nitzan H, Lubin F, Berlin S, Almagor M, Zulty L, Chetrit A, Mishal J, et al. Comprehensive individualised nonpharmacological treatment programme for

hypertension in physician-nurse clinics: two year follow-up. J Hum Hyptertens 1993 Dec;7(6):585-91.

[69]So N, Gotman J. Changes in seizure activity following anticonvulsant drug withdrawal. Neurology 1990 Mar;40(3 Pt1):407-13.

[70]Stults BM. Digoxin use in the elderly. J Am Geriatr Soc 1985;30(3):158.

[71]Hering R, Steiner TJ. Abrupt outpatient withdrawal of medication in analgesic-abusing migraineurs. Lancet 1991 Jun 15;337(8755):1442-3.

[72]Anonymous. The effects of nonpharmacologic interventions on blood pressure of persons with high normal levels. Results of the Trials of Hypertension Prevention, Phase I [published erratum appears in JAMA 1992 May 6;267(17):2330] [see comments]. JAMA 1992 Mar 4; 267(9):1213-20.

[73]Griffin JP, Griffin TD. The economic implications of therapeutic conservatism [see comments]. J R Coll Physicians Lond 1993 Apr;27(2):121-6.

[74]Tjoa HI, Kaplan NM. Nonpharmacological treatment of hypertension in diabetes mellitus [Review]. Diabetes Care 1991 Jun;14(6):449-60.

[75]Pickering TG. Predicting the response to nonpharmacologic treatment in mild hypertension [editorial; comment]. JAMA 1992 Mar 4;267(9):1256-7.

[76]Strasser T. Nonpharmacological treatment [Review]. J Hum Hypertens 1990 Feb;Suppl 1:39-42.

[77]Moriguchi Y, Consoni PR, Hekman PR. Systemic arterial hypertension: results of the change from pharmacological to nonpharmacological treatment. J Cardiovasc Pharmacol 1990;16 Suppl 8:S72-4.

[78]Dall JLC. Maintenance digoxin in elderly patients. Br Med J 1970;2:702.

[79]Packer M, Gheorghiade M, Young JB, et al. Withdrawal of digoxin from patients with chronic congestive heart failure treated with angiotensin-converting-enzyme inhibitors. N Engl J Med 1993;329:1-7.

[80]Akhtar M, Breithardt G, Camm AJ, Coumel P, Janse MJ, Lazzara R, Myerberg RJ, Schwartz PJ, Waldo AL, Wellens HJ, et al. CAST and beyond. Implications of the Cardiac Arrhythmia Suppression Trial. Task Force of the Working Group on Arrhythmias of the European Society of Cardiology [Review]. Circulation 1990 Mar;81(3):1123-7.

[81]Akiyama T, Pawitan Y, Greenberg H, Kuo CS, Reynolds-Haertle RA. Increased risk of death and cardiac arrest from encainide and flecainide in patients after non-Q-wave acute myocardial infarction in the Cardiac Arrhythmia Suppression Trial. CAST investigators. Am J Cardiol 1991 Dec 15;68(17):1551-5.

[82]Anonymous. Randomized antiarrhythmic drug therapy in survivors of cardiac arrest (the CAS-CADE Study). The CASCADE investigators. Am J Cardiol 1993 Aug 1;72(3):280-7.

[83]Mindardo JD, et al. Clinical characteristics of patients with ventricular fibrillation during antiarrhythmic drug therapy. N Engl J Med 1988;319:257.

[84]Peters RW, Mitchell LB, Brooks MM, Echt DS, Barker AH, Capone R, Liebson PR, Greene HL. Circadian pattern of arrhythmic death in patients receiving encainide, flecainide or moricizine in the Cardiac Arrhythmia Suppression Trial (CAST). J Am Coll Cardiol 1994 Feb;23(2):283-9.

[85]Prystowsky EN, Waldo AL, Fisher JD. Use of disopyramide by arrhythmia specialists after Cardiac Arrhythmia Suppression Trial: patient selection and initial outcome. Am Heart J 1991 May; 121(5):1571-82.

[86]Maynard C. Rehospitalization in surviving patients of out-of-hospital ventricular fibrillation (the CASCADE study). Cardiac Arrest in Seattle: Conventional Amiodarone Drug Evaluation. Am J Cardiol 1993 Dec 1;72(17):1295-300.

[87]Morganroth J, Bigger JT Jr, Anderson JL. Treatment of ventricular arrhythmias by United States cardiologists: a survey before the Cardiac Arrhythmia Suppression Trial results were available. Am J Cardiol 1990 Jan 1;65(1):40-8.

[88]Willund I, Gorkin L, Pawitan Y, Schron E, Schoenberger J, Jared LL, Shumaker S. Methods for assessing quality of life in the cardiac arrhythmia suppression trial (CAST). Qual Life Res 1992 Jun;1(3):187-201.

[89]Puech P. Practical aspects of the use of amiodarone [Review]. Drugs 1991;41 Suppl 2:67-73.

[90]Hine LK, Laird NM, et al. Meta-analysis of empirical long-term antiarrhythmic therapy after myocardial infarction. JAMA 1989;262:3037-40.

[91]Malik R, Ellenbogen KA, Stambler BS, Wood MA. Flecainide: its value and danger [Review]. Heart Dis Stroke 1994 Mar-Apr;3(2):85-9.

[92]Reiffel JA, Cook JR. Physician attitudes toward the use of type IC antiarrhythmics after the Cardiac Arrhythmia Suppression Trial (CAST). Am J Cardiol 1990 Nov 15;66(17):1262-4.

[93]Hirsh J. Oral anticoagulant drugs [see comments] [Review]. N Engl J Med 1991 Jun 27;324(26):1865-75.

[94]Hirsh J, Dalen JE, Fuster V, Harker LB, Slazman EW. Aspirin and other platelet-active drugs. The relationship between dose, effectiveness, and side effects [Review]. Chest 1992 Oct;102(4Suppl):327S-36S.

[95]Samuelsson K, Svensson J. Aspirin: optimal dose in stroke prevention [letter; comment]. Stroke 1993 Aug;24(8)1259-61.

[96]vanGijn J. Aspirin: dose and indications in modern stroke prevention. Neurologic Clin 1992 Feb; 10(1):193-207; discussion 208.

[97]Harker LA, Bernstein EF, et al. Failure of aspirin plus dipyridamole to prevent restenosis after carotid endarterectomy. Ann Intern Med 1992;116:731.

[98]Stroke Prevention in Atrial Fibrillation Study Group. Preliminary report of the stroke prevention in atrial fibrillation study. N Engl J Med 1990;322:863-8.

[99]Anonymous. Drugs for treatment of peptic ulcers. Med Lett Drugs Ther 1991 Nov 29; 33(858):111-4.

[100]Sessler CN. Theophylline toxicity: clinical features of 116 cases. Am J Med 1990;88:567-76.

[101]Hamilton RA, Gordon T. Incidence and cost of hospital admissions secondary to drug interactions involving theophylline. Ann Pharmacother 1992 Dec;26(12):1507-11.

[102]Richardson JP. Theophylline toxicity associated with the administration of ciprofloxacin in a nursing home patient. J Am Geriatr Soc 1990 Mar;38(3):236-8.

[103]LaRochelle GE, et al. Recovery of hypothalamic-pituitary-adrenal (HPA) axis in patients with rheumatic diseases receiving low-dose prednisone. Am J Med;95:258-64.

[104]Laan RF, et al. Low-dose prednisone induces rapid reversible axial bone loss in patients with rheumatoid arthritis. Ann Intern Med 1993;119:963-8.

[105]Broadhead WE, Larson DB, Yarnall KS, Blazer DG, Tse CK. Tricyclic antidepressant prescribing for nonpsychiatric disorders. An analysis based on data from the 1985 National Ambulatory Medical Care Survey [see comments]. J Fam Prac 1991 July;33(1):24-32.

[106]Huszonek JJ, Dewan MJ, Koss M, Hardoby WJ, Isphani A. Antidepressant side effects and physician prescribing patterns [Review]. Ann Clin Psychiatry 1993 Mar;5(1):7-11.

[107]Levin GM, DeVane CL. Prescribing attitudes of different physician groups regarding fluoxetine. Ann Pharmacother 1993 Dec;27(12):1443-7.

[108]Katon W, von Korff M, Lin E, Bush T, Ormel J. Adequacy and duration of antidepressant treatment in primary care. Med Care 1992 Jan;30(1):67-76.

[109]Keller MB, et al. Treatment received by depressed patients. JAMA 1982;248(15):1848.

[110]Greenblatt DJ, Miller LG, Shader RI. Benzodiazepine discontinuation syndromes [Review]. J Psychiatr Res 1990;24 Suppl 2:73-9.

[111]Pecknold JC. Discontinuation reactions to alprazolam in panic disorder. J Psychiat Res 1993;27 Suppl 1:155-70.

[112]Rosenbaum JF. Switching patients from alprazolam to clonazepam. Hosp Comm Psychiatry 1990 Dec;41(12):1302, 1305.

[113]Udelman HD, Udelman DL. Concurrent use of buspirone in anxious patients during withdrawal from alprazolam therapy. J Clin Psychiatry 1990 Sep;51 Suppl:46-50.

[114]Swantek SS, Grossberg GT, Neppe VM, Doubek WG, Martin T, Bender JE. The use of carbamazepine to treat benzodiazepine withdrawal in a geriatric population. J Geriatr Psychiatry Neurol 1991 Apr-Jun;4(2):106-9.

[115]Rickels, Schweizer, et al. Long-term therapeutic use of benzodiazepines: Part I, effects of abrupt discontinuation; Part II, effects of gradual taper. Arch Gen Psychiatry 1990;47:899-915.

[116]Anonymous. Anti-anxiety drug usage in the United States, 1989. Statistical Bulletin-Metropolitan Insurance Companies 1991 Jan-Mar;72(1):18-27.

[117]Bolten W, Gomes JA, Stead H, Geis GS. The gastroduodenal safety and efficacy of the fixed combination of diclofenac and misoprostol in the treatment of osteoarthritis. Br J Rheumatol 1992 Nov;31(11):753-8.

[118]MacWalter RS, Lindsay GH. A policy for minimising NSAID induced peptic ulcer. Scott Med J 1992 Feb;37(1):3-4.

[119]Penston JG, Dixon JS, Boyd EJ, Wormsley KG. A placebo-controlled investigation of duodenal ulcer recurrence after withdrawal of long-term treatment with ranitidine. Aliment Pharmacol Ther 1993 Jun;7(3):259-65.

[120]Creutzfeldt W. Risk-benefit assessment of omeprazole in the treatment of gastrointestinal disorders [Review]. Drug Saf 1994 Jan;10(1):66-82.

[121]Falk GW. Omeprazole: a new drug for the treatment of acid-peptic diseases [Review]. Cleve Clin J Med 1991 Sep-Oct;58(5):418-27.

[122]Hetzel DJ. Controlled clinical trials of omeprazole in the long-term management of reflux disease [Review]. Digestion 1992;51 Suppl 1:35-42.

[123]Holt S, Howden CW. Omeprazole. Overview and opinion [Review]. Dig Dis Sci 1991 Apr; 36(4):385-93.

[124]Maton PN. Omeprazole [Review]. N Engl J Med 1991 Apr 4;324(14):965-75.

[125]Ispano M, Fontana A, Scibilia J, Ortolani C. Oral challenge with alternative nonsteroidal anti-inflammatory drugs (NSAIDs) and paracetamol in patients intolerant to these agents. Drugs 1993; 46 Suppl 1:253-6.

[126]Lamy P. Adverse drug effects [Review]. Clin Geriatr Med 1990 May;6(2):293-307.

[127]Sager DS, Bennett RM. Individualizing the risk/benefit ratio of NSAIDs in older patients [Review]. Geriatrics 1992 Aug;47(8):24-31.

[128]World Health Organization. Health care in the elderly: report of the technical group on the use of medications in the elderly. Drugs 1981;22:279.

[129]Prichard P. The management of upper gastrointestinal problems in patients taking NSAIDs. Aust Fam Physician 1991 Dec;20(12):1739-41.

[130]Stalnikowicz R, Rachmilewitz D. NSAID-induced gastroduodenal damage: is prevention needed? A review and metaanalysis. J Clin Gastroenterol 1993 Oct;17(3):238-43.

[131]Gabriel SE, Campion ME, O'Fallon WM. A cost-utility analysis of misoprostol prophylaxis for rheumatoid arthritis patients receiving nonsteroidal anti-inflammatory drugs. Arthritis Rheum 1994 Mar;37(3):333-41.

[132]Walt RP. Misoprostol for the treatment of peptic ulcer and antiinflammatory-drug-induced gastroduodenal ulceration. N Engl J Med 1992;327:1575.

[133]Graham DY, White RH, Moreland LW, et al. Duodenal and gastric ulcer prevention with misoprostol in arthritis patients taking NSAIDs. Ann Intern Med 1993;119:257.

[134]Graham DY, White RH, Moreland LW, Schubert TT, Katz R, Jaszewski R, Tindall E, Triadafilopoulos G, Stromatt SC, Teoh LS. Duodenal and gastric ulcer prevention with misoprostol in arthritis patients taking NSAIDs. Misoprostol Study Group [see comments]. Ann Intern Med 1993 Aug 15;119(4):257-62.

[135]Bussey HI, Force RW, Bianco TM, et al. Reliance on prothrombin time ratios causes significant errors in anticoagulation therapy. Arch Intern Med 1992;152:278-82. See also the editorial by Hirsh J. Substandard monitoring of warfarin in North America. Arch Intern Med 1992; 152:257-8.

[136]Landefeld CS, Goldman, L. Major bleeding in outpatients treated with warfarin: incidence and prediction by factors known at the start of outpatient therapy. Am J Med 1989;87:144-52; Landefeld CS, Rosenblatt MW, Goldman L. Bleeding in outpatients treated with warfarin: relation to prothrombin time and important remediable lesions. Am J Med 1989;87:153-9.

[137]Jahnigens D, Cooper D, La Force M. Adverse events among hospitalized elderly patients. J Am Geriatr Soc 1988;36:65-72.

[138]Brigden ML. Oral anticoagulant therapy. Newer indications and an improved method of monitoring [Review]. Postgrad Med 1992 Feb 1;91(2):285-8, 293-6.

[139]Hirsh J, Dalen JE, Deykin D, Poller L. Oral anticoagulants. Mechanism of action, clinical effectiveness, and optimal therapeutic range [see comments] [Review]. Chest 1992 Oct;102(4 Suppl):312S-26S.

[140]Ansell JE. Oral anticoagulant therapy—50 years later [Review]. Arch Intern Med 1993 Mar 8; 153(5):586-96.

[141]Chapman KR, et al. Effect of a short course of prednisone in the prevention of early relapse after the emergency room treatment of acute asthma. N Engl J Med 1991;324:788.

[142]Aronow WS. Treatment of Ventricular Arrhythmias In Older Adults. JAGS 1995;43:688-95.

[143]Becker RC, Ansell J. Antithrombotic Therapy. An Abbreviated Reference for Clinicians. Arch Intern Med 1995;155:149.

[144]Bussey HI, Force RW, Bianco TM, et al. Reliance on prothrombin time ratios causes significant errors in anticoagulation therapy. Arch Intern Med 1992;152:278-82.

[145]Hirsh J. Substandard monitoring of warfarin in North America. Arch Intern Med 1992;152:257-8.

5

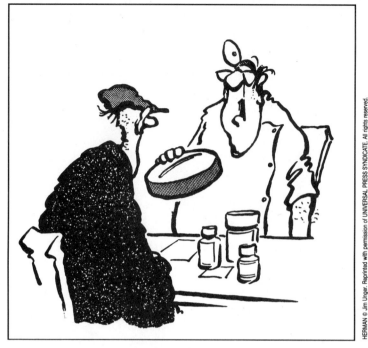

"I want you to take one of these with water every four years."

The DRESC™ Program: Drug Reduction, Elimination, Simplification, and Consolidation

A program of drug reduction, elimination, simplification, and consolidation (DRESC™ program) represents a logical, systematic, and practical approach to streamlining therapeutic regimens and reducing polypharmacy. Based on these guiding principles, the DRESC program is designed for daily use by physicians or pharmacists as they deconstruct and reconstruct drug houses. The principle objective of the DRESC program is to *minimize* medications in order to *maximize* clinical results. Initially, the DRESC program requires a meticulous review of the patient's current drug regimen, including a careful reevaluation of the original indications for medication use (see Figure 5-1). Although this drug streamlining program usually requires several consultations, the elimination of unnecessary medications and dosage reductions, as well as a decrease in drug-related adverse patient events, (DRAPES)[1] will produce long-term cost savings for the patient (see Figure 5-2).[2,3]

Figure 5-1

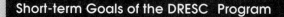

Short-term Goals of the DRESC Program

ELIMINATE
■ **Unnecessary prescription drugs**

SIMPLIFY REGIMEN
■ **Reduce number of drugs and total pill intake**

REDUCTION
■ **Reduction of drug dose**

CONSOLIDATION OF THERAPY
■ **Treat more than one condition with single drug**

Short-term goals of the DRESC program include elimination of unnecessary prescription drugs, reduction in the number of different medications and in the total number of pills taken per day, decreasing the dose of one or more drugs, and, finally, consolidation of drug therapy. The long-term goals of the DRESC program include improvement in quality of life[4-8] and functional status[9,10] of the patient, minimizing the potential for adverse drug reactions and interactions,[11-13] improving patient education,[14-16] and encouraging lifestyle modifications that permit nonpharmacologic management of chronic diseases. Generally speaking, patients who are taking four or more different prescription medications are excellent candidates for drug simplification, elimination, and consolidation. Individuals who take fewer than four drugs are still likely to benefit from dose reduction.

Potential benefits of the DRESC program are listed in Table 5-1. It should be stressed that the DRESC program plays a central role in total pharmacotherapeutic quality management (TPQM™) (see Table 5-2). Specifically, the DRESC program provides a practical, hands-on approach to the simplification and consolidation of complicated, polypharmacy drug regimens. Because the process of drug reduction, simplification, and consolidation requires frequent contact between patients and health care providers, this program promotes patient-physician and patient-pharmacist communication regarding medication-related issues.[14,16,19,20] Moreover, quality assurance objectives are fostered, because the three phases of drug regimen deconstruction and reconstruction—assessment, implementation, and evaluation—require regular reviews of the appropriateness of medication orders. It specifically encourages periodic reassessments of

Figure 5-2

Long-term Goals of the DRESC Program

■ **Improve Quality of Life**

■ **Enhance Functional Status**

■ **Minimize Potential for Adverse Drug Reactions**

■ **Improve Patient Education**

■ **Lifestyle Modification**

the drug regimen to determine whether stepdown therapy is possible. For these reasons, the DRESC program can easily be incorporated into risk management programs designed to evaluate drug safety and utilization. When successful, the DRESC program will promote long-term patient satisfaction with drug therapy, and can also be used as a centerpiece program for drug reduction clinics.

Table 5-1

Benefits of Drug Reduction, Elimination, Simplification and Consolidation (DRESC)	
• Enhance medication compliance	• Screen for redundancy in drug regimen
• Reduce risk for adverse drug reactions	• Reduce overall cost of drug house
• Quality-of-life improvements	• Ensure duration limits for short-term therapy
• Reduces inappropriate medication orders	• Ensure dosage limitations not exceeded
• Reduce risk of polypharmacy	• Promote "smart drug" therapy
• Improve quality of medication selection	

Table 5-2

Total Pharmacotherapeutic Quality Management (TPQM): Role of The DRESC Program
• Provides practical, hands-on approach to simplification and con-solidation of drug regimens
• Promotes patient-physician and patient-pharmacist communication about medication-related issues
• Requires regular reviews of appropriateness of medication orders
• Encourages regular reviews of drug regimens to determine whether step-down therapy is possible
• Can be incorporated into risk-management programs evaluating drug safety and utilization
• Promotes long-term consumer (i.e., patient) satisfaction with drug therapy
• May influence P&T formulary adoptions and reviews
• Centerpiece program for drug reduction clinics

Screening Candidates For The DRESC Program

Although most patients who are taking multiple medications for chronic medical conditions will benefit from DRESC program strategies, not all individuals will benefit equally from attempts to streamline their medication intake. However, there are a number of risk factors, demographic characteristics, medication intake patterns, and clinical conditions that increase the likelihood that a patient will benefit from measures aimed at streamlining their medication intake (see Table 5-3). Programs oriented around TPQM should screen for these risk factors in order to identify patient candidates most likely to benefit from drug regimen redesign.

In particular, any patient who is taking *several* medications simultaneously is an excellent candidate for the DRESC program. In addition, four high-risk patient populations warrant special attention because of their increased risk of incurring drug-related toxicity. In this regard, DRESC strategies should be considered for patients who are critically ill,[21] for the elderly,[22-25] for persons with AIDS, and for substance abusers. Generally speaking the risk of having a drug-related adverse patient event is linked to the number of *diseases* a person is burdened with, as well as the number of different *prescription ingredients* in the drug regimen. Inasmuch as little can be done to reduce disease burden, attention must be focused on *reducing pharmacologic burden* to decrease the risk of drug-related toxicity and associated complications.

Table 5-3

Screening for and Identifying Candidates Appropriate For DRESC Program
PATIENTS WITH THE FOLLOWING DRUG REGIMENS, RISK FACTORS, DEMOGRAPHIC CHARACTERISTICS, AND CLINICAL CONDITIONS SHOULD BE CONSIDERED FOR DRUG REDUCTION, ELIMINATION, SIMPLIFICATION, AND CONSOLIDATION.

- Patients taking three or more drugs
- 65 years of age and older
- A history of unexplained fatigue, sexual dysfunction, sleep disturbance, depression, mood disturbance, cough.
- Six or more physician visits within a 1-year period
- A history of adverse drug reactions or interactions
- Perception that drug regimen is too costly
- Regimen contains drugs dosed at multiple daily dose frequencies
- Medications with only one end-organ salvage function
- Medications considered inappropriate for age group (e.g., the elderly)
- Medications consumed at highest recommended dose
- Patients taking more than 9 doses per day
- Patients taking medications beyond normally accepted duration limits (H2 blockers, antibiotics, corticosteroids, etc.)
- Regimen consists of primarily generic medications
- Complaints of medication side effects

Patient Factors. Patients who complain of unexplained fatigue, sexual dysfunction, sleep disturbance, depression, mood disturbance, or cough, require meticulous screening of their drug intake to determine whether any of these symptoms are the result of pharmacologic toxicity.[10] Agents used to treat neuropsychiatric disorders, hypertension, and cardiovascular diseases require special scrutiny.[26-29] Studies show that individuals who make six or more physician visits within a one-year period also are at increased risk for having drug-related toxicity. In addition, when these physician encounters occur with more than one practitioner, the risk of pharmacologic mismanagement is even greater. Hence, patients taking multiple medications who have made more than six physician visits within a one-year period, and who acknowledge that they have multiple prescribing sources, will almost always benefit from streamlining programs aimed at reduction, simplification, and consolidation.

In addition, individuals with a history of adverse drug reactions,[13,30] medication compliance problems,[20,31-33] or drug interactions require careful evaluation. These patients may be extremely susceptible to pharmacologic intervention, and therefore, DRESC program strategies can help reduce the risk of drug-related problems. In addition, if patients perceive that their drug regimen is too costly, the practitioner should determine whether medication compliance has been affected by drug cost. In this patient subgroup, simple alterations that reduce drug acquisition costs for the patient can produce dramatic improvements in compliance, and, therefore, enhance therapeutic outcomes.

Drug Factors. Most drug regimens require careful screening and assessment to uncover suboptimal drugs, dosing patterns, combinations, or prescribing practices. For example, a regimen that contains many medications given at multiple daily dose frequencies will usually be less than satisfactory from a compliance perspective. In these cases, a streamlining program aimed at consolidating the regimen with primarily once-daily medications may improve drug compliance and, in the process, enhance therapeutic results. The regimen should also be screened to determine if medications with only one function are being used. For example, if a patient with diabetes is taking one medication to treat high blood pressure, a different medication to treat congestive heart failure, and yet another drug to treat renal dysfunction, it may be more appropriate to consolidate this patient's drug regimen with a single agent, such as an ACE inhibitor, which is able to service several target organs simultaneously. Similarly, if a patient is consuming one drug to treat angina, another drug to treat high blood pressure, and another medication to treat esophageal spasm, it may be therapeutically far more effective to identify a *single* agent, such as a calcium channel blocker, that can provide both symptomatic relief and treatment for hypertension using only one medication.

As a general rule, patients who have multiple clinical disorders and are being treated with many different medications—each of which is targeted at only *one* disease or clinical problem—are likely to benefit from DRESC program *consolidation* strategies; whenever possible, the objective is to treat multiple conditions with a single prescription drug (see Table 5-4). Drug regimens should also be screened for medications considered to be inappropriate or unsuitable for use in the elderly. In particular, drug houses that include sedative or hypnotic agents, tricyclic antidepressants, nonsteroidal anti-inflammatory drugs (NSAIDs), unproven dementia therapies, muscle relaxants, and bronchodilators will almost always benefit from DRESC program modifications.

The need for drug house deconstruction and reconstruction is also suggested when treatment regimens contain medications prescribed at levels that approach their highest recommended daily dose. In these cases, DRESC program strategies aimed at selecting drugs that are dosed at lower levels will usually improve side effect profiles and medication compliance. DRESC program strategies also deserve application in patients who are taking more than 10 pills per day, in individuals who are taking medications that are frequently prescribed beyond their normally accepted duration limits (e.g., H_2 blockers, antibiotics, corticosteroids), and in persons whose drug houses consist primarily of *generic medications*. Finally, any patient complaining of side effects or quality-of-life impairments that may be attributable to their medication intake requires a careful review of the drug house to see whether DRESC program strategies are indicated.

Table 5-4

CONSOLIDATION OF REGIMENS WITH SMART DRUGS	
SMART DRUG	**CONDITIONS/SYMPTOMS**
AMLODIPINE	
	Angina
	Hypertension
	Renal dysfunction
AMLODIPINE	
	Hypertension
	Angina
VERAPAMIL OR DILTIAZEM	
	Hypertension
	Supraventricular tachycardia
PROPRANOLOL OR VERAPAMIL	
	Hypertension
	Migraine prophylaxis
ATENOLOL	
	Hypertension
	Secondary prevention of myocardial infarction
ENALAPRIL, LISINOPRIL OR HYDROCHLOROTHIAZIDE	
	Hypertension
	Congestive heart failure
ENALAPRIL, LISINOPRIL	
	Hypertension
	Diabetes with microalbuminuria
	Congestive heart failure
AMLODIPINE	
	Hypertension
	Angina
	Diabetes (no microalbuminuria)
DOXAZOSIN	
	Hypertension
	Mild hypercholesterolemia
DOXAZOSIN, TERAZOSIN	
	Hypertension
	Benign prostatic hypertrophy (symptomatic relief, surgery not indicated)
DOXAZOSIN	
	Hypertension
	Mild hypercholesterolemia
	Benign prostatic hypertrophy

Table 5-4

CONSOLIDATION OF REGIMENS WITH SMART DRUGS — cont'd.	
SMART DRUG	**CONDITIONS/SYMPTOMS**
DIGOXIN	
	Chronic atrial fibrillation Congestive heart failure
ENALAPRIL, LISINOPRIL	
	Cardioprevention following MI Congestive heart failure
ENALAPRIL, LISINOPRIL	
	Cardioprevention following MI Congestive heart failure Hypertension
ASPIRIN	
	Secondary prevention of MI Stroke prevention
ESTROGEN REPLACEMENT THERAPY (WITH PROGESTERONE IF NECESSARY)	
	Cardioprevention Osteoporosis prevention Amelioration of postmeno- pausal symptoms
SEROTONIN SELECTIVE REUPTAKE INHIBITORS (E.G., SERTRALINE) OR TRICYCLIC ANTIDEPRESSANTS	
	Depression Panic attacks Pain syndromes
TRICYCLIC ANTIDEPRESSANT	
	Diabetic neuropathy Depression Sleep disorder
SERTRALINE OR TRICYCLIC ANTIDEPRESSANT	
	Depression Sleep disorder Pain management
SHORT-ACTING BENZODIAZEPINE	
	Insomnia Panic attacks Chronic anxiety

Establishing Patient Confidence and Cooperation

Practitioners with substantial clinical experience understand that streamlining a patient's drug house is much easier said than done. No matter how logical, practical, or pharmacologically justified a program of drug reduction, simplification, and consolidation may be, it always requires the patient's cooperation to put such a program into practice, and although many drugs probably do more harm than good, patients don't always perceive it that way. In fact, patients often depend heavily on their medications for reasons that may not be logical or scientific. Consequently, implementation of the DRESC program requires patient confidence and cooperation, two barriers that can be difficult to overcome. For example, older patients who have been taking multiple medications for many years often believe that drugs help them feel secure and control symptoms that otherwise might be incomprehensible, painful, or frightening. Consequently, these individuals may resist attempts at pharmacologic weaning.

Stemming the tide of pills may be the first problem that a practitioner encounters. However, the tendency to overuse drugs is not entirely the fault of patients. On occasion, a practitioner may be too busy to review medication-related information from the patient's chart. Insufficient time spent taking a case history is also a risk factor for polypharmacy. For example, a physician may fail to associate the onset of a new symptom with the introduction of a new medication into the therapeutic regimen. Patients who suffer from anxiety, somatization disorder, depression, and multiple medical conditions also are prone to the pitfalls of polypharmacy. These individuals often consult various physicians about vague and numerous complaints. Consequently, they may have a tendency to accumulate drugs. The patient may still be taking a number of these medications, perhaps intermittently, according to his or her own appraisal of symptoms and general state of health.

Successful implementation of the DRESC program requires planning, education, and patience. As a preliminary step to drug regimen simplification, the patient's current medications should be grouped into three categories: (1) drugs that are clearly not needed and can be toxic in normal doses or lethal in overdose, thus giving them the greatest potential for harm. These would include most sedative hypnotics, barbiturates, narcotics, and certain cardiovascular agents; (2) drugs that are probably unnecessary but in normal doses are not harmful. This category includes ordinary medical preparations such as thyroid replacement drugs, pain relievers such as ibuprofen, and psychotropic drugs; (3) those drugs that are reasonably safe and for which there is some medical indication. Drugs used to treat hypertension, diabetes, asthma, arthritis, and HIV-related disorders usually fall into this category.

Physician Factors. Preparing a patient to comply with the DRESC program is often a delicate process. Too often, physicians or pharmacists may simply tell their patients what to do, rather than explain why they want them to do it. In general, a patient is more likely to comply with a streamlining program if a credible reason is offered for discontinuing certain drugs. For example, the practitioner may point out that not only are some of the medications in the drug house potentially harmful, but they also may not have worked as well as expected, and a different pharmacologic approach should be tried. If the patient has more than one physician, it is imperative that all participate in the DRESC program. Usually however, the primary care practitioner or consulting pharmacist will be the liaison person for all individuals involved in writing prescriptions for the patient. Ideally, only one physician should write prescriptions. If this is not possible, all participating physicians should write prescriptions only in their specialty fields, and each should notify the others when medications are added, changed, or deleted. In addition, all medications should be filled at one pharmacy. This will reduce the likelihood that multiple or duplicate medications are prescribed for the same symptom or clinical disorder. In general, patient cooperation will be facilitated if physicians and other prescibers are collaborating on a drug reduction program.

Patient Factors. Despite initial patient reluctance to consider modifications in the drug regimen, a number of strategies are useful for informing, reassuring, and guiding patients through the DRESC program. As a prelude to drug house redesign, the patient should be educated about the risks associated with inappropriate drug prescribing and the necessity for constant reevaluation of drug house building blocks. Specifically the patient should be taught that many medications once considered state-of-the-art therapy for a particular condition have been replaced by better drugs that are dosed less frequently and produce fewer side effects. Interestingly, many patients feel insecure about reducing daily dose frequency of a medication because they think that drugs taken more frequently are better equipped to treat their condition. Physicians and pharmacists should reassure patients that medications with a long half-life, when indicated, can produce around-the-clock coverage with simpler dosing regimens. In this regard, many patients need special reassurance that *once-daily* medications used to manage high blood pressure, inflammatory osteoarthritic conditions, pain-producing syndromes, and depression are proven to be just as effective as medications previously dosed on a more frequent basis (see Table 5-5). Reassurance and education are especially necessary for patients who suffer from symptomatic clinical disorders because these individuals may tend to associate pain relief with consumption of many pills throughout the day. Informing the patient that medications dosed less frequently are able to achieve constant blood levels throughout the day, therefore, providing adequate protection against pain, may be all that is necessary to induce patient acceptance of and compliance with once-daily medications.

Reluctance to permit streamlining of drug therapy is also observed in patients who are accustomed to taking a 10- to 14-day course of antibiotic therapy to treat common infectious diseases such as pneumonia, sinusitis, cellulitis, and sexually transmitted diseases. In such cases, it may be helpful for the clinician to point out that "less is more," and that one-dose or short-duration therapeutic courses treat these infections just as effectively as older regimens (see Table 5-6).

Program Factors. As previously mentioned, patients should be reassured that the DRESC program is a *collaborative* process between physician, pharmacist, and patient (see Table 5-7). It is especially helpful to stress the importance of

Table 5-5

DRESC Strategies: Once-A-Day Drug Therapy Selected Medications With Clinical Effectiveness	
ONCE-DAILY DRUG	**COMMENTS AND ANALYSIS**
SULFONYLUREAS	
Glipizide GITS Glyburide	24-hour effectiveness
H₂ BLOCKERS	
Famotidine Ranitidine Nazatidine	Minimal risk of drug interactions
BETA-BLOCKERS	
Atenolol Acebutolol	Useful for secondary prevention of MI
PERIPHERAL ALPHA-BLOCKER	
Doxazosin	Useful in patient with high blood pressure who also has benign prostatic hypertrophy or mild elevations in blood cholesterol level.
CALCIUM CHANNEL BLOCKERS	
Amlodipine Nifedipine GITS	These agents are approved for both angina and hypertension. Amlodipine does not cause myocardial suppression.
Diltiazem CD	Diltiazem can inhibit AV node conduction and cause myocardial suppression, especially in patients with preexisting conduction disease and/or who are taking beta-blockers concurrently.
ACE INHIBITORS	
Enalapril Lisinopril	Useful for diabetic renal disease, hypertension, and congestive heart failure.
LIPID LOWERING DRUGS	
Lovastatin Parvastatin	
ANTIDEPRESSANTS	
Sertraline	Selective serotonin reuptake inhibitor with minimal inhibition of P₄₅₀ cytochrome oxidase system.

maintaining both patient-physician and patient-pharmacist communication regarding drug-induced side effects and concerns about drug costs. Cooperation is more likely if the patient is informed that only drugs deemed to be unnecessary, redundant, outdated, prescribed for excessive duration, or prescribed at inappropriately high doses will be considered for deletion or modification. Once again, education and reassurance are essential for establishing patient confidence and cooperation. It is also useful to stress that the patient's overall clinical status, as well as such parameters as blood pressure, symptom level, and pain patterns will be carefully monitored during the DRESC program.

Sometimes, patient cooperation is facilitated if individuals are presented with opportunities for lifestyle modification that will enable nonpharmacologic management of their chronic conditions. Patients frequently welcome the opportunity to be a coparticipant in a drug streamlining program, especially if they can be convinced that drug reduction and elimination will be facilitated by lifestyle modifications that include weight loss, regular physical activity, and cessation of cigarette smoking.

In general, individuals do not respond well to *precipitous* changes in their therapeutic regimen. Consequently, it is often helpful to reassure the patient that the DRESC program will be a *gradual* process, involving no more than one to two drug substitutions per 12-week cycle (see Chapter 6). Initial patient enthusiasm for a drug streamlining program frequently can be generated by stressing that significant cost savings may result from drug elimination or substitution. In those cases in which *increased* drug expenditures are required, the patient should be reassured that benefits such as quality-of-life improvements, simplified dosing, enhanced compliance, and reduced risk of drug interactions are well worth the price. Finally, it should be stressed that gaining patient confidence and cooperation for participation in a drug simplification program can be a time-consuming process. In the long run, however, laying the groundwork that will make the patient a full-fledged collaborator in the DRESC program is essential for maximizing pharmacotherapeutic results.

Cost Considerations and Potential Risks

One of the principal objectives of the DRESC program is to *reduce* overall medical expenditures associated with a long-term therapeutic regimen (see Table 5-8). To achieve this objective, however, increased *short-term* costs associated with multiple consultations may be required. It is important to remember, however, that the purpose of these visits is to identify medications that are unnecessary and can be eliminated, thereby producing *long-term cost savings* to the patient. In general, when generic medications are replaced by brand-name products, increases in drug costs can be expected. However, the newer, more expensive medications may be associated with better compliance, dose stability, regimen durability, and fewer side effects. Often these advantages will justify the increased costs. There are many opportunities for offsetting the costs associated with introducing more expensive and better-tolerated agents into the drug house.

Table 5-6

DRESC PROGRAM: ONE DOSE/SHORT DURATION THERAPEUTIC OPTIONS FOR INFECTIONS	
Condition/Disease	**One Dose/Short Course Option**
Nonspecific bacterial vaginosis	Metronidazole, 2 g PO
Trichomoniasis	Metronidazole, 2 g PO (contraindicated during first trimester of pregnancy)
Chancroid	Azithromycin 1 g PO or ceftriaxone, 250 mg IM
Candida vaginitis	Fluconazole, 150 mg PO or tioconazole 6.5% vaginal ointment
Gonorrhea	Ceftriaxone, 125 mg IM or cefixime, 400 mg PO or ciprofloxacin, 500 mg PO or ofloxacin, 400 mg PO
Chlamydia (uncomplicated) (cervicitis, urethritis)	Azithromycin 1 g PO
Cellulitis *(Staphylococcus aureus, Streptococcus)*	Azithromycin, 500 mg PO day 1, 250 mg PO gel x 4 days
Otitis media (children)	Ceftriaxone, 50 mg/kg IM once
Urinary tract infection (uncomplicated)	TMP/SMZ 4 tabs PO once (high relapse rate, 35%) TMP/SMZ 1 tab PO bid × 3 days (relapse rate reduced to 15%)
Whipworm Infection *(Truchuris trichiuria)*	Albendazole, 400 mg PO
Pinworm Infection *(Enterobius vermicularis)*	Mebendazole, 100 mg PO and repeat after 2 weeks
Hookworm *(Necator Americanus)*	Albendazole, 400 mg PO or mebendazole, 100 mg PO
Scabies/Mites *(Sarcoptes scabei)*	Permethrin (5%) massage from head to soles; wash off after 8-14 hours
Body Lice *(Pediculus huanus coporis)*	Pyrethrin with piperonyl butoxide; apply lotion for 10 minutes, then bathe
Corticosteroid taper (asthma, allergic reactions)	5-7 day tapering of drug as effective as longer tapering courses

Table 5-7

The DRESC Program:
Establishing Patient Confidence and Cooperation

THE FOLLOWING STRATEGIES WILL HELP INFORM, REASSURE, AND GUIDE PATIENTS THROUGH REGIMEN STREAMLINING:

- Educate patient about risks associated with inappropriate drug prescribing and necessity of evaluation of drug house building blocks

- Emphasize that DRESC program is a collaborative process between physician, pharmacist, and patient

- Stress that significant cost savings may be accomplished with DRESC changes

- Inform patient that original indications for using certain drugs may have changed and that it is possible that medications can be deleted without adverse effects

- Reassure patient that clinical status and parameters (blood pressure, symptom level, pain patterns, etc.) will be carefully monitored during DRESC program

- Reassure patient that only drugs deemed to be unnecessary, redundant, outdated, prescribed for excessive duration, or at inappropriately high doses will be considered for modification

- Inform patient of opportunities for nonpharmacologic management (weight loss, dietary modifications, etc.) for certain disorders

- Emphasize importance of medication compliance and its relation to daily dose frequency

- Stress advantages of simplified drug regimens

- Reassure patient that DRESC program is a gradual process, involving no more than 1-2 drug substitutions per cycle

- Stress importance of patient-physician communication regarding drug-induced side effects and lifestyle changes noted during DRESC process

Clearly, the most desirable approach is to selectively eliminate medications that are unnecessary from the therapeutic regimen, consolidate two or more drugs with the use of a single agent, and/or introduce better agents that are of similar cost. Nevertheless, it should be stressed that if the improved drug regimen is, indeed, more costly than the original regimen, this increase in drug cost may be justified.

Although the DRESC program is designed to produce more streamlined, better tolerated pharmacotherapeutic regimens, there are potential risks (see Table 5-9). For example, the practitioner may discontinue a medication that is needed by the patient. Naturally, precautions should be taken to avoid elimination of necessary medications. Discontinuation of medications such as digoxin, theophylline, antidepressants, or corticosteroids requires careful clinical monitoring and evaluation. Inappropriate elimination of medications can be prevented by establishing strict criteria for drug discontinuation. For example, digoxin should not be discontinued in patients who have documented congestive heart failure. However, it may be appropriate to attempt discontinuation of this agent in individuals who have normal sinus rhythm and who have echocardiographic confirmation of normal ventricular function.

Table 5-8

Cost Considerations Associated With DRESC Program
• Increased short-term cost of multiple physician/pharmacist consultations will be more than offset by reduction in long-term cost savings associated with a streamlined drug regimen
• Potential increases in cost of some drug substitutions may be offset by reduction in total outcome costs produced by better medication compliance
• Post-DRESC program (i.e., reconstructed) drug regimen may be less costly than original therapeutic regimen
• If post-DRESC program drug regimen is more costly than original therapeutic regimen, these potential increases in drug cost may still be associated with reduced costs associated with return visits, drug monitoring costs, and therapeutic failures caused by poor compliance

Table 5-9

Potential Risks of the DRESC Program
• Elimination of necessary medications
• Clinical deterioration caused by reduction of drug dosage
• Erosion of patient confidence in drug regimen
• Introduction of unexpected side effects
• Introduction of unexpected drug interactions
• Reduced clinical efficacy of reconstructed drug regimen
• Increased cost of reconstructed drug regimen

Discontinuation of antidepressants may precipitate episodes of severe clinical depression. Elimination of these agents is more likely to be successful in patients with limited, situational depression and in those persons who have had no more than one episode of serious depression in the last 5 years. Clinical deterioration can result not only from drug cessation but from reduction of drug dosage. Many of these problems can be avoided by careful screening and clinical monitoring of drugs that are withdrawn (see Tables 5-10 and 5-11).

Other potential risks of the DRESC program include introduction of unexpected side effects from the addition of new agents or the precipitation of unexpected drug interactions. As a rule, however, the purpose of DRESC program drug substitutions is to identify medications with fewer side effects and drug interactions. Nevertheless, sometimes the reconstructed drug regimen may produce undesirable side effects, in which case other therapeutic alternatives should be considered. Whenever drug deletions, substitutions, or additions are made, it is always possible that the reconstructed drug house will not be as clinically effective as the original regimen. For example, a patient who is taking a thiazide diuretic and beta-blocker for the management of hypertension may find that his blood pressure is not as well controlled with the ACE inhibitor that is substituted for the two original antihypertensive agents. In such cases, it may be worth considering the use of another antihypertensive agent, such as a calcium blocker, instead of the ACE inhibitor, before returning the patient to the original drug regimen. The point is, reduction of clinical efficacy is a potential liability of any reconstructed drug house, and, therefore, careful clinical monitoring is mandatory whenever drug substitutions or consolidations are made.

ELIMINATION OF UNNECESSARY PRESCRIPTION DRUGS

Elimination of unnecessary prescription drugs is one of the cornerstones of the DRESC program. The process of drug elimination begins with a careful review of the patient's current medication list. There are many opportunities and indications for cessation of prescription medications, all of which deserve careful consideration (see Table 5-12). For example, some commonly used medications can be discontinued simply because the initial indications for starting the drug were insufficient in the first place. In other cases, drugs can be eliminated because they are being used for a duration of time that extends beyond the window of therapeutic opportunity (see Table 5-11). For example, maintenance therapy with H_2 blockers beyond 12 months duration is usually not required for patients with mild peptic ulcer disease, especially those with no history of gastrointestinal hemorrhage. Similarly, short-acting benzodiazepines should initially be prescribed for brief duration courses only. The original indications for initiating drugs from this class should always be reviewed, and unless there are continuing indications for long-term maintenance therapy, drug discontinuation should be considered. Sometimes a drug can be eliminated because new clinical trials demonstrate that the agent is not useful in the condition for which it was thought to be effective. For example, dipyridamole is commonly used in patients with cerebrovascular disease, despite the fact that a number of well-designed clinical trials confirm that it offers no advantages over aspirin in the prevention of transient ischemic attacks, stroke, or myocardial infarction. Similar justifications can be given for discontinuing cyclandelate and isoxsuprine, both of which have been shown to be ineffective for the treatment of chronic dementia. Antiarrhythmic agents represent some of the most dramatic examples of medications

Table 5-10

Medications That May Be Suitable For Elimination Because of Inappropriate or Questionable Indications For Clinical Use	
DRUG	**COMMENTS AND ANALYSIS**
DIGOXIN	
	Useful in patients with *documented* CHF and for rate control in chronic atrial fibrillation. Digoxin is overused in patients with normal sinus rhythm and a presumptive diagnosis of CHF, which should be confirmed with objective criteria such as echocardiography.
MISOPROSTOL	
	Should not be used just because patient is over 65 years of age and is on long-term NSAID therapy. Cost-effective therapy is limited to patients who require NSAIDs and who also have a documented history of peptic or gastric ulcer disease.
DIPYRIDAMOLE	
	Aspirin is more effective at lower cost for prevention of secondary MI, TIAs, and stroke. Persantine may have role as adjunct therapy in patients with prosthetic heart valves.
CHOLESTYRAMINE	
	Noncompliance is extremely common and undermines clinical efficacy of the drug. Alternatives such as lovastatin are generally preferrable.
THEOPHYLLINE	
	This drug is overused in treatment of bronchospastic pulmonary disease, COPD, and asthma. Prior to inclusion of theophylline in a drug regimen, inhaled beta-agonists or inhaled corticosteroids (in asthmatic patients) should be tried, and compliance with metered-dose inhalers should be ensured by providing instructions to patients or using spacer.

Table 5-10

Medications That May Be Suitable For Elimination Because of Inappropriate or Questionable Indications For Clinical Use — cont'd.

DRUG	COMMENTS AND ANALYSIS
PROPOXYPHENE	
	Equally effective analgesics available with less toxicity.
BENZODIAZEPINES	
Diazepam Chlordiazepoxide Clonazepam Flurazepam Oxazepam Lorazepam	Review original indications for drug. Many patients can have benzodiazepines slowly discontinued over several weeks.
ANTIARRHYTHMICS	
Flecainide Quinidine	Generally not indicated for outpatient management of nonlife-threatening arrhythmias. Use of quinidine in patients with atrial fibrillation.
OMEPRAZOLE	
	Long-term safety may soon be established, but this agent is sometimes introduced into regimen for treatment of erosive esophagitis or peptic ulcer disease before attempting more conservative, less costly therapy with H_2 blockers.
PENTOZIFYLLINE	
	Efficacy in conditions other than severe claudication not established.
TACRINE	
	Efficacy of tacrine in patients with Alzheimer's disease is limited to patients with mild to moderate disease.
NSAIDS	
	Acetaminophen should be tried for analgesia before committing patients to long-term NSAID use.

Table 5-11

DRESC Screening For Drugs With Established or Possible Duration Limits	
DRUG	**COMMENTS AND ANALYSIS**
HISTAMINE ANTAGONISTS	
Cimetidine Ranitidine Famotidine Nizatidine	Maintenance therapy for 12 months is indicated in patients with documented peptic or gastric ulceration. Long-term maintenance therapy (i.e., > 12 months) is generally not indicated, except in patients who continue to be at high risk for complications such as hemorrhage.
SHORT-ACTING BENZODIAZEPINES	
	Therapy for sleep disorders, anxiety, and panic attacks should initially be short-term. Patients with panic attacks who are symptom-free for at least 6 months are appropriate candidates for gradual discontinuation of alprazolam.
OMEPRAZOLE	
	Not recommended for long-term maintenance therapy.
ORAL ANTIBIOTICS	
	Long-term suppressive therapy rarely indicated except in patients with HIV infection.
PHENYTOIN	
	Patients who have an idiopathic seizure disorder and are seizure-free for 3 years or longer may be tapered off the drug and monitored.
ANTIHYPERTENSIVE AGENTS	
	Step-down therapy may be attempted in patients with mild hypertension who have excellent control with monotherapy. Tapering dose and/or elimination of antihypertensive agents is encouraged, especially in patients who have implemented lifestyle changes (i.e., weight reduction, increased exercise, etc.) for nonpharmacologic management of hypertension.

Table 5-11

DRESC Screening For Drugs With Established or Possible Duration Limits — cont'd.	
DRUG	**COMMENTS AND ANALYSIS**
ANTIDEPRESSANTS	
	Step-down therapy may be advisable in patients with self-limited, situational depression, and in those individuals with no more than one episode of serious depression in the last 3 years. Lifetime maintenance *usually* is required in patients who are 50 years old or more at the onset of their first major depressive episode, aged 40 or more at onset with two or more depressive episodes, or with more than three prior episodes at any age.
ORAL SULFONYLUREAS	
	Dose reduction or discontinuation may be possible in patients who pursue active lifestyle modifications (weight reduction, exercise, etc.) known to lower blood glucose.
BETA-BLOCKERS	
	Beta-blockers are useful for preventing myocardial reinfarction, but studies suggest this cardioprotective effect is demonstrable for no longer than 24 months following acute myocardial infarction.
CORTICOSTEROIDS	
	Short duration tapering course of 7-10 days are as effective as long tapering courses (i.e., 2-3 weeks) in preventing exacerbations of asthma.

Table 5-12

Opportunities and Indications For Possible Elimination of Unnecessary Prescription Drugs
• Inadequate initial indications for beginning medication (example: digoxin, benzodiazepine, misoprostol etc.)
• Drug can be eliminated because it has been used for duration that extends beyond window of opportunity (example: H2 blocker)
• Drug can be eliminated because new clinical trials show it is not useful in condition for which it was thought to be effective (example: dipyridamole, isoxsuprine, hydergine)
• Drug can be eliminated because less toxic agents are available that produce equivalent clinical result (example: theophylline, indocin, indomethacin)
• Drug may be eliminated because patient is clinically stable for long periods without exacerbations of disease state (example: dilantin, corticosteroids)
• Drug can possibly be eliminated because condition has stabilized and pharmacologic therapy is no longer required for clinical maintenance (example: antihypertensive medications, antiulcer drugs, theophylline)
• Drug can be eliminated because less expensive, equally effective agents are available (ticlodipine, dipyridamole)
• Drug can be eliminated because it is associated with noncompliance (example: cholestyramine)

that now can be eliminated based on recent clinical trials that show this drug class does not prevent morbidity or mortality in patients who have nonlife-threatening ventricular ectopy.

In some cases, medications can be eliminated because less toxic agents are available that produce equivalent clinical results. For example, a prescriber may eliminate theophylline in an asthmatic patient experiencing gastrointestinal side effects and replace it with an inhaled beta-agonist, producing equivalent relief with far less toxicity. Drug cessation may be especially successful in individuals who are clinically stable for long periods of time and have no exacerbations of their disease. For example, a patient with an idiopathic seizure disorder who is epilepsy-free for three or more years while taking dilantin may be a candidate for drug discontinuation. Similarly, patients who remain clinically stable for long periods while taking corticosteroids, NSAIDs, and benzodiazepines should be considered for drug discontinuation. Naturally, drug substitution should be attempted when less expensive, equally effective agents are available. Finally, some drugs can be eliminated simply because they are associated with patient noncompliance.[33] Although cholestyramine, when taken as prescribed, will lower serum cholesterol levels, few patients are able to tolerate a drug with the consistency of liquid sand. There are many other drugs which, because they require a complicated dosing schedule, produce virtually intolerable side effects, or are associated with extraordinary financial expenditures, may require evaluation for drug cessation or substitution, simply because they are associated with poor compliance patterns that undermine therapeutic efficacy.

Drug Discontinuation in the Elderly

The opportunities and indications for medication discontinuation in the *elderly* warrant special attention (see Table 5-13). Individuals aged 65 years or older account for about 25% of all prescription drug use in the United States and are at high risk for adverse drug effects. Polypharmacy, which is common in the geriatric population, sharply increases the risk of side effects.

In 1991, a comprehensive set of explicit criteria was published for inadequate drug-prescribing practices in the elderly based on the following three concepts: (1) prescription medications that should be entirely avoided in the elderly; (2) excessive dosage; and (3) excessive duration of treatment. Using these criteria, a recent investigation developed conservative estimates of the incidence of potentially inappropriate prescribing practices for community-dwelling elderly persons in the United States.[34]

The investigators reported an alarming incidence of prescriptions in the elderly for 20 potentially inappropriate drugs, using explicit criteria previously developed by Canadian and American geriatric experts. In particular, this landmark study demonstrated that a total of 23.5% of people aged 65 years or older living in the community, or about 6.64 million Americans, received *at least one* of the 20 contraindicated drugs. While 79.6% of the people receiving potentially inappropriate medications received only one such drug, about 20% received two or more of these contraindicated agents. Among the drugs considered inappropriate in this population, the most commonly prescribed medications were dipyridamole, propoxyphene, amitriptyline, chlorpropamide, diazepam, indomethacin, and chlordiazepoxide, each of which was taken by at least 600,000 individuals aged 65 years or older. If one includes three controversial cardiovascular agents (propranolol, methyldopa, and reserpine) in the list of contraindicated drugs, the incidence of inappropriate medication use rose to 32%, or 9 million people. The study concluded that physicians prescribed potentially inappropriate medications for nearly a quarter of all older people living in the community, placing them at risk for adverse drug effects such as cognitive impairment and sedation.[34-36]

Inappropriate Medications

Anxiolytics. Medications considered to be inappropriate include those that ought to be entirely avoided, those used in excessive dosages, and drugs used for an excessive duration. Among the sedative or hypnotic agents, diazepam, chlordiazepoxide, flurazepam, and meprobamate should generally be considered inappropriate for use in the elderly patient. Many of these benzodiazepines have a prolonged half-life, produce increased daytime sedation, and are associated with an increased risk of falls and hip fractures. When benzodiazepine use *is* indicated

Table 5-13

DRESC Program Summary of Inappropriate Medication Use: Drugs To Be Avoided In The Elderly	
DRUG CLASS	**REASON FOR AVOIDANCE**
SEDATIVE OR HYPNOTIC AGENTS	
Diazepam Chlordiazepoxide Flurazepam	Prolonged half-life, increased daytime sedation, increased risk of falls and hip fractures. Shorter acting benzo-diazepines such as lorazepam, temazepam, etc. considered safer.
Meprobamate	Considered to be less safe than short-acting benzodiazepines for treatment of anxiety and sleep disturbance.
SHORT-DURATION BARBITURATES	
Pentobarbital	Shorter-acting benzodiazepines safer for sedation in the elderly and phenobarbital preferable in epilepsy
TRICYCLIC ANTIDEPRESSANTS	
Amitriptyline Doxepin	Anticholinergic side effects, orthostatic hypotension, and sedation more pronounced than with serotonin selective reuptake inhibitors (i.e., ser-traline, flouxetine, etc.,) that are preferrable in the elderly
COMBINATION ANTIDEPRESSANTS/ANTIPSYCHOTICS	
	Geriatric doses are difficult to titrate in fixed-dose combinations
NONSTEROIDAL ANTIINFLAMMATORY DRUGS (NSAIDS)	
Indomethacin	Greater CNS, gastrointestinal, and renal toxicity, than other NSAIDs. Indomethicin may also cause coronary vasocon-striction and interfere with antianginal effects of beta blockers. The drug may be indicated for treatment of acute gout, but colchicine may be a better option in the elderly.

Table 5-13

DRESC Program Summary of Inappropriate Medication Use: Drugs To Be Avoided In The Elderly — cont'd.	
DRUG CLASS	**REASON FOR AVOIDANCE**
PROPIONIC ACID NSAIDS	
Ibuprofen Ketoprofen Fenoprofen	Some evidence to suggest these drugs are more likely to cause renal deterioration in the elderly than other NSAIDs, such as those in the oxicam (piroxicam) or indole acetic acid (sulindac) groups.
ORAL SULFONYLUREAS	
Chlorpropamide	Long half-life and binding to serum proteins increases risk of hypoglycemia; risk of syndrome of inappropriate antidiuretic hormone secretion increased with chlor-propamide. Glipizide GITS and glyburide are better options in the elderly.
ANALGESICS	
Propoxyphene	Relatively ineffective (perhaps no better pain relief than acetaminophen) and low toxic-to-therapeutic ratio may cause CNS and cardiac toxicity from accumulation of toxic metabolites.
Pentazocine	Overdose is associated with seizures and cardiotoxicity.
DEMENTIA THERAPIES	
Cyclandelate Isoxsuprine	No demonstrated efficacy for these drugs.
PLATELET INHIBITORS	
Dipyridamole	Useful only as adjunct to warfarin therapy in patients with artificial heart valves. Use for prophylaxis in other conditions not substantiated. Can cause headache, dizzi-ness, and CNS disturbances at higher doses.

Table 5-13

DRESC Program Summary of Inappropriate Medication Use: Drugs To Be Avoided In The Elderly — cont'd.	
DRUG CLASS	**REASON FOR AVOIDANCE**
MUSCLE RELAXANTS/ANTISPASMODICS	
Cyclobenzaprine Orphenadrine Methocarbamol Carisoprodol	Potential CNS toxicity outweighs benefits
ANTIEMETIC AGENTS	
Trimethobenzamide	Less effective than other agents and may cause drowsiness, rash, diarrhea, and extrapyramidal reactions.
ANTIHYPERTENSIVES	
Propranolol Methyldopa Reserpine Verapamil	Better agents available with fewer side effects
BRONCHODILATORS	
Theophylline Terbutaline	Toxicity increased in the elderly. Inhaled beta agonists should be tried first.
H$_2$ BLOCKERS	
Cimetidine	Inhibits P$_{450}$ cytochrome oxidase system and, therefore, it has the potential to cause drug interactions with a wide range of commonly used therapeutic agents. Although not strictly contraindicated in the elderly, H$_2$ blockers (e.g., famotidine) that do not inhibit drug metabolism are preferrable, especially in patients on polypharmacy.

in an elderly patient, shorter-acting agents such as lorazepam, temazepam, or oxazepam are considered to be safer. Meprobamate is considered to be less safe than short-acting benzodiazepines for the treatment of anxiety and sleep disturbances. Short duration barbiturates such as pentobarbital and secobarbital are generally not advised for the geriatric patient, in whom shorter-acting benzodiazepines have proven safer for sedation. In general, patients should be converted from long-acting to short-acting benzodiazepine therapy. In many cases, benzodiazepine therapy may be eliminated altogether, and if gradual tapering programs are followed, withdrawal symptoms can be minimized.[17,26,40]

The decision to discontinue use of a benzodiazepine can be difficult. After all, patients frequently take these anxiolytic agents for many years and depend on them for behavioral and emotional stability. On the other hand, these drugs are frequently started for management of short-term, situational crises and then become permanent fixtures in the drug house. On occasion, the patient is unaware that physical or psychological addiction has occurred and may pressure the physician into long-term maintenance therapy.[26,43] These cases can be difficult to manage because the patient believes that the anxiolytic agent is still required for symptomatic relief. Also, the physician may be reluctant to withdraw a drug that has the potential for producing withdrawal symptoms.

Despite these obstacles to benzodiazepine cessation, physicians and pharmacists should carefully evaluate the original reasons for prescribing drugs in this class. Ideally, this review is conducted in collaboration with the patient, who may provide valuable information. Patients often express their own willingness to attempt a program of drug cessation under careful physician supervision. Benzodiazepines that should be targeted for elimination, when appropriate, include diazepam, chlordiazepoxide, flurazepam, oxazepam, lorazepam, and alprazolam. Success rates are improved when the tapering process is extremely gradual (over 3 to 6 months), if the patient is informed about the likely withdrawal symptoms and if supportive counseling is provided.

The elimination of amitriptyline and doxepin is usually justified in this age group because anticholinergic side effects such as orthostatic hypotension, sedation, and confusion are more pronounced with tricyclic antidepressants than with serotonin selective reuptake inhibitors (SSRI) (e.g., sertraline, fluoxetine), which are preferable in the elderly. Use of combination antidepressant/antipsychotic agents are discouraged because geriatric doses are difficult to titrate in fixed-dose combinations.[37,38] If behavioral disturbances, symptoms related to anxiety, aggressive behavior, and sleep patterns are well-controlled it is appropriate to consider incremental elimination or dosage reduction of psychotropic medications. (See Table 5-14)[39] This is especially true if excessive sedation or lethargy is a problem. In addition, it is reasonable to reduce antidepressant drug use to 50% of the recommended dose and evaluate the patient for clinical deterioration. If antidepressant medications *are* needed, it is usually preferable to convert patients from tricyclic antidepressants to SSRIs. In those patients on polypharmacy regimens who are already taking fluoxetine, a case can be made for substitution of sertraline, which has less pronounced effects on the P450 cytochrome oxidase system.

NSAIDs. The use of NSAIDs remains controversial, and all opportunities for eliminating this drug class from a patient's regimen should be pursued. In particular, indomethacin and phenylbutazone are inappropriate medications for the geriatric patient. Indomethacin is associated with greater central nervous system, gastrointestinal, and renal toxicity than other NSAIDs. Indomethacin may also cause coronary vasoconstriction and interfere with the antianginal

Table 5-14

DRESC PROGRAM STRATEGIES FOR REDUCTION AND CONSOLIDATION OF PSYCHOTROPIC MEDICATIONS
• Review original indications for psychotropic drug use: if behavioral disturbance, symptoms,
• In elderly, reduce antidepressant to 50% of recommended dose and evaluate for clinical deterioration
• Convert patient from long-acting to short-acting benzodiazepines (if benzodiazepine therapy is still required)
• Convert patient from tricyclic antidepressant to serotonin selective reuptake inhibitor, if there are no contraindications
• In elderly patient on multiple medications, consider converting from fluoxetine (P450 cytochrome oxidase inhibitor) to sertraline (minimal P450 cytochrome oxidase inhibition).
• Alprazolam: Patients with panic attacks who have been symptom-free for at least six months are appropriate candidates for gradual discontinuation of alprazolam.

effects of beta blockers. Although this drug is indicated for the treatment of acute gout, colchicine may be a better, less toxic option. Phenylbutazone, which is no longer available in the U.S., is more likely than other NSAIDs to cause bone marrow toxicity and renal deterioration and should be eliminated from the drug houses of all older patients. There is even some evidence to suggest that propionic acid group NSAIDs such as ibuprofen, ketoprofen, and fenoprofen are more likely to cause renal deterioration in the elderly than other NSAIDs. The decision to eliminate an NSAID from the therapeutic regimen of an older patient requires consideration of multiple clinical factors. If an agent from this drug class is indicated, phenylbutazone and indomethacin should be avoided, and preference should be given to once-daily NSAIDs that cause less GI toxicity. Finally, some patients may achieve adequate symptomatic or pain relief with acetaminophen.

Analgesics. The appropriateness of analgesic drug use in the elderly requires evaluation on a case-by-case basis. It should be stressed that patients with chronic pain, terminal malignancy, and other disabling inflammatory disorders should not be deprived of narcotic pain medication. In fact, there are many studies that indicate that pain medications are *underused* in older patients. Nevertheless, there are better and worse choices when it comes to selecting analgesics in this patient population. Propoxyphene should be avoided because it is relatively ineffective. When taken in excessive quantities, propoxyphene can cause central nervous system, hepatic, and cardiac toxicity due to accumulation of toxic metabolites. Similarly, pentazocine should be avoided in the elderly because overdose is associated with seizures and cardiotoxicity. Consequently, when either propoxyphene or pentazocine appear in the drug regimen of an older individual, strong consideration should be given to their elimination. If pain relief is needed, therapy with either codeine or hydrocodone is preferable.

Neuromuscular Agents. Although there are strong pressures to use therapies aimed at improving cognitive and behavioral function in patients with chronic dementia, there is no justification for maintaining patients on medications that have no demonstrated efficacy in this condition. Therefore, cyclandelate and isoxsuprine can be eliminated from the drug houses of older patients. Although their toxicity may be minimal, ineffective treatments are difficult to justify. Dipyridamole, which is prescribed for many patients with cerebrovascular disease, does not improve clinical outcomes in patients with transient ischemic attacks, strokes, carotid stenosis, or cardiovascular disease. Its use for prophylaxis in these conditions cannot be substantiated, and, therefore, the drug should be eliminated from nearly all drug regimens. It may, however, be useful as an adjunct to warfarin therapy in patients with artificial heart valves. Elimination of this drug is justified not only because it can cause headache, dizziness, and central nervous system disturbances at higher doses, but also because it is relatively expensive.

There are a number of reasons to discontinue use of muscle relaxants and antispasmodic drugs such as cyclobenzaprine, orphenadrine, methocarbamol, and carisoprodol. Several of these agents have anticholinergic side effects. In others, the potential central nervous system toxicity of the agent outweighs its potential benefits. Trimethobenzamide should be avoided in older patients because it is less effective than other antiemetic agents, and may cause drowsiness, rash, diarrhea, and extrapyramidal reactions.

Antihypertensive Agents. The elimination of specific antihypertensive agents from the drug houses of older individuals is a highly controversial topic. Most geriatric experts agree that propranolol, methyldopa, reserpine, and verapamil should be avoided in the majority of elderly patients. Propranolol is a lipophilic agent, and, therefore, is more likely to penetrate the central nervous system and cause such symptoms as lethargy, fatigue, and depression. Methyldopa and reserpine also can cause sedation, sexual dysfunction, and mood disturbances. Verapamil should be avoided because of its propensity to produce bradyarrhythmias, AV node conduction disturbances, and myocardial suppression that can sometimes lead to congestive heart failure. Naturally, caution is required when eliminating these medications from a drug regimen.[41,42] Precipitous withdrawal of a beta blocker such as propranolol can precipitate rebound angina; therefore, if discontinuation of one beta blocker is contemplated, substitution with another agent from the same therapeutic class is usually recommended. When antihypertensive medications are withdrawn, the patient should be monitored closely, and if blood pressure rises, new agents may be required.

As a rule, drugs used to treat hypertension are used for appropriate reasons.[44-46] However, because the decision to start antihypertensive therapy has long-term implications, it is prudent to review the original indications for beginning blood pressure-lowering medications. Patients who have normal or subnormal blood pressure recordings on *multiple* clinic visits while taking medication may be candidates for discontinuation of treatment. An examination of the medical records should attempt to establish that the diagnosis of hypertension was not made on the basis of a single measurement. Patients on monotherapy who are consistently normotensive over a one-year period should have their records reviewed to ensure that their initial elevated blood pressure measurements were confirmed on at least two subsequent visits over a period of several weeks. In addition, patients who were not given a 3- to 6-month trial of nonpharmacologic therapy (i.e., lifestyle changes and modifications known to reduce blood pressure) should: (1) be instructed in a weight reduction program if the patient is overweight; (2) be encouraged to engage in aerobic exercise regularly; and (3) be persuaded to limit alcohol intake. Although discontinuation of antihypertensive medications is oftentimes *not* possible, those patients who are taking a single drug, who are consistently normotensive, and whose records fail to confirm multiple elevated blood pressure measurements at the onset of therapy, constitute the best candidates for discontinuation of blood pressure lowering medications (see Table 5-15).

Bronchodilators. Bronchodilators such as theophylline and terbutaline should be eliminated from the drug regimens of older patients whenever possible. Side effects associated with these agents are increased in the elderly, in whom life-threatening toxicity is not uncommon. In general, inhaled beta agonists are preferable to theophylline for the management of bronchospastic pulmonary disease. Finally, elimination of cimetidine and substitution with another H_2 blocker is recommended in all older patients who are taking three or more different prescription ingredients.

Gastrointestinal Agents. Among drugs used to treat gastrointestinal disorders, a careful evaluation of medications such as misoprostol, H_2 blockers, and omeprazole may reveal situations in which these agents were started for inappropriate or questionable reasons. For example, misoprostol should not be used just because a patient is over the age of 65 and is taking long-term NSAID therapy. Therapy with misoprostol should be limited to patients who require NSAID therapy and who *also* have a documented history of peptic or gastric ulcer disease. And although omeprazole is a highly effective treatment for erosive esophagitis and peptic ulcer disease, this agent should not be used until more conservative, less costly therapy with H_2 blockers is attempted. Finally, the use of H_2 blockers should be limited to short-term therapy for those individuals with suspected peptic ulcer disease. Long-term maintenance therapy is justified only in patients with recurrent disease, as well as those who are at high risk for incurring complications such as gastrointestinal hemorrhage.

Digoxin. Although cardiovascular drugs are important for the management of patients with congestive heart failure, hypertension, and cardiac arrhythmias, a number of medications used for these conditions can be eliminated. Unfortunately, there is still considerable confusion about the role of digoxin therapy in patients with congestive heart failure. Digoxin is a useful agent for patients with left ventricular dysfunction. In fact, numerous trials show that when digoxin is discontinued in patients with mild to moderate congestive heart failure, clinical deterioration is likely. Therefore, patients whose medical records contain diagnostic studies that confirm the presence of left ventricular systolic dysfunction

Table 5-15

·DRESC PROGRAM STRATEGIES FOR ANTIHYPERTENSIVE THERAPY: Indications for treatment, step-down therapy, discontinuation, and lifestyle modifications

Step 1: Ensure that blood pressure requires therapy before initiating pharmacotherapeutic intervention

- Hypertension should *not* be diagnosed on the basis of a single measurement
- Blood pressure ≥ 140/90 justifies treatment
- Initial elevated readings should be confirmed on at least two subsequent visits during one to several weeks (unless systolic BP > 210 mm Hg and/or diastolic BP > 120 mm Hg, in which case immediate therapy is justified)
- When readings are obtained, two or more measurements separated by two minutes should be recorded and averaged. If the first two readings differ by more than 5 mm Hg, additional readings should be obtained.
- Measurements should be taken after 5 minutes at rest, and it is important to ensure that patient has not ingested caffeine, a phenylpropanolamine-containing compound, or smoked cigarettes 30 minutes prior to recording.
- Blood pressure characterized by systolic readings in the 130-139 mm Hg range and diastolic blood pressure in the 85-89 mm Hg range should be rechecked in 1 year; systolic readings in the 140-159 mm Hg range and diastolic blood pressure in the 90-99 mm
  Hg range should be confirmed within 2 months; systolic readings in the 160-179 mm Hg range and diastolic blood pressure in the 100-109 mm Hg range require evaluation and referral to definitive source of care within 1 month.
- The presence of target organ disease is an indicate for evaluation, prompt referral, and treatment.

Step 2: Attempt a 3-6 month trial of nonpharmacologic therapy (i.e., in cases of mild to moderate hypertension, vigorously encourage the following lifestyle modifications known to reduce blood pressure)

- Instruct patient in weight reduction program if the patient is overweight
- Limit alcohol intake to < 1 oz per day of ethanol (24 oz beer, 8 oz of wine, or 2 oz of 100 proof whiskey)
- Aerobic exercise regularly
- Reduce sodium intake to < 100 mmol/d (< 2.3 g of sodium or approximately < 6 g of sodium chloride)
- Stop smoking
- Reduce dietary intake of saturated fat and cholesterol for overall cardiovascular health.

Table 5-15

DRESC PROGRAM STRATEGIES FOR
ANTIHYPERTENSIVE THERAPY:
Indications for treatment, step-down therapy, discontinuation, and
lifestyle° modifications — cont'd.

Step 3: If measures outlined under Step 2 above produce inadequate blood pressure control, then lifestyle modifications should continue and pharmacologic therapy should be initiated.

- Initial choice of agent is controversial, but in general, unless cost is an absolute deterrent to medication acquisition, therapy with a calcium blocker, ACE inhibitor, or alpha-blocker is recommended (See Table 3-4). This agent should be started at the lowest recommended daily dose.
- When cost is the sole barrier to drug acquisition and compliance, therapy with a thiazide diuretic or beta-blocker is indicated.
- If an inadequate response is observed, it is preferable to maintain a single agent at a higher dose level, but only if no side effects are observed at this dose.
- If side effects are observed at any dose, substitute another agent or reduce dose of the drug and start additional agent at low dose.

Step 4: Situations in which automated, noninvasive ambulatory blood pressure monitoring devices may be useful

- "Office" or "white-coat" hypertension (i.e. blood pressure is repeatedly elevated in office or clinic setting but is repeatedly normal in other environments).
- Unexplained drug resistance
- Unexplained nocturnal blood pressure changes
- Episodic hypertension

Step 5: Is ongoing drug therapy still required for hypertension?

- "Step Down" approach is encouraged, which includes elimination of drug or dose reduction if blood pressure is controlled for more than 1 year.

should not have digoxin discontinued from their therapeutic regimen. In addition, patients who require digoxin for ventricular rate control are also suitable candidates for long-term maintenance therapy with digoxin. Occasionally, however, congestive heart failure is overdiagnosed in the outpatient population. If physicians rely *solely* on physical examination and history to diagnose congestive heart failure in the ambulatory patient, approximately 25% of these individuals will be inappropriately treated with digoxin because subsequent echocardiography will reveal normal left ventricular function. It is this overdiagnosis of congestive heart failure that is primarily responsible for the excessive prescribing of digoxin. Therefore, if a careful review of the medical records of a patient who is taking digoxin therapy fails to turn up objective, confirmatory evidence for congestive heart failure, and the patient is in normal sinus rhythm, attempts to discontinue digoxin therapy are indicated.

Antiarrhythmic Agents. Antiarrhythmic agents such as encainide, flecainide, and others are generally not indicated for outpatient management of nonlife-threatening ventricular arrhythmias. Even the use of quinidine to maintain patients in normal sinus rhythm after being pharmacologically cardioverted from atrial fibrillation has been seriously questioned. There is now strong evidence to suggest that patients with coronary heart disease and congestive heart failure who once had atrial fibrillation but are now maintained in normal sinus rhythm with quinidine, have twice the mortality rate as patients who remain in atrial fibrillation and have their ventricular rates controlled with digoxin alone. Therefore, physicians and pharmacists should review the original reasons for initiating quinidine therapy. If medical records indicate that quinidine was started to maintain normal sinus rhythm after atrial fibrillation, careful consideration should be given to discontinuing the drug, observing the patient for recurrence of the arrhythmia, and, if ventricular rate problems emerge, treating them with AV node blocking agents such as digoxin.

Drugs with Duration Limits

One of the principal objectives of the DRESC program is to screen for drugs that can be eliminated because they are being used beyond their established *duration limits*. There are many reasons that drugs are not withdrawn from a drug regimen even though they no longer serve a useful purpose. Often, the patient will continue to fill the prescription because he or she is not aware that the medication has duration limits. In other cases, physicians maintain individuals on drugs as a preventive measure, even though continued therapy with the drug is not strictly indicated. Sometimes patients are lost to follow-up and continue filling the prescription, assuming that this is what their physician would have recommended.

H₂ Blockers. Regardless of the reasons for prolonged, unnecessary, and sometimes costly drug use, a number of medications can be identified that are frequently used beyond their customary duration limits. For example, individuals who are taking cimetidine, ranitidine, famotidine, or nizatidine should be carefully screened to ensure that their medication is cost effective and clinically useful. In general, high dose therapy for 6 to 12 weeks is recommended for the management of acute peptic or gastric ulceration. Maintenance therapy at lower doses is appropriate for 12 months in patients with documented peptic or gastric ulceration. Long-term maintenance therapy (i.e., greater than 12 months) is generally not indicated, except in patients who continue to be at high risk for complications such as hemorrhage.

Proton Pump Blockers. Omeprazole, which is useful for the management of both ulcer disease as well as erosive esophagitis, is generally not recommended for long-term maintenance therapy. However, there are recent studies that suggest that the safe use of this drug extends beyond the acute 12-week period for which this medication is approved.[48,49] The use of omeprazole for the management of gastroesophageal reflux disease (GERD) deserves special consideration. The last few decades provided major advances in the pharmacologic options available for patients with chronic GERD, including omeprazole, which can virtually eliminate all gastric acid secretions via selective and profound inhibition of the proton pump in the gastric parietal cell. In numerous trials,[48] omeprazole was proven to be superior to H_2-receptor antagonists in the short-term management of reflux esophagitis, but after discontinuation of therapy, esophagitis recurs in most cases. At present, omeprazole is approved in the United States only for short-term use, primarily because of the uncertain significance of increased gastrin levels during omeprazole therapy, and because of animal data that raise concerns about the increased potential for gastric tumors associated with increased gastrin secretion. Nevertheless, long-term use of omeprazole is approved in Europe and other parts of the world.

Recent investigations[49] have helped to clarify the potential risks and benefits of long-term therapy with omeprazole. Researchers at seven referral centers in the Netherlands conducted a trial on patients with erosive reflux esophagitis diagnosed by endoscopy who had not responded to high-dose H_2-receptor antagonists. Eligible patients (91) had endoscopic lesions ranging from noncircumferential erosions of the esophagus to circumferential erosions with deep ulcer or stricture, to Barrett's esophagus (32 subjects). All patients were given 40 mg of omeprazole once daily for 4 to 16 weeks, until endoscopic examinations indicated healing. At that time, a maintenance dose of 20 mg daily was continued. For patients who relapsed, the daily dose was increased to 40 mg. Serum gastrin levels were monitored, and gastric biopsies were obtained at 3-month intervals during the first year of maintenance therapy and at 6-month intervals thereafter. Of the 91 subjects enrolled in the trial, esophagitis was healed in 64% of patients after 4 weeks of treatment with 40 mg of omeprazole daily; it healed in 18% of cases after 8 weeks of therapy and in 13% after 12 weeks. Four patients were healed only after acute treatment was extended to 16 weeks, and one patient healed only after the dose was increased to 60 mg per day. The time for healing in patients with Barrett's esophagus coexistent with esophagitis was the same as it was for other patients.

All these subjects were followed at least 36 months; 67 were followed for 48 months, and 27 patients were followed for 16 months or longer. Relapse occurred in 47% of patients receiving maintenance therapy with 20 mg of omeprazole; but all patients with relapse healed within 3 months of increasing the daily dose of the drug by 20 mg. Median gastrin levels increased from 60 ng/L before study entry to 162 ng/L with treatment and reached a plateau during maintenance therapy. A very small subgroup of patients (11%) developed very high serum gastrin levels. No dysplasia or neoplasia was detected on biopsy specimens obtained during the study. Mild adverse events occurred in 19% of patients during therapy, and three patients died during the trial from illnesses unrelated to GERD.

Long Term Safety. This trial is important because it confirms the efficacy of omeprazole in healing severe manifestations of reflux esophagitis and the high rate of relapse when this potent therapy is *discontinued*. The major purpose of this open, nonrandomized study was to assess the long-term efficacy and safety of omeprazole. Fortunately, important conclusions that affect clinical practice can be gleaned from this trial. Therapy was well tolerated and effective during a monitoring period of up to 60 months, with all patients remaining in remission with doses up to 60 mg per day. Not surprisingly, serum gastrin levels were significantly increased with omeprazole therapy, but there was no evidence on biopsy specimens that these levels were stimulating tumor growth. There was also a progression toward atrophic gastritis and micronodular hyperplasia during long-term treatment with omeprazole, the significance of which is uncertain.

As far as implications for clinical practice and discontinuation of omeprazole therapy, this trial provides some reassuring information for physicians and pharmacists regarding the long-term safety and efficacy of this drug for patients with severe GERD. It is important to remember, however, that the vast majority of individuals with GERD respond to conservative, nonpharmacologic measures (dietary modification, elevation of head of the bed, etc.) and standard pharmacologic therapy with antacids or H_2-receptor antagonists. For the approximately 10% of patients with severe GERD, including erosive esophagitis, strictures, or Barrett's esophagus, and perhaps those with refractory symptoms, omeprazole is appropriate therapy. Based on this trial, it appears that the efficacy and safety of long-term omeprazole treatment outweigh the risks in appropriately selected patients with severe disease. Although elevation of serum gastrin occurs in all patients treated with omeprazole, very few have marked elevation to the range where inducement of gastric or other tumors is a serious concern. Therefore, discontinuation of this medication depends primarily on the necessity to manage severe symptoms and at the present time, cessation of the drug is not warranted based on arbitrary duration limits.

Antiseizure Medications. With respect to antiepileptic drug therapy, when a drug is ineffective or causes troublesome side effects, it should be tapered gradually, while an alternative drug is simultaneously introduced. Benzodiazepines and barbiturates should always be withdrawn slowly because rapid discontinuation often precipitates withdrawal seizures. Although other antiepileptic drugs can be withdrawn more rapidly, abrupt discontinuation is not recommended unless clinically indicated by toxic effects.

When idiopathic seizures are well-controlled (i.e., absent) with drug therapy for two to four years, many patients can safely discontinue medications such as carbamazepine, valproic acid, or phenytoin.[47] The relapse rate after medication withdrawal is 20% to 35% in children and 30% to 65% in adults. Recurrence during or after medication withdrawal is more common in patients with: (1) abnormalities on EEG, especially elliptoform discharges; (2) progressive EEG abnormalities documented while medication is being discontinued; (3) abnormalities on neurologic examination; (4) mental retardation; or (5) frequent seizures before adequate control. Social considerations, such as driving needs and employment, should be included in the decision to discontinue antiepileptic medications.

Antidementia Therapy. Constructing drug houses that are fit for individuals who suffer from chronic dementia is one of the most important challenges facing American physicians and pharmacists.[43,50] Alzheimer's disease is the most common cause of chronic dementia, affecting approximately 2.5 million people older than 65 years of age in the United States and Canada. Not surprisingly, the pressures to pharmacologically manage behavioral disturbances, cognitive dysfunction, and memory loss associated with this devastating illness are intense. Patients may require significant levels of care, and intensive pharmacotherapy for many years, resulting in a tremendous toll for patients, family, and society as a whole. Aggressive pharmacologic management with antipsychotic medications such as haloperidol and prochlorperazine, as well as anxiolytics, has been the mainstay of drug therapy for many years.[17,39]

Recent studies discussed in previous sections provide encouraging data that suggest these medications can often be discontinued without adversely affecting behavioral functions in this chronic condition. Recently, neuropathologic studies that demonstrate selective loss of cholinergic neurons focused interest on medications capable of enhancing cholinergic activity. One such agent, tacrine hydrochloride (Cognex®), helps some patients when used in low doses, although the response is not universal. Strategies for initiating, maintaining, and discontinuing this drug in patients with Alzheimer's disease are a fiercely debated clinical issue. Considering the pressures put on physicians and pharmacists by family members and institutions, the climate is conducive to overprescribe this expensive medication. Consequently, practical but strict parameters regarding tacrine use, as well as cessation of therapy when appropriate, are advisable.

Patients with *mild to moderate* Alzheimer's disease who are motivated and otherwise reasonably healthy may have disease progression slowed or modestly reversed for 6 months or more by use of low-dose tacrine. These encouraging results have prompted interest in evaluating the safety and efficacy of even higher doses. To address these issues, a recent trial[50] evaluated the safety and efficacy of tacrine at a dosage as high as 160 mg per day for 30 weeks for 663 patients with Alzheimer's dementia. It should be emphasized that all subjects were at least 50 years old, met established criteria for the diagnosis of Alzheimer's dementia, and had mild to moderate symptoms for at least one year. Patients previously exposed to tacrine, and those who were taking psychotropic medications, cimetidine, or theophylline (the latter two because of possible drug interactions with tacrine) were excluded, as were those with other significant medical problems.

The study has important pharmacotherapeutic implications, because it successfully evaluated the efficacy of various dosage schedules and approaches to drug discontinuation. Group 1 in this study received a placebo for the entire 30 weeks. Groups 2, 3, and 4 received 40 mg per day of tacrine for 6 weeks, followed by 80 mg per day for 6 weeks. Group 2 remained on 80 mg per day through week 30. Group 3 received 120 mg per day for the last 18 weeks of the study, and Group 4 increased to 120 mg per day for 6 weeks, and then to 160 mg per day for the final 12 weeks of the study. The success of these various drug regimens was measured using validated instruments for mental, social, and global functioning.

Based on this trial, the ability of patients with Alzheimer's disease to comply with long-term tacrine therapy is marginal, at best. Of the original 663 patients enrolled, 384 individuals withdrew before week 30; 285 (74%) did so because of adverse events, 5% because of lack of compliance, 5% for lack of efficacy, and approximately 16% of patients withdrew for other reasons. Interestingly, the 80 mg per day dose was *not* statistically more effective than placebo. Statistically significant dose-related improvements were noted at 18 weeks and persisted at 30 weeks *only* for patients who ultimately received 160 mg per day of tacrine. In addition, elevations of liver transaminase was a well-recognized effect of tacrine therapy, and in this trial 54% of tacrine-treated subjects had at least one alanine-transaminase (ALT) value that exceeded the upper limit of normal; 29% had values that exceeded three times normal, and 6% had values more than 10 times normal. The vast majority of elevations occurred within the first 12 weeks of therapy, were unaccompanied by clinical signs or symptoms of liver injury, and were transient and reversible.

This study provides favorable evidence to support the efficacy and safety of tacrine therapy for selected patients with Alzheimer's dementia. It is the first such trial to use dosages as high as 160 mg per day. Although this dose produced greater treatment effects, it should be stressed that a significant percentage of subjects initially enrolled did not complete the trial. Based on this study, tacrine, although clearly not a cure for Alzheimer's disease, can cause objective improvements in cognitive function tests and quality-of-life measures in some patients. Unfortunately, there is no good way to predict which patients will be among the 50% of those treated who respond favorably to this drug. It appears that a total of 160 mg daily in four divided doses should be the goal of therapy, and the titration schedule outlined above provides a reasonable direction for clinicians to follow. The persistence of benefit demonstrated at 30 weeks in this trial is also a reasonable period to use to determine whether an individual responds to tacrine, although that decision should be individualized and decided jointly by patient, clinician, and family. As a rule, however, the drug should not be initiated in patients who have *severe* Alzheimer's disease, should be used only in patients who are relatively early in the course of their illness, and probably should be discontinued if no objective or subjective indication of clinical improvement is noted by 30 weeks of therapy.

Discontinuation of tacrine may also be prompted by elevation of liver transaminases, which occurs in about 50% of all patients, and is generally not accompanied by clinical symptoms. Most elevations return to normal when the medication is discontinued. Unfortunately, it is not possible to predict which patients will develop hepatic enzyme changes. In approximately 90% of those with enzyme elevations greater than three times normal, hepatic enzyme changes will develop within the first 12 weeks of therapy. Therefore, liver enzymes should be monitored periodically in all patients receiving tacrine, particularly during the first 3 months of therapy. The drug should be discontinued in those patients whose serum transaminase values are greater than three times normal. Retreatment with tacrine is possible in many patients. This usually results in an immediate, but mild, enzyme elevation, but there is no exaggerated liver toxicity. Most patients have normalization of liver enzymes despite ongoing therapy, often tolerating doses higher than those which originally caused toxicity. In the small proportion of patients (2% to 5%) in whom marked enzyme elevations develop (10 to 20 times above normal), retreatment should not be attempted. The same is true for patients on tacrine who develop clinical jaundice (bilirubin 3 mg/dl), fever, rash, or marked peripheral eosinophilia.

HIV Infection. Decisions regarding discontinuation of medications in patients with HIV infection presents a particularly vexing and difficult clinical problem. Most of these patients require polypharmacy, both for the purpose of antiretroviral therapy, and as preventive therapy for a number of opportunistic infections. It is not uncommon for a patient with advanced HIV infection to tolerate a drug house consisting of trimethoprim/sulfamethoxazole, pentamidine isethionate, fluconazole, clarithromycin, and one of a number of antiretroviral agents, including zidovudine, didanosine, or zalcitabine. Discontinuation of medications used for prophylaxis and antiretroviral therapy is not recommended. Unfortunately, however, a large percentage of patients with AIDS develop toxicity from their medication regimens and discontinuation of drugs becomes absolutely necessary. The decision to discontinue a drug is always based on laboratory parameters, the patient's previous clinical course, and symptomatic complaints related to pharmacotherapy. (See Tables 5-16 through 5-18 for dosages and adverse effects requiring possible discontinuation for drugs used to treat HIV disease).

PHARMATECTURAL STRATEGIES FOR SHORT-DURATION ANTIBIOTIC THERAPY

Because of the vast number of options available among antimicrobial agents, the pharmatectural approach to drug selection is especially useful for outpatient antibiotic prescribing where resistance barriers play an important role in compromising clinical outcomes. To facilitate antibiotic selections that are cost-effective and address "real world" parameters affecting drug compliance, pharmatectural principles have been used to generate drug prescribing systems that can be used in day-to-day clinical practice.

The PPD™ (Prescription Resistance, Patient Resistance, and Drug Resistance) Approach to Antimicrobial Drug Selection: The Journey from Prescription Pad to Clinical Cure system is used for antibiotic drug selection. The PPD approach to antibiotic drug selection uses visual architecture to illustrate "real world" barriers—*prescription resistance, patient resistance, and drug resistance*—that can impede the journey down the outcome highway from prescription pad to clinical cure. By using a simple, direct, easily assimilated pharmatectural foundation in which prescription resistance refers to the cost of the medication; patient resistance refers to compliance, side effect, and duration of therapy issues; and drug resistance refers to the spectrum of antibiotic coverage, the PPD approach can help physicians and pharmacists make choices among drugs with respect to achieving desirable clinical outcomes.

Table 5-16

	Dosages and Adverse Effects of Medications Used For PCP Prophylaxis		
Medication	**Dosage Adult/Tanner stage IV and V Adolescents[3]**	**Dosage Infants/children/ Tanner stage I and II adolescents**	**Adverse Effects**

Trimethoprim-Sulfamethoxazole
 	
(TMP-SMZ)
Bactrim®
Septra®
 	
Formulations:
Single-strength tablet:
  80 mg TMP
  400 mg SMZ
 	
Double-strength tablet:
  160 mg TMP
  800 mg SMZ
 	
Pediatric suspension:
(per 5 ml)
  40 mg TMP
  200 mg SMZ
	Most commonly used regimens: one double-strength tablet taken orally three times per week on alternate days or daily 7 days per week.	150 mg/m^2 TMP
		750 mg/m^2 SMZ
		Total oral daily dose given 3 times/week
		
		Can be divided into two doses or administered as a single daily dose and given on 3 consecutive days or 3 alternate days per week
		
		This same oral daily dose divided into 2 doses can be given 7 days per week
			Drug allergy:
			Skin rash
			Stevens-Johnson syndrome
			Fever
			Arthralgia
			Toxic epidermal necrolysis
			
			Hematologic:
			Anemia
			Neutropenia
			Thrombocytopenia
			
			Gastrointestinal:
			Elevation of serum transaminase
			Nausea
			Vomiting
			Anorexia
			Fulminant hepatic necrosis (rare)

Table 5-16

Dosages and Adverse Effects of Medications Used For PCP Prophylaxis — cont'd.

Medication	Dosage Adult/Tanner stage IV and V Adolescents[3]	Dosage Infants/children/ Tanner stage I and II adolescents	Adverse Effects
Pentamidine Isethionate NebuPent® 300 mg The vial must be dissolved in 6 ml sterile water and used with Respirguard® nebulizer	Aerosolized pentamidine (AP) (NebuPent®) is given as single 300 mg (one vial) dose every 4 weeks. Nebulized dose given over 30-45 min at a flow rate of 5-9 liters/min from a 40-50 lb per square inch air or oxygen source Alternative: If a Fisons ultrasonic nebulizer is used, dose of pentamidine is 60 mg given every 2 weeks after a loading dose of five treatments given over 2 weeks	Children over 5 yr can receive same inhalation dose as adults	Pulmonary: Bronchospasm with cough Pneumothorax Other: Extrapulmonary *P. carinii* infection Increased risk of environmental transmission of *M. tuberculosis*

Table 5-16

	Dosages and Adverse Effects of Medications Used For PCP Prophylaxis — cont'd.		
Medication	**Dosage Adult/Tanner stage IV and V Adolescents[3]**	**Dosage Infants/children/ Tanner stage I and II adolescents**	**Adverse Effects**
Dapsone Formulation: 25 and 100 mg tablets	50-100 mg total daily dose divided into two doses or administered as a single daily dose given 2-7 times per week daily dose given 7 days per week	1 mg/kg administered orally as a single daily dose given 7 days per week	Hematologic: Agranulocytosis Aplastic anemia Hemolytic anemia in G6PD deficiency Methemoglobinemia Cutaneous reactions: Bullous and exfoliative dermatitis Erythema nodosum Erythema multiform Peripheral neuropathy Gastrointestinal: Nausea Vomiting

Table 5-17

Dosages and Adverse Effects Requiring Possible Discontinuation of Antiretroviral Drugs Used in HIV Infection — cont'd.

Medication	Dosage Adult/Tanner Stage IV and V adolescents[3]	Dosage Infants/children/Tanner stage I and II adolescents[3]	Adverse effects
Didanosine (ddI) (dideoxyinosine) Videx® Formulation: 25, 50, 100, 150 mg tablets Pediatric powder for oral solution 10 mg/ml	Patients under 45 kg: 100 mg/dose orally given every 12 hours 7 days/week Patients over 45 kg: 200 mg/dose administered orally every 12 hours given 7 days/week (Tablet should be chewed and taken on an empty stomach)	200 mg/m²/day administered orally every 12 hours given 7 days per week	Pancreatitis, potentially fatal Peripheral neuropathy Peripheral retinal atrophy (in children only) Nausea Diarrhea Confusion Seizures
Zalcitabine (ddC) (dideoxycitidine) Formulation: 0.375 mg tablets 0.750 mg tablets Pediatric 0.1 mg/ml syrup	Patients under 45 kg: 0.375 mg/dose administered orally every 8 hours given 7 days/week Patients over 45 kg: 0.750 mg dose administered orally every 8 hours given 7 days/week	0.005-0.01 mg/kg/dose administered orally every 8 hours given 7 days/week	Aphthous ulcers Esophageal ulcers Peripheral neuropathy Stomatitis Cutaneous eruptions Thrombocytopenia Pancreatitis

Table 5-17

Dosages and Adverse Effects Requiring Possible Discontinuation of Antiretroviral Drugs Used in HIV Infection

Medication	Dosage Adult/Tanner Stage IV and V adolescents[3]	Dosage Infants/children/Tanner stage I and II adolescents[3]	Adverse effects
Zidovudine (ZDV) formerly azidothymidine (AZT) Retrovir® Formulation: 100 mg capsules Pediatric syrup 50 mg/5 ml	100 mg/dose administered orally every 4 hours or 5 doses given 7 days/week	180 mg/m² dose administered orally every 6 hours given 7 days/week	Granulocytopenia Anemia Nausea Headache Confusion Myositis Anorexia Hepatitis Seizures Nail discoloration

Table 5-18

Dosages and Adverse Effects Requiring Possible Discontinuation For Antimycobacterial Drugs Used in HIV Infection

Medication	Dosage Adult/Tanner stage IV and V adolescents[3]	Dosage Infants/children/Tanner stage I and II adolescents[3]	Adverse Effects[4]
Isoniazid INHR Nydrazid® Formulation: 50 mg, 100 mg, 300 mg tablets 1 gram vial Syrup 50 mg/5 ml	300 mg administered orally as a single daily dose given 7 days/wk for 12 mo or 900 mg administered orally as a single daily dose given 2 days/week for 12 mo	10-15 mg/kg/day (max 300 mg/day) administered orally as a single daily dose given 7 days/wk for 12 mo	Gastrointestinal: Hepatotoxicity (rare in children) Nausea, vomiting, anorexia Neurologic: Peripheral neuropathy Neuritis, fatigue Weakness

Table 5-18

Dosages and Adverse Effects Requiring Possible Discontinuation For Antimycobacterial Drugs Used in HIV Infection — cont'd.

Medication	Dosage Adult/Tanner stage IV and V adolescents[3]	Dosage Infants/children/Tanner stage I and II adolescents[3]	Adverse Effects[4]
Isoniazid (cont'd)			Hematologic: Agranulocytosis Hemolytic and aplastic anemia Thrombocytopenia Eosinophilia Drug allergy: Skin rash Fever Lymphadenopathy and vasculitis (SLE-like syndrome)

Figure 5-3

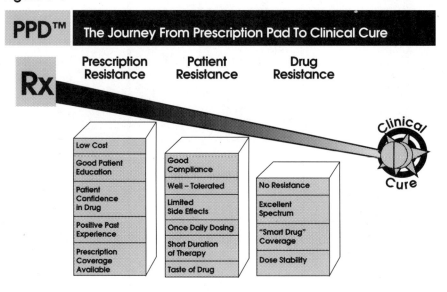

The PPD™ Approach: Rationale In Clinical Practice

The PPD system is easily adapted to clinical practice. Specifically, the PPD approach uses architectural barriers (green in color when favorable; red when obstructive) to indicate when the outcome highway is "blocked" and when it is "clear" for passage. The PPD approach outlines a logical framework for evaluating and comparing the cost-effectiveness and therapeutic success rate of different antibiotics. In its fully schematized format (i.e., PPD™ Profiles), the PPD approach to drug selection permits physicians and pharmacists to evaluate and compare the clinical success profiles (CSP™) of one antibiotic versus another, according to established specifications and parameters such as price, daily dose frequency, duration of therapy, side effect profile, and spectrum of coverage.

In order for the antibiotic to journey down the "outcome highway" from prescription pad to clinical cure, the antimicrobila regimen will have to overcome prescription, patient, and drug resistance barriers to achieve an optimal clinical outcome. Using this outcome-based, cost-effectiveness oriented, and "real world" approach, some antibiotics will fare well, whereas others will encounter resistance barriers on the outcome highway.

The antibiotic's *clinical success profile* is determined by the architecture of the resistance barriers. For example, if all resistance barriers are sufficiently low to permit passage of the antibiotic, it will complete the journey to clinical cure. On the other hand, when barriers poke through (and obstruct) the outcome highway and impede passage, the antibiotic is prevented from completing its journey to therapeutic success. These barrier-mediated obstructions are associated with less-than-optimal, real world cure rates.

This system, which can be used for ensuring Total Pharmacotherapeutic Quality Management (TPQM™), relies on a comprehensive data base that takes into account several parameters: Pharmacoeconomic and cost considerations, compliance issues, clinical outcome-oriented parameters, and FDA-approved drug information (eg, daily dose frequency, side effects, spectrum of coverage, discontinuation rates, drug-drug interactions). Organizing this raw information into an application-oriented approach presents a value-oriented analysis of antibiotics that can be used by physicians, pharmacists, quality assurance managers, and formulary directors. It is especially well-adapted to physicians and pharmacists operating within prescribing protocols in managed care systems, HMOs, VA hospitals, and large institutional settings whose formularies are driven by PharmD managers.

The utility of the PPD system is derived from its easy-to-analyze, visual approach to antibiotic selection and from practical, day-to-day clinical needs, and it relies on cost and compliance factors routinely used by pharmacists and physicians to make antibiotic prescribing and formulary adoption decisions. It reframes and systematizes time-honored evaluation criteria pharmacists and physicians have used into a *drug selection system* that guides them toward medications associated with low prescription, patient, and drug resistance barriers. Moreover, the system is enhanced by incorporating concepts and terminology that are part of the current managerial/quality assurance catechism driving formulary decisions. These PPD concepts include: "Outcome Highway", cost, compliance, side effects, resistance barriers, and Clinical Success Profiles (CSP).

PPD™ Resistance Barriers for Oral Antibiotic Therapy

It must be stressed that each of the three resistance barriers are *equally* important in determining if the antibiotic can complete the journey to clinical cure. Each of the three PPD barriers (prescription resistance, patient resistance, and drug resistance) can either be large enough to impede movement of the antibiotic toward the clinical outcome target, or the barrier will be sufficiently low to permit easy passage toward the outcome target. If any single resistance barrier is large enough to obstruct the outcome highway, a less-than-optimal outcome should be anticipated. Finally, a specific set of parameters is used to determine the size of the resistance barriers. They are discussed in the following sections.

Prescription Resistance. Prescription resistance refers to the likelihood that a patient will actually *fill* the prescription. The greater the patient's acquisition costs for a course of therapy, the less likely the prescription will be filled. Studies show that up to 25% of patients given a prescription for an antibiotic never fill the prescription, and the risk of non-filling increases with the medication cost. Accordingly, the primary determinant of prescription resistance is the cost of the medication. In general, courses of therapy that exceed $60 are associated with less-than optimal fill rates (75%), courses costing $40 to $60 produce adequate filling rates (80%-85%), whereas courses of therapy costing less than $40 yield optimal prescription filling rates (>90%).

In addition to the cost of the antibiotic, other factors affecting the patient's propensity for filling the prescription include: (1) the clinical provider's persuasiveness in convincing the patient that he or she needs the antibiotic as part of the therapeutic program; (2) the "word of mouth" about the drug, i.e., is it perceived by the community as a tolerable or poorly tolerated medication; (3) previous experiences with the medication; and (4) the patient's perception of the seriousness of his or her condition.

When cost of a course of therapy is high, or the physician or pharmacist has not taken the time to persuade the patient of the importance of filling the prescription, or the patient perceives his or her illness as mild in nature, prescription resistance barriers are high and may impede movement of the antibiotic down the outcome highway.

Patient Resistance. Patient resistance refers to the likelihood that the patient will actually take the medication, assuming that the prescription resistance barrier was low enough to induce the patient to fill the prescription. Once filled, however, there are a number of factors that determine how likely it is that the patient will be compliant with his or her medication.

The principal factors determining patient resistance include the daily dose frequency of the medication, duration of therapy, side effect profile, and discontinuation rate of the medicine. Not surprisingly, the antibiotic with the lowest patient resistance profile would be characterized by a well-tolerated, single-dose therapy administered under supervision. Examples of low patient resistance regimens include a single 2 gm dose of metronidazole for nonspecific bacterial vaginosis, a single 400 mg dose of cefixime for gonorrhea, a single 1 gm dose of azithromycin for uncomplicated chlamydial cervicitis, or a single 150 mg dose of fluconazole for Candida vaginitis. These approaches satisfy the criteria for Universal Compliance Precautions (UCP™) because, in general, administration of single-dose therapy prevents noncompliance-mediated therapeutic failure from undermining the success of a drug regimen.

Generally speaking, patient resistance is acceptable, although less than perfect, for therapeutic courses based on antibiotics dosed on a once-daily basis, given for 5 days or less, and which have a low incidence of side effects (usually, gastrointestinal in origin). Patient resistance becomes an important barrier to clinical cure for medications given on a BID or greater daily dose frequency, for 7 or more days, and for agents which have gastrointestinal side effects severe enough to produce drug discontinuation.

The effect of patient resistance (i.e., compliance profile) barriers on clinical outcomes in outpatient infections should never be underestimated. Even when the cost of the medication is sufficiently low to encourage prescription fulfillment, the pill will be impeded in its journey down the outcome highway if patient resistance factors are sufficiently imposing.

Drug Resistance. Drug resistance refers to the spectrum of coverage (i.e., antimicrobial activity) provided by the antibiotic against the most likely organisms encountered in the specific infection. For example, organisms targeted for empiric therapy in community-acquired respiratory infections include *Strep-tococcus pneumoniae, Haemophilis influenzae, Mycoplasma pneumoniae,* and *Moraxella cattarhalis.* An antibiotic with proven activity against all four organisms would provide optimal coverage and would be associated with a low drug resistance barrier. On the other hand, an antibiotic with activity against only three (or fewer) of these organisms might produce therapeutic failures in a significant percentage of cases and would be associated with a prescription resistance barrier obstructing the outcome highway.

Drug resistance must always be considered when selecting an antibiotic. Even when the medication is inexpensive and well-tolerated (i.e., prescription and patient resistance barriers are low), if the drug has a poor spectrum of coverage against anticipated organisms at the site of infection, the antibiotic's journey to the targeted outcome (i.e., cure) will be compromised by the presence of a large drug resistance barrier.

Optimal PPD™ Profiles. Optimal PPD profiles are characterized by antibiotics with low prescription, patient, and drug resistance. The most desirable agent or the antibiotic producing the greatest likelihood of clinical success is inexpensive enough to encourage prescription filling, well-tolerated enough by the patient to promote compliance, and active against all anticipated pathogens so that its empiric use will provide appropriate coverage without the necessity for retreatment due to resistance organisms.

PPD™ Profiles for Selected Oral Antimicrobial Agents

Using parameters outlined in the previous sections, it is possible to generate PPD profiles for commonly used antibiotics. It is important to emphasize that the following PPD profiles have been generated for the purpose of evaluating the usefulness of these oral agents for empiric therapy of community-acquired respiratory infections. These profiles do not provide information about the appropriateness of their use in non-respiratory conditions such as urinary tract infections, prostatitis, STDs, etc. Accordingly, the drug resistance barrier is low (i.e., optimal) only if the antibiotic has been shown to be active *in vitro* against all four organisms which, according to the American Thoracic Society Guidelines, are commonly encountered in these infections, i.e., *Streptococcus pneumoniae, Haemophilis influenzae, Mycoplasma pneumoniae,* and *Moraxella cattarhalis.* If the antibiotic fails to cover any one or more of these etiologic agents, its drug resistance barrier is considered less-than-optimal. As a result, it will obstruct the outcome highway, indicating possible deficiencies in spectrum of coverage.

Finally, the following PPD™ profiles are based on FDA-approved information regarding dosing frequency, duration of therapy, side effects, and possible drug-drug interactions for the most commonly used antibiotics. The pricing information is based on Average Wholesale Price (AWP) data provided by pharmaceutical wholesalers. It should be stressed that, from the perspective of drug selection, PPD™ profiles are intended to provide only an overview of some of the factors influencing antibiotic use. These analyses are not intended to imply that antibiotic profiles with fewer barriers are preferable to others in all situations.

As with other drug classes, pharmatectural choices should always be patient-specific.

In this regard, it should be stressed that even antibiotics with significant prescription, patient, or drug resistance barriers will emerge as drugs of choice in specific patient subgroups. From a pharmatectural perspective, therapy must always be individualized to the patient and condition, and the PPD™ profile suggests a set of possible guideposts for making these pharmacotherapeutic choices. For example, even though amoxicillin-clavulanate has significant PPD™ barriers, it is a useful and appropriate agent for patients with cat bites, resistant otitis media with effusion, and chronic sinusitis complicated by anaerobic infection. Similarly, although second-generation cephalosporins such as cefuroxime may be more expensive than other antibiotics used to treat lower respiratory tract infections; however, they (in combination with a macrolide) are extremely useful for treating older patients with community-acquired pneumonia who are deemed suitable candidates for outpatient therapy. Similar considerations apply for the other drugs analyzed by this system, including trimethoprim-sulfa, quinolones, clarithromycin, and azithromycin.

Erythromycin. The PPD profile for erythromycin reflects the drug's attractive acquisition cost. Consequently, the prescription resistance barrier is green, permitting easy passage. However, the antibiotic may be impeded at the patient resistance barrier because compliance is frequently compromised by the following factors: significant incidence of gastrointestinal side effects; QID dosing; and 10-day duration of therapy. The drug resistance barrier is high because erythromycin fails to cover *Haemophilus influenzae;* a window of bacterial vulnerability that compromises its usefulness in community-acquired respiratory infections.

Figure 5-4

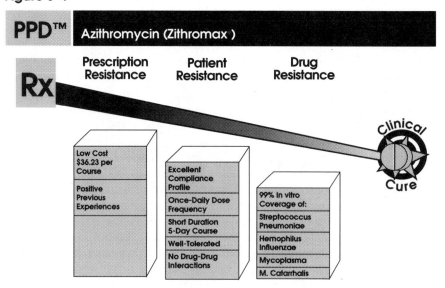

Azithromycin. The PPD profile for azithromycin reflects low prescription, patient, and drug resistance barriers. The average cost for a full course of therapy is $39 and medication compliance is enhanced by its once-daily dosing and 5-day duration of therapy. With respect to drug resistance, azithromycin provides *in vitro* activity against *Streptococcus pneumoniae, Haemophilis influenzae, Mycoplasma pneumoniae,* and *Moraxella cattarhalis.*

Clarithromycin. Clarithromycin when used at the 500 mg BID dose provides activity against *Streptococcus pneumoniae, Haemophilis influenzae, Mycoplasma pneumoniae,* and *Moraxella cattarhalis.* Hence, its drug resistance barrier is non-obstructive, reflecting an optimal spectrum of coverage for empiric therapy of community-acquired respiratory infections. In contrast to the profile for azithromycin, however, the cost of a course of therapy ($52-$60) for clarithromycin can produce prescription resistance. As a result, this barrier is obstructive. Moreover, the drug requires BID daily dosing, a 7-10 day course of therapy, and is associated with gastrointestinal side effects (including metallic taste) that cause discontinuation in a significant percentage of patients. The obstructive patient resistance barrier reflects these features.

Trimethoprim-Sulfa. Because the acquisition cost of trimethoprim-sulfa is attractive ($12-$15), the prescription resistance barrier is low. Although it is dosed BID for 10 days, the drug is well-tolerated with respect to side effects; therefore, the patient resistance barrier is designated as non-obstructive. Its spectrum of coverage is well-suited for urinary tract infections, but trimethoprim-sulfa does not cover *Mycoplasma pneumoniae,* a deficiency that makes it less-than-optimal for empiric therapy of community-acquired respiratory infections.

Amoxacillin-Clavulonate. Amoxacillin-clavulanate is useful as first-line therapy for cat bites, recurrent otitis media with effusion (OME), and chronic sinusitis in which anaerobic organisms are suspected. Nevertheless, its clinical success profile as empiric therapy for community-acquired infections involving the respiratory tract is compromised by the following: cost for a course of therapy is relatively expensive ($75-$85) compared to other agents; it is dosed on a TID basis for 10 days and has a high frequency of gastrointestinal side effects (diarrhea, cramps, etc); and this agent is not active against *Mycoplasma pneumoniae.* These drawbacks are reflected in the high resistance barriers appearing in the PPD profile for amoxicillin-clavulanate.

Fluoroquinolones. Fluoroquinolones are costly, reasonably well-tolerated, but provide only fair coverage against *Streptococcus pneumoniae* and no activity against *Mycoplasma pneumoniae.* The high patient and drug resistance barriers reflect these deficiencies as they apply to pulmonary infections. Despite their less-than-optimal status, compared to the macrolide azithromycin, as agents of first choice for community-acquired respiratory infections, this class is appropriate for initial therapy in the following conditions: complicated urinary tract infections in which *Pseudomonas sp.* are suspected, prostatitis, diabetic vasculopathic ulcers, invasive enteropathic *E. coli* infections with prolonged duration of gastrointestinal symptoms, malignant otitis externa, gonorrhea, and some cases of gram-negative osteomyelitis.

Cefuroxime. The second generation cephalosporins such as cefuroxime, cefixime, and cefaclor are all reasonably well-tolerated. Accordingly, their compliance/patient resistance profiles are designated as non-obstructive. With regard to prescription resistance, however, these agents are costly ($68-$85) for a course of therapy, especially as compared to the macrolides. In addition, although these cephalosporins provide excellent coverage against *Streptococcus pneumoniae* and *Haemophilus influenzae,* they are not effective against *Mycoplasma pneumoniae.* This deficiency in antimicrobial activity explains the high drug resistance barrier appearing in the PPD profile for cefuroxime.

Finally, it should be stressed that cefuroxime provides excellent coverage against a number of gram-negative pathogens (*E. coli, Klebsiella sp.,* etc) implicated in community-acquired respiratory infections in older patients. Consequently, many experts recommend using both a second-generation oral cephalosporin such as cefuroxime and a macrolide (azithromycin, clarithromycin) for initial therapy in this patient subgroup (i.e., patients over the age of 60 years in whom outpatient antimicrobial therapy for community-acquired respiratory infections is being considered).

REDUCTION OF DRUG DOSE

Screening drug houses for opportunities to lower drug dosage is one of the most important guiding principles of the DRESC program. It is staggering to think how many medications are used today at far lower doses than they were in the past, without any compromise in clinical efficacy. In fact, a number of medications are presently used at doses far lower than originally recommended and are more *effective* at these lower doses because they are associated with fewer side effects. For example, when the anxiolytic triazolam was introduced into the market, the manufacturer recommended using this medication at a dose of about 0.5 mg at night for sleep. After sufficient clinical experience with the drug, it became clear that doses of this magnitude, especially in the elderly, could produce a number of undesirable side effects, including memory loss, confusion, and disorientation. When dosage recommendations were lowered to 0.125 mg, the safety and side effect profile of the drug improved considerably, and the drug maintained its therapeutic efficacy for management of sleep disorders and anxiety-related conditions.

Anticoagulants. Unfortunately, despite rigorous FDA mandates governing clinical trials of new pharmaceuticals, drugs are still introduced into the market at doses that exceed what is necessary to produce excellent clinical outcomes. For example, there was a time when physicians and pharmacists believed that to achieve adequate thromboembolic prophylaxis in patients with venous occlusive disease, stroke, and atrial fibrillation, that warfarin doses producing prothrombin times that were 2 to 2.5 times the control value were needed for clinical efficacy. Subsequently, we have learned that equally effective outcomes are obtained when warfarin is dosed to achieve prothrombin times that are 1.3 to 1.5 times the control value. In the process of reducing the drug's dose, therapeutic efficacy is maintained, but the devastating hemorrhagic complications are reduced dramatically.

Interestingly, there is now strong evidence to suggest that low-dose warfarin therapy can prevent deep venous thrombosis in patients with metastatic breast cancer. Clearly, confirmation that very low dose warfarin therapy can be used at a fixed dosage of 1 mg per day without monitoring the prothrombin time, has important clinical implications. Although numerous methods are used to prevent venous thromboembolism in hospitalized patients, these methods are often impractical for outpatients. Standard warfarin therapy carries a risk of bleeding that may outweigh any potential benefit as a prophylactic agent. Studies are published, however, in outpatients with indwelling central venous catheters, demonstrating that 1 mg per day of warfarin safely prevents subclavian vein thrombosis without the need to monitor prothrombin time.

In a study[51] that illustrates just how low warfarin doses can go, patients with stage IV breast cancer who had recently begun chemotherapy were randomized to placebo and low-dose warfarin groups. The groups were similar in terms of age and a variety of clinical factors related to thrombogenic risk. Warfarin was initially administered at a fixed dosage of 1 mg per day. International Normalized Ratio (INR) monitoring and warfarin adjustments were made. For the first 6 weeks of therapy, adjustments in warfarin dose were made only if the INR exceeded 2. After that, the warfarin dose was adjusted to obtain an INR between 1.3 and 1.9 (which generally corresponds to a prolongation of partial thromboplastin time of 1 to 3 seconds). The mean dose of warfarin eventually administered was 2.6 mg. The mean duration of treatment was 6 months and was interrupted during periods when the patients' platelet count was below 50 to 109/L.

The results of the study suggested that warfarin produced an 85% reduction in the risk of venous thromboembolism. Although this is not the first study to demonstrate the safety and efficacy of very low-dose warfarin in the prophylaxis of venous thromboembolism, it does suggest that this low dosage regimen may have wide applicability in patients with advanced malignancy. Based on the results of this study, patients with metastatic breast cancer who are receiving chemotherapy should be considered for therapy with very low-dose warfarin to prevent venous thromboembolism, starting at 1 mg per day. The INR should be measured in 2 weeks and then approximately once per month. If the INR is less than 1.3, the dosage of warfarin should be increased by 1 mg per day; if the INR is between 2 and 3, the dosage should be decreased by 1 mg. If the INR exceeds 3, warfarin should be temporarily discontinued and the patient monitored closely for bleeding.

Patients with indwelling subclavian catheters should also be considered for very low-dose warfarin therapy in the outpatient setting. The randomized, controlled trial that supports this recommendation used a fixed dosage of 1 mg per day, without monitoring the prothrombin time. Although it is tempting to generalize these dosage recommendations to other patients with thromboembolic disease, it is not advisable until more studies are performed that confirm the usefulness of this regimen in specific clinical disorders. Nevertheless, these trials are extremely important because they demonstrate the possibility that thromboembolic prophylaxis can be accomplished with far lower doses of warfarin than thought possible.

H₂ Blockers

When cimetidine, the first H₂ blocker approved for use in the management of peptic ulcer disease, was introduced into the market, daily doses as high as 1,600 mg to 2,000 mg were advocated for routine clinical management of acute or recurrent peptic disease. These levels were associated with a significant incidence of central nervous system toxicity including confusion, that frequently necessitated discontinuation of the medication. Subsequent experience demonstrated that doses as low as 400 mg were sufficient for achieving desired therapeutic objectives, such as ulcer healing and symptomatic relief. Because the H_2-receptor antagonists produce several direct side effects, there are powerful incentives for screening these agents to ensure that the lowest acceptable doses are prescribed. As mentioned, the most important adverse reaction seen with H₂ blockers is mental confusion, which is related to high blood levels, especially in children and elderly patients. Antiandrogenic effects (such as breast tenderness, gynecomastia, and impotence) develop in about 1% of patients who take the usual therapeutic dose (1,200 mg per day) of cimetidine and as many as 50% of patients who take the high dose (about 5 g per day) required for therapy of gastronoma. Because adverse effects are documented with the use of all H_2-receptor antagonists, including cimetidine, ranitidine, famotidine, and nizatidine, it is recommended that regimens containing these drugs are reviewed carefully to ensure that the lowest effective daily dose is being administered to the patient.

Cardiovascular Drugs. Some of the most dramatic effects of lowering medication dosage are observed with drugs used to treat hypertension. When ACE inhibitors were introduced, captopril doses as high as 25 mg to 50 mg three times daily were recommended. Not surprisingly, a significant minority of patients developed acute renal failure. Subsequent experience with this drug demonstrated that far lower doses (i.e., 12.5 mg of captopril t.i.d.) could achieve the desired clinical results without the risk of renal toxicity. Recent studies suggest that dose reduction is especially important for thiazide diuretics. As recently as 10 years ago, it was not uncommon for patients to be treated with hydrochlorothiazide doses in the range of 100 to 150 mg per day. Although these dosages were clearly effective in lowering blood pressure and managing congestive heart failure, they were also notorious for producing a number of side effects, ranging from hypokalemia and other electrolyte disturbances to hypercholesterolemia and sudden death.

In fact, recent trials using high dose thiazide diuretics in patients with coronary heart disease and hypertension have revealed an unexpected increase in rates of cardiac sudden death. In fact, the increased risk of sudden cardiac death negated more than 50% of the expected cardiovascular benefit from improved blood pressure control. The suspected thiazide-related precipitants of cardiac arrest have included reductions in serum potassium and magnesium. In a recent study designed to assess the relationship between thiazide treatment for hypertension and occurrence of primary cardiac arrest, a dose-response relationship between thiazide dose and risk of primary cardiac sudden death was confirmed. Compared to low-dose thiazide therapy (25 mg/day), high-dose therapy (100 mg/day) was associated with the greatest risk of sudden death. For intermediate-dose thiazide therapy (50 mg/day), the risk of sudden death compared to low dose therapy was still elevated, but less so. Patients prescribed a potassium-sparing diuretic in conjunction with thiazide treatment manifested a reduction in risk for cardiac death. Similarly, adding a potassium-sparing agent to preexisting thiazide therapy also reduced the risk of sudden death. Potassium supplementation, however, did little to reduce the risk.

This study demonstrates the importance of DRESC program strategies aimed at evaluating dosage levels of commonly prescribed medications such as thiazide diuretics, which are not as innocuous as they may seem. When appropriate, initial therapy for hypertension should begin with a low-dose thiazide diuretic, (i.e., 12.5 to 25 mg per day). If higher thiazide doses are required (50 to 100 mg/day), consideration should be given to adding a potassium-sparing diuretic to the program or switching to another agent. High-dose thiazide therapy may not be a benign therapeutic intervention; whenever possible, regimens containing this agent should be screened to ensure that the lowest effective dose is being used.

Other Drugs. The wisdom of using lower doses has been confirmed for a number of other medications, including heparin, beta agonists, misoprostol, antidepressants, levothyroxine, and NSAIDs (see Table 5-19).

Table 5-19

Reduction of Drug Dose: Medications That Produce Therapeutic Results At Lower Doses Than Originally Prescribed	
• Aspirin	• Cimetidine
• Triazolam	• Misoprostol
• Warfarin	• Heterocyclic antidepressants
• Heparin	• H2 Blockers
• Hydrochlorothiazide	• NSAIDs
• Beta-agonists	• Synthroid
• Estrogen (i.e., in birth control pills)	• Digoxin
• ACE Inhibitors	• AZT
	• SSRIs

As discussed earlier, the risk of producing gastrointestinal toxicity with aspirin and NSAIDs is dose-related, and therefore it is imperative that regimens be reviewed to confirm that these medications are prescribed at the *lowest* effective maintenance dosage. Given the widespread use of antidepressants, ascertaining the appropriate dosage for this drug class presents a particularly difficult problem. Initial trials evaluating dosage requirements for such drugs as fluoxetine, sertraline, and paroxetine were conducted in individuals who were diagnosed as having major affective clinical disorders. In other words, dosage requirements for SSRIs were evaluated based on outcomes in patients who had suffered a major episode of depression. However, these antidepressants are now widely used in patients who would never have qualified for entry into the original studies evaluating the appropriate dosage requirements.

Both the medical literature, as well as the lay press—the best selling book, *Listening to Prozac,* drives the point home—have documented widespread use of antidepressants in younger and middle-aged individuals who complain of chronic anxiety, lack of energy, and mild sleep disturbances. Although the majority of these individuals would not satisfy the criteria for a major affective disorder, they nevertheless are being treated with SSRIs. There is mounting evidence that individuals who do not suffer from a depressive disorder, but who are nonetheless taking an SSRI antidepressant, can achieve desired effects with dosages far less than the recommended minimum dose currently advised by the package insert. Specifically, patients with mood disorders or functional disturbances that may benefit from antidepressant treatment, but who do not meet the *strict* criteria for a major affective disorder, should be started on a very low dose of an SSRI (i.e., 10 mg of fluoxetine or 25 mg of sertraline daily).

DRESC program strategies aimed at dosage reduction are designed not only to produce less expensive therapeutic regimens, but to improve the overall side effect profile of the drug house. In general, adverse side effects are a function of drug dose. Consequently, when a review of the regimen uncovers medications that are being used at the maximal dosage, the possibility that patient symptoms or complaints might reflect drug-induced side effects should be strongly considered. Because side effects tend to be dose related, it is frequently difficult to decide which is preferable: to maintain a patient on a high dose of a single agent, or to prescribe two medications, each of which is given at the lowest recommended dose. The latter approach has the benefit of producing excellent clinical results using medications that are dosed in a range that is unlikely to produce bothersome side effects. On the other hand, converting a patient from monotherapy to two-drug therapy may involve increasing the cost of the therapeutic regimen. In the end, the decision to use a single agent at a maximal dose versus two drugs, each of which is prescribed at a very low dose, depends on a number of factors including side effect profiles, cost issues, and medication compliance patterns. It should be emphasized that patients are just as likely to comply with their drug therapy program if they are taking two different medications once daily as they would on a regimen consisting of only one drug given once daily.

SIMPLIFICATION OF DRUG REGIMENS

Simplifying the drug regimen is a DRESC program strategy designed to prevent and treat noncompliance, as well as reduce the risks of drug interactions. To implement these changes, physicians and pharmacists should examine each regimen and make sure that it represents the safest, simplest and most effective therapy available. Every effort should be made to simplify scheduling. When appropriate, medications with a long half-life that can be given on a once daily basis will offer significant advantages over drugs dosed three or four times daily. When several once-daily medications can be taken simultaneously, at the same time of day, compliance will be enhanced. Medications that require special precautions (i.e., food intake) should be avoided. In general, the total number of pills consumed on a daily basis should be kept to a minimum (see Table 5-20).

Universal Compliance Precautions. Measures aimed at simplifying the drug regimen are part of a DRESC program strategy called Universal Compliance Precautions (UCP™). UCPs are necessary because studies show that physicians and pharmacists are very poor at predicting which patients will take their medications as prescribed.[20,33] Consequently, the most prudent approach for ensuring medication compliance is simply to assume that all patients are noncompliant, and to implement UCP. The most important features of Universal Compliance Precautions include: (1) once-daily dosing; (2) short duration therapies; (3) one-dose therapy (if available); (4) patient education; (5) selecting medications with tolerable side effects; and (6) providing follow-up to ensure medications are taken as prescribed (see Table 5-21).

Table 5-20

Opportunities and Strategies For Simplifying Drug Regimens
• Reduce the total number of pills consumed on a daily basis
• Attempt to construct regimen using once-daily medications consumed simultaneously at the same time of day
• Decrease daily dose frequency of medication
• Avoid medications that require special precautions (i.e., food intake considerations)
• Avoid medications with complex dosing schedules
• Avoid medications that are known to produce drug interactions

Table 5-21

Universal Compliance Precautions UCP™	
• Once daily dosing	• Patient education
• Short duration therapy	• Tolerable side effect profile
• One-dose therapy (if available)	• Follow-up

Once-Daily Therapy. Not surprisingly, identifying once-daily medications with proven clinical effectiveness is an important objective of the DRESC program. The DRESC program always advocates once-daily medications, *except* in cases in which side effects produced by a long half-life are likely to cause complications that require prolonged management until drug levels return to normal limits. For example, the use of once-daily verapamil is not recommended in older patients with cardiovascular disease because if the drug produces symptomatic, life-threatening bradycardia, intensive monitoring and management is required for up to 24 hours. On the other hand, there is no particular advantage to using a short-acting NSAID dosed four times a day, as opposed to a long half-life NSAID which is dosed once daily because if either drug results in gastrointestinal hemorrhage, the treatment is the same and independent of the half-life of the medication.

Within each drug class, some once-daily preparations appear to offer more advantages than others (see Table 5-5). Among the sulfonylureas, chlorpropamide should be avoided because of its long half-life. Oral hypoglycemics such as glipizide and glyburide offer 24-hour effectiveness and fewer side effects than are seen with chlorpropamide. All H_2 blockers are equally effective, but famotidine and nizatidine have the lowest risk of drug interactions. Among the beta blockers, hydrophilic agents such as atenolol are preferable to drugs that penetrate the central nervous system, such as propranolol. Among the calcium channel blockers, amlodipine, nifedipine GITS, and diltiazem are all useful for the management of both angina and hypertension. In older patients who have underlying congestive heart failure, amlodipine may be preferable because it does not cause clinically significant suppression of myocardial pump function. Once-daily ACE inhibitors such as enalapril and lisinopril are useful for the management of hypertension, congestive heart failure, and for preventing progression of diabetic renal disease.

Selection of a once-daily antidepressant presents a unique clinical challenge. The primary care physician now has five distinct classes of antidepressant medications that may be used for treating depression, including tricyclic antidepressants (TCAs); monoamine oxidase inhibitor (MAOIs); SSRIs (e.g., fluoxetine, sertraline, and paroxetine); aminoketones (bupropion); and triazolopyridines (trazodone). Although all these medications are effective antidepressants, recent studies suggest that the SSRI drug class may be the best for treating elderly depressed patients and for those in whom maintenance of work and psychomotor function are important considerations. In particular, the SSRIs have a broad range of antidepressant activity, a wide therapeutic index, and are free of many of the adverse effects associated with other antidepressants, such as cardiovascular toxicity, orthostatic hypotension, and sedation. Although the clinically significant advantages of SSRIs are acknowledged and well documented, there is still debate concerning the relative advantages of specific once-daily drugs within this class of antidepressants. Many experts have begun to analyze and compare the pharmacokinetic, pharmacodynamic, and side effects profiles of sertraline, fluoxetine, and paroxetine to identify which agent or agents might offer unique advantages for middle-aged or older patients.

A multicenter study evaluated sertraline versus fluoxetine in the treatment of patients with major depression.[52] The purpose of the study was to evaluate the comparative efficacy and safety of these two commonly used agents in outpatient depression. Overall, 67.3% of the patients in the sertraline group completed the

8-week study, compared to 44.6% of the fluoxetine group. The frequency of adverse effects during the study was similar between the two treatment groups. The severity of these adverse events was different for the two drugs. In the sertraline-treated group, the adverse drug-related events were usually described as mild, whereas in the fluoxetine group the severity was described as moderately severe. The nature of adverse events also differed between the two drug classes: agitation, anxiety, and insomnia predominated in fluoxetine-treated patients, whereas irritability, headache, and somnolence were more frequent in the sertraline patients.

The rate of discontinuation for the sertraline group was 34%, in contrast to 55% for fluoxetine. Among those discontinuing sertraline, 13.5% discontinued use because of clinical improvement, and 9.6% discontinued because of therapy failure. In contrast, 10% of patients in the fluoxetine group discontinued because of clinical improvement, while 20% discontinued because of therapy failure. Interestingly, benzodiazepine treatment was initiated during the study in 30% of the fluoxetine group, but in only 12.5% of the sertraline group. The increased propensity to add sedative hypnotic agents such as a benzodiazepines may reflect the increased agitation, anxiety, and insomnia reported with fluoxetine.

Despite the small numbers in this trial, this study suggests that although both drugs have side effects sertraline overall is the better tolerated antidepressant. It produces fewer side effects, is less likely to necessitate concurrent hypnotic drug use, and is associated with a lower discontinuation rate in middle-aged, and especially elderly patients, than is fluoxetine.

In addition to the results of this study suggesting that sertraline is better tolerated, there are other potentially important differences between SSRIs. Unlike fluoxetine and paroxetine, sertraline has linear pharmacokinetics in both young and old patients, which means special dosing requirements are less often necessary with this drug in older individuals. Second, the longer elimination half-life of norfluoxetine (active metabolite of fluoxetine) requires a significantly longer wash-out period when a patient is switched from fluoxetine than from sertraline or paroxetine. Finally, sertraline may be less likely to produce clinically meaningful inhibition of the hepatic P450 IID6 cytochrome oxidase system than is fluoxetine. This means that it may be less likely to produce adverse drug interactions. This is especially important in older patients taking drugs such as warfarin or phenytoin.

In addition to once-daily medications, the DRESC program also encourages the use of one-dose/short-duration therapies as part of its simplification strategy. The rationale for using one-dose/short-duration therapies is supported by a large number of studies that show noncompliance-mediated therapeutic failures are not only a problem for long-term management of chronic conditions, but also short-term therapy. A number of one-dose therapies are now available for treating many common infections (see Table 5-6).

Simplification of drug regimens takes many forms, from once-daily dosing and reduction of daily pill consumption, to implementation of UCP and use of one-dose therapies. It should be stressed that simplification strategies are useful for both long-term and short-term drug regimens. Finally, identifying once-daily medications which are best suited to a particular patient is a process that takes into account a number of factors, including cost of the medication, side effect profile, and the risk for drug interactions (see Chapter 3).

CONSOLIDATION OF DRUG REGIMENS

From a pharmatectural perspective, consolidating therapeutic regimens is an essential strategy for minimizing medications in order to maximize results. Fortunately, there are many opportunities for treating multiple conditions, symptoms, and disease states with a single active prescription ingredient (see Table 5-4). In general, opportunities for implementing consolidation strategies are most easily recognized by listing all the patient's conditions, abnormal laboratory values, and symptoms on one side of the page, and then trying to match this list with the fewest number of drugs possible to treat these clinical abnormalities.

Consolidating therapeutic regimens will be facilitated by gaining familiarity with those drugs that have established indications for treating *more than one* clinical disorder. For example, the patient who has hypertension, angina, and requires enhanced renal perfusion is most appropriately treated with a calcium channel blocker such as amlodipine, which is indicated for the treatment of angina and high blood pressure, and which has the additional property of improving renal plasma blood flow. On the other hand, for younger patients who have recurrent episodes of supraventricular tachycardia and hypertension, the calcium channel blocker verapamil has the advantage of both lowering blood pressure and being useful for the prevention of supraventricular tachyarrhythmia. When hypertension must be treated in a patient who also requires secondary prevention of myocardial infarction, a beta blocker such as atenolol is a reasonable choice. However, when hypertension is encountered along with congestive heart failure or diabetes with microalbuminuria, an ACE inhibitor such as captopril, enalapril, or lisinopril is most appropriate for consolidating the drug regimen.

A significant percentage of patients who have hypertension also have mild elevations in their serum cholesterol level. As a rule, these mild elevations in serum cholesterol are most appropriately managed with lifestyle modification. However, in many cases, patients fail to comply or cholesterol levels remain elevated despite lifestyle changes. In these situations, a peripheral alpha blocker such as doxazosin has the advantages of both lowering serum cholesterol level treating hypertension. Similarly, older patients who have high blood pressure *and* benign prostatic hypertrophy also benefit from the use of a peripheral alpha blocker such as doxazosin or terazosin. The postmenopausal woman who requires prophylaxis against cardiovascular disease, osteoporosis prevention, and amelioration of postmenopausal symptoms is best managed with estrogen replacement therapy. In the case of neuropsychiatric disorders, the combination of insomnia, panic attacks, and chronic anxiety is best managed with a short-acting benzodiazepine or SSRI, whereas the combination of diabetic mononeuropathy, depression, and a sleep disorder can be consolidated by using a tricyclic antidepressant.

Although attempts at consolidating drug therapy are an important part of the DRESC program, it should be emphasized that streamlining drug regimens is not always successful. Some patients may simply require two or three different prescription ingredients to manage their constellation of clinical disorders. This is the exception, however, rather than the rule. In the majority of cases in which a drug has approved indications for managing more than one condition, consolidation strategies that match single drugs to multiple clinical abnormalities or symptoms will be successful. Consolidation strategies are most likely to succeed if withdrawal symptoms are prevented, if medications are tapered within accepted duration limits, and if the patient becomes an active participant in the streamlining process. Finally, when replacing two, three, or more medications with a single drug, it may be necessary to introduce the consolidating agent at its mid-dosage range. In other words, it is sometimes necessary to use monotherapeutic regimens at higher doses to achieve the same therapeutic goals that were previously maintained by two or more drugs. When this is the case, the physician or pharmacist will have to weigh the potential disadvantages of possible side effects that are incurred at higher dosage ranges against the potential advantages of a simplified and consolidated drug regimen. The final decision is best made through a collaborative process that includes patient, physician, and pharmacist.

DRESC PROGRAM DRUG SURVEILLANCE

Screening for and identifying patient candidates who are appropriate for the DRESC program requires a meticulous review of the safety of pharmacologic building blocks that constitute the patient's drug house. A number of risk factors, demographic characteristics, and clinical conditions have been highlighted that suggest drug streamlining will be of benefit. Patients on polypharmacy, the elderly, individuals who are receiving medications from more than three physicians, and drug regimens consisting primarily of generic medications are just some of the risk factors that should prompt physicians and pharmacists to evaluate the integrity of the therapeutic regimen. However, no risk factor is more important than the presence of medications that are known to cause drug interactions (see Tables 5-22 and 5-23).

Table 5-22

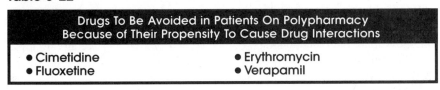

Drugs To Be Avoided in Patients On Polypharmacy Because of Their Propensity To Cause Drug Interactions	
• Cimetidine	• Erythromycin
• Fluoxetine	• Verapamil

For example, drugs known to inhibit the P450 cytochrome oxidase system, including cimetidine, fluoxetine, and erythromycin, should at least raise a red flag in patients who are on polypharmacy. When one or more anticholinergic agents are in a single regimen, careful evaluation should be made for anticholinergic signs and symptoms. Anticholinergic drugs that are frequently encountered in the drug houses of older individuals include tricyclic antidepressants, scopolamine-containing anti-diarrheal agents, antihistamines such as diphenhydramine, muscle relaxants, antiparkinsonian drugs, and antipsychotic agents such as phenothiazines. Sedative hypnotics in the benzodiazepine class can produce sedation, drowsiness, memory disturbance, and confusion in both younger and older patients. If patients on long-term benzodiazepine therapy have agitation, diaphoresis, or dehydration, the physician or pharmacist should consider the possibility of withdrawal syndrome.

Among cardiovascular agents, the calcium channel blockers verapamil and diltiazem can cause bradycardia, AV node conduction inhibition, myocardial suppression, constipation, and congestive heart failure in vulnerable individuals. It should be stressed that the adverse effects of these calcium channel blockers are potentiated by concurrent use of beta blockers and central sympatholytics such as clonidine. Special vigilance when using these agents is required, especially in older patients with underlying cardiovascular disease characterized by conduction disturbances or congestive heart failure. When beta blockers are in a therapeutic regimen, the history should focus on symptoms related to depression, fatigue, sexual dysfunction, or sleep disturbances. ACE inhibitors, which are frequently used in diabetic patients with hypertension, produce cough that is serious enough to prompt discontinuation of this drug in up to 15% of all patients. ACE inhibitor-induced cough is more likely to occur in elderly females with hypertension. Not infrequently, it may be difficult to distinguish between ACE inhibitor-induced cough, and coughing symptoms that reflect progression of underlying disease. Consequently, cigarette smokers, and patients with asthma, chronic obstructive pulmonary disease, or occupational lung disease are not ideal candidates for ACE inhibitor therapy because it may be difficult to distinguish between drug-induced cough and disease-induced cough. Nevertheless, when there are strong indications for the use of ACE inhibitors, the drug should not be denied to those patients who need them, even if they have underlying conditions known to cause cough.

The presence of any antihypertensive drug in a patient's drug house should prompt the physician or pharmacist to look for symptoms of sexual dysfunction.[53-56] Not surprisingly, many patients are reluctant to complain about sexual function, unless asked directly. Virtually all antihypertensive drugs are associated with sexual dysfunction (see Figure 5-6), and, therefore, when any of these agents are encountered in the patient's drug house, a careful sexual history is mandatory. Spironolactone, alpha methyldopa, clonidine, and propranolol are among those most likely to cause sexual problems. In general, the calcium channel blockers, ACE inhibitors, and peripheral alpha blockers are relatively preserving of sexual function.

Table 5-23

DRESC PROGRAM DRUG SURVEILLANCE: Common Drug Interactions	
Drug or Drug Class	**Side Effects/Drug Interaction**
NSAIDS	
	Gastrointestinal hemorrhage, gastritis, renal deterioration, hyperkalemia, azotemia. Adverse effects potentiated by concurrent thiazide use and presence of renal disease, coronary artery disease, or diabetes.
CORTICOSTEROIDS	
	Psychosis, confusion, fluid retention, hyperglycemia, GI hemorrhage (especially when used in combination with NSAIDs or aspirin, osteoporosis, etc.)
DIGOXIN	
	Nausea, visual disturbances, conduction disturbances, arrhythmias. Blood levels increased by quinidine and some calcium channel blockers.
CALCIUM CHANNEL BLOCKERS	
Verapamil Diltiazem	These calcium blockers can cause bradycardia, AV node conduction inhibition, myocardial suppression, constipation, and congestive heart failure in vulnerable individuals. Adverse effects are potentiated by concomitant use of beta-blockers and in older patients with underlying cardiovascular disease (i.e., conduction disturbances, CHF).
BETA-BLOCKERS	
Propranolol Atenolol Metoprolol Acebutolol	May produce depression, fatigue, sexual dysfunction, and sleep disturbances. Alone, but especially in combination with calcium blockers such as verapamil or diltiazem, beta-blockers may produce bradycardia, AV node blocker, myocardial suppression, or congestive heart failure.

Table 5-23

DRESC PROGRAM DRUG SURVEILLANCE: Common Drug Interactions — cont'd.	
Drug or Drug Class	**Side Effects/Drug Interaction**
ANTIDEPRESSANTS	
Tricyclics Heterocyclics	Anticholinergic side effects, including dry mouth, visual disturbance, orthostatic hypotension, urinary retention, low-grade fever, and disorientation can result from such agents as amitriptyline, doxepin, nortriptyline, etc. These effects can be potentiated by concomitant use of other drugs with anticholinergic properties, including diphenhydramine, muscle relaxants, antipsychotics (phenothiazines), and scopolamine-containing antidiarrheal agents.
SELECTIVE SEROTININ REUPTAKE INHIBITORS (SSRIs)	
Sertraline Fluoxetine	These agents can cause anxiety, headache, edginess, sleep disturbances, and gastrointestinal complaints.
ANTIPSYCHOTICS	
	Phenothiazines are noted for their anticholinergic side effects, whereas haloperidol-like agents are more likely to cause tardive dyskinesia. Both classes can cause CNS sedation and other mental status changes.
ANTICHOLINERGIC MEDICATIONS	
Tricyclic antidepressants Scopolamine Diphenhydramine Muscle relaxants Phenothiazines	When one or more of these agents is in a single regimen, careful evaluation should be made for anticholinergic signs and symptoms (i.e., dry mouth, confusion, excessive sedation, orthostatic hypotension, urinary retention, etc.)

Table 5-23

DRESC PROGRAM DRUG SURVEILLANCE: Common Drug Interactions — cont'd.	
Drug or Drug Class	**Side Effects/Drug Interaction**
SEDATIVE HYPNOTICS	
	Sedation, drowsiness, memory disturbance, and confusion can be seen in both younger and older patients. Long-acting agents (diazepam, flurazepam, and chlordiazepoxide) are to be avoided in older patients, because there is an increased risk of falling, daytime sleepiness, and hip fractures associated with their use. If patient on long-term benzodiazepine therapy presents with agitation, diaphoresis, and dehydration, consider withdrawal syndrome.
CIMETIDINE	
	This drug is potent inhibitor of the P450 cytochrome oxidase system and, therefore, can potentially elevate the blood levels of a number of commonly used medications including: theophylline, warfarin, narcotics, antidepressants, beta-blockers, verapamil, and many others. Antiulcer therapy with ranitidine, famotidine, or nizatidine is preferred because of their relative lack of effect on hepatic drug metabolism.
ERYTHROMYCIN/CLARITHROMYCIN	
	Theophylline levels can be elevated and, therefore, careful monitoring of drug levels during concurrent administration is advisable. Erythromycin and clarithromycin should not be used in conjunction with such nonsedating antihistamines as terfanidine and astemizole, because cardiac arrhythmias may result. Erythromycin can produce clinically important elevations in carbamazepine (*Tegretol*®) blood levels.

Table 5-23

DRESC PROGRAM DRUG SURVEILLANCE: Common Drug Interactions — cont'd.	
Drug or Drug Class	**Side Effects/Drug Interaction**
KETOCONAZOLE	
	Potentiates cyclosporine renal toxicity, can cause cardiac arrhythmias with nonsedating antihistamines, and potentiate quinidine toxicity.
QUINIDINE	
	May potentiate toxic effects of digoxin, amiodarone, beta-adrenergic blockers (including ophthalmic medications), procainamide, and others.
THEOPHYLLINES	
	These drugs can produce gastrointestinal upset, seizures, cardiac arrhythmias, and mental status changes. Their action is potentiated by concurrent use with erythromycin, cimetidine, fluoroquinolones, neuromuscular blocking agents, thiabendazole, and other agents.

The presence of NSAIDs, corticosteroids, and aspirin could cause gastrointestinal side effects. In addition to producing gastric erosions and ulceration, NSAIDs also can produce renal deterioration, hyperkalemia, and azotemia. These adverse effects are potentiated by concurrent thiazide use and by the presence of renal disease, coronary artery disease, or diabetes. When corticosteroids are added to a regimen consisting of nonsteroidal drugs, the risk of GI tract hemorrhage is increased by fourfold. As a result, NSAIDs and corticosteroids should not be used concurrently unless absolutely indicated.

SUMMARY

The three main objectives of the DRESC program are to be simple, to be safe, and to be certain. In most patients taking multiple medications, a meticulous review of the drug regimen and a thorough history that includes the patient's social, cognitive, and sexual well-being will usually uncover opportunities for making alterations that will enhance medication compliance, reduce the risk of adverse drug interactions, improve quality of life, and in many circumstances, reduce the overall cost of the therapeutic regimen.

[1]Ahronheim J. Practical pharmacology for older patients; avoiding adverse drug effects. Mt Sinai J Med 1993 Nov;60(6):497-501.

[2]Bailey RA, Ashcraft NA. Pharmacist-physician drug fair for educating physicians in cost-effective prescribing. Am J Hosp Pharm 1993 Oct;50(10):2088-9.

[3]Jolicoeur LM, Jones-Grizzle AJ, Boyer JG. Guidelines for performing a pharmacoeconomic analysis. Am J Hosp Pharm 1992 July;49(7):1741-7.

[4]Bulpitt CJ, Fletcher AE. Drug treatment and quality of life in the elderly [Review]. Clin Geriatr Med 1990 May;6(2):309-17.

[5]Coons SJ, Kaplan RM. Assessing health-related quality of life: application to drug therapy. Clin Ther 1992;14(6):850-8; discussion 849.

[6]Fletcher AE, Battersby C, Adnitt P, Underwood N, Jurgensen HJ, Bulpitt CJ. Quality of life on antihypertensive therapy: a double-blind trial comparing quality of life on pinacidil and nifedipine in combination with a thiazide diuretic. European Pinacidil Study Group. J Cardiovasc Pharmacol 1992 July;20(1):108-14.

[7]Limouzin-Lamothe MA, Mairon N, Joyce CR, Le Gal M. Quality of life after the menopause; influence of hormonal replacement therapy. Am J Obstet Gynecol 1994 Feb;170(2):618-24.

[8]Wiklund I, Karlberg J, Mattsson LA. Quality of life of postmenopausal women on a regimen of transdermal estradiol therapy; a double-blind placebo-controlled study. Am J Obstet Gynecol 1993 Mar;168(3 Pt 1):824-30.

[9]deBoer JB, van Dam FS, Sprangers MA, Frissen PH, Lange JM. Longitudinal study on the quality of life of symptomatic HIV-infected patients in a trial of zidovudine versus zidovudine and interferon-alpha. AIDS 1993 July;7(7):947-53.

[10]LeMay P. Quality of life—measuring outcomes of pharmaceutical management. Summary of workshop proceedings. Can J Public Health 1992 May-June;83(3):S5-16.

[11]Hallas J, Harvald B, Worm J, Beck-Nielsen J, Gram LF, Grodum E, Damsbo N, Schou J, Kromann-Andersen H, Frolund F. Drug related hospital admissions. Results from an intervention program. Eur J Clin Pharmacol 1993;45(3):199-203.

[12]Hallas J, Worm J, Beck-Nielsen J, Gram LF, Grodum E, Damsbo N, Brosen K. Drug related events and drug utilization in patients admitted to a geriatric hospital department. Dan Med Bull 1991 Oct;38(5):417-20.

[13]Lamy P. Adverse drug effects [Review]. Clin Geriatr Med 1990 May;6(2):293-307.

[14]De Geest S, Abraham I, Gemoets H, Evers G. Development of the long-term medication behavior self-efficacy scale: qualitative study for item development. J Adv Nurs 1994 Feb;19(2):233-8.

[15]Mawhinney H, Spector SL, Heitjan D, Kinsman RA, Dirks JF, Pines I. As-needed medication use in asthma usage patterns and patient characteristics. J Asthma 1993;30(1):61-71.

[16]Opdycke RA, Ascione FJ, Shimp LA, Rosen RI. A systematic approach to educating elderly patients about their medications. Pat Ed Coun 1992 Feb;19(1):43-60.

[17]Carlyle W, Ancill RJ, Sheldon L. Aggression in the demented patient: a double-blind study of loxapine versus haloperidol. Intern Clin Psychopharmacol 1993 Summer;8(2):103-8.

[18]Thomas DR. "The brown bag" and other approaches to decreasing polypharmacy in the elderly. N C Med J 1991 Nov;52(11):565-6.

[19]Barry K. Patient self-medication: an innovative approach to medication teaching [Review]. J Nurs Care Qual 1993 Oct;8(1):75-82.

[20]McNally DL, Wertheimer D. Strategies to reduce the high cost of patient noncompliance. Md Med J 1992 Mar;41(3):223-5.

[21]Nielson C. Pharmacologic considerations in critical care of the elderly [Review]. Clin Geriatr Med 1994 Feb;10(1):71-89.

[22]Anonymous. Medication use and the elderly. Can Med Assoc J 1993 Oct 15;149(8):1152A-D.

[23]Gainsborough N, Powell-Jackson P. Prescribing for the elderly. Practitioner 1990 Mar 8; 234(1484):246-8.

[24]Harris R. Pharmacological and nonpharmacological approaches to the treatment of cardiovascular disease in the geriatric patients. Geriatr Med Today 1982;1(3):47.

[25]Newton PF, Levinson W, Maslen D. The geriatric medication algorithm; a pilot study. J Gen Intern Med 1994 Mar;9(3):164-7.

[26]Busto UE, Sellers EM. Anxiolytics and sedative/hypnotics dependence. Br J Addict 1991 Dec; 86(12):1647-52.

[27]Morss SE, Lenert LA, Faustman WO. The side effects of antipsychotic drugs and patients' quality of life; patient education and preference assessment with computers and multimedia. Proceedings - the Annual Symposium on Computer Applications in Medical Care 1993; :17-21.

[28]Amir M, Cristal N, Bar-On D, Loidl A. Does the combination of ACE inhibitor and calcium antagonist control hypertension and improve quality of life? The LOMIR-MCT-IL study experience. Blood Pres 1994;Suppl 1:40-2.

[29]Palmer AJ, Fletcher AE, Rudge PJ, Andrews CD, Callaghan TS, Bulpitt CJ. Quality of life in hypertensives treated with atenolol or captopril: a double-blind crossover trial. J Hyptertens 1992 Nov;10(11):1409-16.

[30]Sager DS, Bennett RM. Individualizing the risk/benefit ratio of NSAIDs in older patients [Review]. Geriatrics 1992 Aug;47(8):24-31.

[31]Buchanan N. Noncompliance with medication amongst persons attending a tertiary referral epilepsy clinic: implications, management and outcome. Seizure 1993 Mar;2(1):79-82.

[32]Phillips SL, Carr-Lopez SM. Impact of a pharmacist on medication discontinuation in a hospital-based geriatric clinic. Am J Hosp Pharm 1990 May;47(5):1075-9.

[33]Weintrub M. Compliance in the elderly. Clin Geriatr Med 1990 May;6(2):445-52.

[34]Wilcox SM, Himmelstein DU, Woolhander S. Inappropriate drug prescribing for the community-dwelling elderly. JAMA 1994 July 27;272(4):292-6.

[35]Burris JF. Hypertension management in the elderly [Review]. Heart Dis Stroke 1994 Mar-Apr;3(2):77-83.

[36]Report of the Royal College of General Physicians: Medication for the elderly. J R Coll Physicians Lond 1984;18:7.

[37]Anonymous. Medication use and the elderly. Canadian Medical Association. Can Med Assoc J 1993 Oct 15;149(8):1152A-D.

[38]Cadieux RJ. Geriatric psychopharmacology. A primary care challenge [Review]. Postgrad Med 1993 Mar;93(4):281-2, 285-8, 294-301.

[39]Ancill RJ, Carlyle WW, Liang RA, Holliday SG. Agitation in the demented elderly: a role for the benzodiazepines? Int Clin Psychopharmacol 1991 Winter;6(3):141-6.

[40]Burrows GD, Norman TR, Judd FK, Marriott PF. Short-acting versus long-acting benzodiazepines: discontinuation effects in panic disorders. J Psychiatr Res 1990;24 Supp 2:65-72.

[41]Frank T. Tapering antihypertensives: avoiding the rebound. Senior Patient. 1990 16, June.

[42]Frishman WH. Beta-adrenergic blocker withdrawal. Am J Cardiol 1987;59:26F-32F.

[43]Coccaro EF, Kramer E, Zemishlany Z, Thorne A, Rice CM 3d, Giordani B, Duvvi K, Patel BM, Torres J, Nora R, et al. Pharmacologic treatment of noncognitive behavioral disturbances in elderly demented patients. [see comments]. Am J Psychiatry 1990 Dec;147(12):1640-5.

[44]Amery A, et al. Mortality and morbidity results from the European working party on high blood pressure in the elderly. Lancet 1985;1:1349-54.

[45]Applegate WB, Rutan GH. Advances in management of hypertension in older persons [see comments] [Review]. J Am Geriatr Soc 1992 Nov;40(11):1164-74.

[46]Avanzini F, Alli C, Bettelli G, Corso R, Colombo F, Mariotti G, Radice M, Torri V, Tognoni G. Antihypertensive efficacy and tolerability of different drug regimens in isolated systolic hypertension in the elderly. Eur Heart J 1994 Feb;15(2):206-12.

[47]Jenck MA, Reynolds MS. Anticonvulsant drug withdrawal in seizure-free patients [Review]. Clin Pharm 1990 Oct;9(10):781-7.

[48]Hetzel DJ. Controlled clinical trials of omeprazole in the long-term management of reflux disease [Review]. Digestion 1992;51 Suppl 1:35-42.

[49]Maton PN. Omeprazole [Review]. N Engl J Med 1991 Apr 4;324(14):965-75.

[50]Eagger SA, Levy R, Sahakian BJ. Tacrine in Alzheimer's disease [see comments]. Lancet 1991 Apr 27;337(8748):989-92.

[51]Levine M, Hirsh J, Gent M, et al. Double blind randomized trial of very-low-dose warfarin for prevention of thromboembolism in stage IV breast cancer. Lancet 1994;343:886-9.

[52]Aguglia E, Casacchi GB, et al. Double blinded study of the efficacy and safety of sertraline versus fluoxetine in major depression. Int Clin Psychopharmacol 1994;8:197-202.

[53]Avanzini F, Alli C, Bettelli G, Corso R, Colombo F, Mariotti G, Radice M, Torri V, Tognoni G. Antihypertensive efficacy and tolerability of different drug regimens in isolated systolic hypertension in the elderly. Eur Heart J 1994 Feb;15(2):206-12.

[54]Borland C, et al. Biochemical and clinical correlates of diuretics therapy in the elderly. Age Ageing 1986;15:357-63.

[55]Coope J, Warrender TS. Randomized trial of treatment of hypertension in elderly patients in primary care. BMJ 1986;293:1145,1148.

[56]Wassertheil-Smoller S, Blaufox DM, et al. Effect of antihypertensives on sexual function and quality of life: The TAIM study. Ann Intern Med 1991;114:613-20.

6

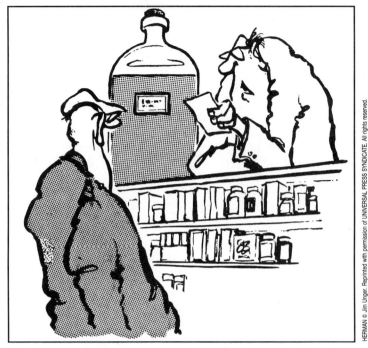

"That's what it says: 'one tablespoonful, 300 times a day.'"

ADRESC™: Applying Drug Reduction, Elimination, Simplification, and Consolidation

It is now time to put the DRESC program into practice. This requires not only specific information regarding opportunities for drug reduction, elimination, simplification, and consolidation as outlined in previous chapters, but a practical step-by-step approach that can be implemented in an outpatient setting.

The most common questions asked when implementing the DRESC program are the following: (1) which medications should be discontinued first; (2) how rapidly medication additions, substitutions, or deletions should be made; (3) how many physician visits or telephone consultations are required to monitor the effects of, and establish the effectiveness of, DRESC program strategies; (4) what instruments can be used to measure patient satisfaction and response to the reconstructed drug regimens; and (5) what endpoints should be monitored to ensure that the remodeled drug house is stable.[1]

Figure 6-1

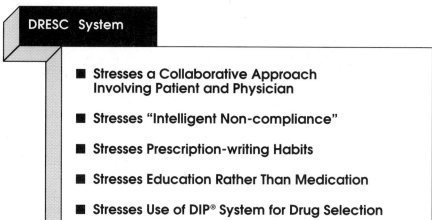

DRESC System

■ Stresses a Collaborative Approach
   Involving Patient and Physician

■ Stresses "Intelligent Non-compliance"

■ Stresses Prescription-writing Habits

■ Stresses Education Rather Than Medication

■ Stresses Use of DIP® System for Drug Selection

Because establishing patient confidence is an important priority, physicians and pharmacists should *first* identify those medications that can be discontinued *without* adversely affecting the patient's clinical condition. In other words, before discontinuing a medication that can produce significant exacerbations of the underlying disease if *inappropriately* discontinued, it is preferable to start with a medication that has a *low* probability of producing clinical deterioration if deleted from the regimen.

In general, a 12-week period is required to implement, monitor, and fully assess the clinical effectiveness of any single-drug deletion, substitution, or addition. This 12-week period is divided into three phases: (1) assessment; (2) implementation; and (3) evaluation. Following the initial encounter, a physician visit is required at week 4, week 8, and week 12. If, at that time, alterations in the drug regimen have produced the desired therapeutic effects, the physician can begin a second 12-week cycle for modifications that apply to a second drug, and so on. As a rule, only one drug deletion, alteration, or substitution is made per 12-week period. This incremental approach encourages careful patient monitoring for side effects, measurement of clinical goals, and opportunities to evaluate dosages. Because the step-by-step approach to drug house remodeling is gradual, it may take several weeks, or months to complete the entire process of deconstruction and reconstruction.[2-4] In the process, however, not only will more durable drug regimens result, but physicians and pharmacists will be able to better assess patient attitudes and responses to changes in their medication regimens.

Figure 6-2

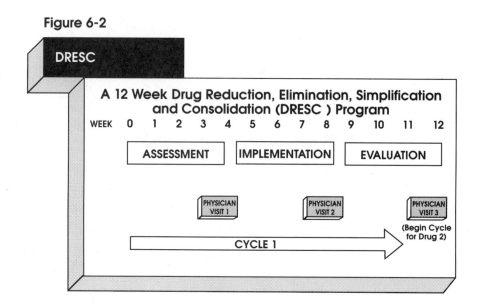

PHASE I: ASSESSMENT

The first phase of the DRESC program is a 4-week period of comprehensive assessment of the patient's drug house (see Figure 6-2).[3] During this 4-week period, the physician or pharmacist explores a number of features related to the patient's drug regimen. Thorough questioning is necessary to assess the current regimen's side effects, compliance pattern, and quality-of-life issues. A careful history will reveal the patient's overall well-being, preferences regarding medication intake, and provide information that will help construct a drug chronicle.

The purpose of the assessment phase is to help the physician or pharmacist determine just how comfortable the patient is with the current medication regimen and how well the pharmacotherapeutic program is meeting its objectives. As part of the assessment, inquiries should be made about a wide range of symptoms and patient concerns (see Table 6-1). For example, the patient should be asked whether he or she has noticed any significant changes in energy levels while on the current drug regimen. Have there been problems sleeping through the entire night? Quality-of-life issues are important in making drug selections. Consequently, questioning regarding the patient's sex life is appropriate. The physician should ask whether the patient's desire for sex has decreased significantly since beginning the current regimen and whether there are specific impairments in the performance of sexual activities.

Figure 6-3

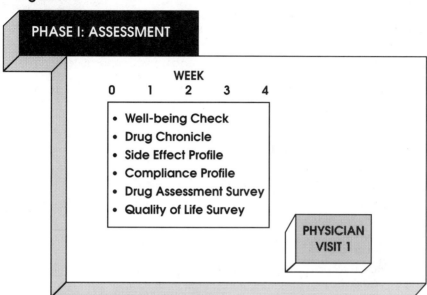

Because older patients are treated with a wide range of anticholinergic medications, questions regarding the presence of dry mouth, visual disturbances, difficulty voiding, constipation, or excessive daytime sleepiness are appropriate. Does the patient have excessive fatigue, lethargy, or lack of energy, and is the patient still interested in participating in hobbies, work activities, or social functions while on the current medication? Finally, the patient should be asked to document any skin changes, peripheral edema, changes in appetite, or unexplained headaches.

Before DRESC program strategies are implemented, it is sometimes helpful to ask patients which specific drugs they might feel comfortable doing without and which medications they feel are particularly valuable. This assessment phase also requires the patient to document drug intake in the form of a chronicle. Table 6-1 suggests one scheme that is useful for documenting medication intake.[5] Finally, the drug chronicle should also include any over-the-counter drugs the patient is taking.

Table 6-1

DRESC Program Drug Regimen/Assessment Questionnaire
Well-Being Check and Side-Effect Profile Assessment
1. Have you noticed significant changes in your energy level while on the current drug regimen?
2. Are you sleeping the entire night? Do you have problems going to sleep or awakening in the morning?
3. Has your desire for sex decreased significantly since beginning your current drug regimen?
4. Have you noted any of the following symptoms: dry mouth, visual disturbances, difficulty voiding, constipation, excessive daytime sleepiness, or light-headedness?
5. Have you noticed an unexplained cough since starting your medication?
6. Have you experienced shakiness, palpitations, anxiety, or rapid heart rate?
7. Have you experienced excessive fatigue, lethargy, or lack of energy?
8. Do you still have the desire and energy to engage in hobbies and social activities since beginning your current medications?
9. Have you experienced any unusual, undesirable, or unexplained tastes in your mouth?
10. Have you had any unexplained headaches or difficulty concentrating?
11. Have you noticed any burning in your stomach, nausea, constipation, diarrhea, or abdominal discomfort while on the current drug regimen?
12. Have you noticed any unusual swelling in your legs?
13. Are there any medications in the drug regimen that you feel might be responsible for producing undesirable side effects?
14. Are there any medications you are taking that do not agree with you?
15. Has your appetite either increased or decreased significantly?

Table 6-1

DRESC Program Drug Regimen/Assessment Questionnaire — cont'd.
Drug Chronicle and Assessment Survey

1. Please list the medications you are currently taking, and the time of day you take them. (You may use your medication bottles or any other sources you require to provide this information.)

    Medication 1 _____

    Time of Day Taken _____

    Medication 2 _____

    Time of Day Taken _____

    Medication 3 _____

    Time of Day Taken _____

2. Do you regularly take any over-the-counter drugs? If so, which ones and when do you take them? What do you take for a headache? How often? When was last time?

    OTC Medication 1 _____

    Time of Day Taken _____

    OTC Medication 2 _____

    Time of Day Taken _____

    OTC Medication 3 _____

    Time of Day Taken _____

3. Are there any medications in your drug regimen that you would prefer not to take? If so, which one(s) and why?
4. Are you happy with your current drug regimen? If not, please explain why.
5. Are there any medications in your regimen that you feel are too expensive? If so, which ones?
6. Would you be interested in trying other medications that are just as effective for your medical problem, but are much less likely to cause side effects?
7. Would you be interested in being on medications that are less expensive than the ones you are currently taking?
8. Would you be willing to make regular visits to the physician over the next several weeks to make medication adjustments that would help streamline your drug regimen?
9. Is there any single medication you feel you absolutely must stay on because it has produced such dramatic improvements in your condition?
10. Is there any single medication you feel you should absolutely stop taking because it has produced such a dramatic worsening in your medical condition?

Table 6-1

DRESC   Program Drug Regimen/Assessment Questionnaire — cont'd.
Quality-of-Life Survey
1. In general, do you feel better or worse than you did before starting your current medication regimen?
2. Do you think you would feel better or worse if you were taken off all your medications?
3. Do you think the quality of your life would improve if you were taking smaller doses of the medications?
4. In general, what makes you feel worse—your medical condition or your medications?

Patient Perspective. Although drug substitutions, eliminations, additions, and deletions should be based on sound pharmacologic principles, important information can be gleaned, and a sense of collaboration is fostered, if patients are asked *their preferences* about how they want their drug house to be remodeled. For example, it is valuable to ask if there are any medications in the drug regimen that the patient would prefer *not* to take. If so, which medications and why? Financial considerations can be a deterrent to drug intake; therefore, patients should be asked to identify any medications that are too expensive. Does the patient indicate an interest in trying medications that are much less expensive than the ones they are currently taking? Occasionally, patients perceive that some of their medications as extremely valuable and dislike others. Finally, a valuable index of the patient's willingness to cooperate with the DRESC program can be gleaned from the following question: "Would you be willing to visit your physician regularly over the next several weeks or months to make medication adjustments that would help streamline your drug regimen?" This important question reveals the physician's intentions and educates the patient as to the sacrifices and cooperation necessary to implement a program of drug house reconstruction.

Compliance Profile. Compliance is also necessary to set the stage for remodeling the therapeutic regimen. Patients should be asked whether or not they take their medications as prescribed. Those patients who acknowledge that their medication compliance is less than perfect should fill out a compliance profile assessment questionnaire (Table 6-2) that can reveal specific reasons for poor medication intake. The purpose of this questionnaire is to uncover both objective and subjective features of the current drug house that deter patients from taking their medications as prescribed. For example, the patient is asked if the medications are too expensive, whether they are taken too frequently, how the patient feels after taking the medication, and whether or not they think the medication is working. In addition, patients are encouraged to indicate whether or not they have received adequate instructions regarding medication intake, whether or not they believe better medications are available to treat their condition, and if they know of undesirable side effects. As part of the compliance profile assessment, patients should be asked directly whether or not they would be interested in trying other medications that might produce the same or better results with fewer side effects and a reduction in their total pill intake.

Table 6-2

DRESC Program Drug Regimen/Assessment Questionnaire
Compliance Profile Assessment

1. For the most part, do you take your medications exactly as prescribed?

   (If your answer to Question 1 was "No," "Maybe," "Some of the time," or something similar, please complete Question 2)

2. In your view, the failure to take your pills as prescribed is best explained by the following factors (Please check all the answers that apply to your situation):
   ( ) The medications are too expensive
   ( ) I have to take them too often
   ( ) I don't like the way they make me feel
   ( ) They don't seem to be working
   ( ) The medication(s) seem to make me feel worse than I did before starting them
   ( ) I don't think I need as much medication as I once did
   ( ) The medication(s) seem(s) not to work as well as it once did
   ( ) I am a forgetful person
   ( ) It is too complicated to take them the way they are prescribed
   ( ) I haven't been told exactly how these medications should be taken
   ( ) I haven't been given written instructions on how to take my medications
   ( ) In general, I just don't like taking pills
   ( ) I believe there may be better medications available to treat my medical problem
   ( ) I have heard that this medication produces undesirable side effects

3. Would you be interested in having your medications adjusted so that you could take fewer pills less frequently?

4. Would you be interested in trying other medications that might produce fewer side effects?

The first follow-up visit occurs approximately 4 or 5 weeks after the patient has stabilized on an established drug regimen. Preferably, patient assessment should occur after the patient is stabilized on a regimen for at least 2 to 3 months. Based on the information, perceptions, and impressions collected during this first phase, specific drug additions, deletions, or substitutions can be made. Implementation of DRESC program strategies can occur during either the first or second follow-up visit. If the physician or pharmacist feels there is enough information to initiate a single drug elimination, substitution, or addition, this modification to the drug house can be made after the first 4-week assessment phase.

PHASE II: IMPLEMENTATION

DRESC program strategies are implemented in a systematic fashion, but only after the assessment phase of the program is completed.[6,7] The assessment phase, if successful, provides the physician and pharmacist with valuable information about the patient's willingness to cooperate with a drug streamlining program, about medications thought to be troublesome, and about side effect issues that may be undermining medication compliance or patient well-being. During the implementation phase, which includes weeks 5 through 8, the physician or pharmacist should discuss the drug assessment survey, as well as opportunities for making changes in the therapeutic regimen that are tailored to the specific patient. The patient should be reassured that implementation of DRESC strategies will require ongoing collaboration between physician, patient, and pharmacist. Both oral and written instructions regarding drug changes must be provided during the implementation phase. The patient should be encouraged to immediately report any side effects from medication discontinuation, substitution, or additions.

If one medication is being tapered while another drug is gradually being introduced, explain to the patient the rationale of slow medication tapering. If tapering a medication is known to cause withdrawal symptoms, the patient should be alerted to expect these symptoms and reassured that reintroduction of the drug is always possible if withdrawal symptoms are intolerable. During the implementation phase, the physician or pharmacist has the option of either gradually decreasing the dose of a medication or stopping the drug immediately. This decision depends on specific pharmacologic and pharmacokinetic properties of the drug and how strongly the physician believes that the patient does not need the medication to maintain clinical stability.

If changes to the drug regimen are made during the first follow-up visit (i.e., after 4 weeks into the DRESC program cycle), the purpose of the next visit is to evaluate the clinical response to these changes and to make necessary changes. By the end of the second follow-up visit, a specific strategy for drug reduction, simplification, and consolidation should be formulated. It is preferable to begin with drug elimination or dose reduction. If there are no opportunities for drug elimination or dosage reduction, it is appropriate to proceed with consolidation of the drug regimen, (i.e., identifying a single prescription ingredient that can substitute for two or three different drugs currently in the regimen). After alterations are made as part of the implementation phase, the patient undergoes an evaluation phase lasting for an additional 4 weeks to determine if remodeling strategies have proved beneficial to the patient's clinical condition and well-being.

Figure 6-4

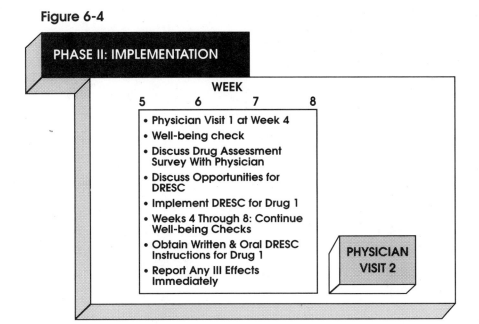

PHASE II: IMPLEMENTATION

WEEK

| 5 | 6 | 7 | 8 |

- Physician Visit 1 at Week 4
- Well-being check
- Discuss Drug Assessment Survey With Physician
- Discuss Opportunities for DRESC
- Implement DRESC for Drug 1
- Weeks 4 Through 8: Continue Well-being Checks
- Obtain Written & Oral DRESC Instructions for Drug 1
- Report Any Ill Effects Immediately

PHYSICIAN VISIT 2

PHASE III: EVALUATION

The purpose of Phase III is to evaluate the patient's clinical, psychological, and symptomatic response to modifications in the drug regimen. During this phase, the patient is asked to report any subjective or objective changes that seem related to modifications made in the drug house. This is the time to assess the need for minor DRESC program changes, adjustments, and drug house repairs. For example, should the tapering of a medication occur over a longer duration than originally planned? By the tenth week, it should be apparent whether or not the patient is tolerating changes in the drug regimen. At this point in the DRESC Program, it is also useful to review the well-being medication profile and quality-of-life assessment questionnaire that was completed during phase I. During the third physician visit, the patient might be asked to complete an additional questionnaire, and the results from each phase of the DRESC program cycle can be compared. The purpose of this comparison, which can be conducted either through a formal, written questionnaire or as a part of the patient's history, is to determine if the patient's attitudes about his or her reconstructed drug regimen have improved since the first visit. If changes to the drug house meet with patient approval, opportunities for additional medication changes should be presented at this time.

Figure 6-5

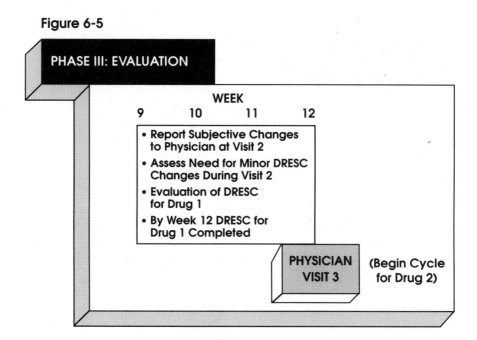

By the end of week 12, the physician and patient can assess whether or not symptoms, clinical condition, side effects, and the patient's overall sense of well-being have improved or deteriorated as a result of DRESC program strategies. If significant benefits are observed from the first DRESC program cycle, it is appropriate to start a new three-phase DRESC cycle for another drug. In general, one 12-week DRESC program cycle is required for each significant drug elimination, substitution, or consolidation. Simplification of the drug regimen and reductions in dosage can occur at any time during the course of this cycle.

ADRESC : APPLYING DRUG REDUCTION, ELIMINATION, SIMPLIFICATION AND CONSOLIDATION

Not surprisingly, the opportunities for implementing DRESC program strategies are wide and varied. It is helpful, however, to evaluate some actual case studies to fully appreciate the benefits that can be derived from streamlining pharmacotherapeutic regimens.

DRESC PROGRAM CASE STUDY NUMBER 1

Figure 6-7

ORIGINAL DRUG REGIMEN	RECONSTRUCTED DRUG REGIMEN
■ PROPRANOLOL: 80 mg P.O. T.I.D. ■ HYDROCHLOROTHIAZIDE: 50 mg P.O. q.D. ■ NITROGLYCERIN: 4 mg sublingual PRN ■ K-LOR: 40 meq. P.O. B.I.D.	■ AMLODIPINE 10 mg P.O. q.D.
1. Seven pills per day consumed to treat angina and hypertension. 2. Compliance profile is about 45%. 3. Risk of drug-related adverse patient event (DRAPE) increased by ten-fold. 4. Nine potential adverse side effects, metabolic sequelae, or interactions. 5. Quality of life impaired. 6. Exercise capacity compromised.	1. One pill capable of treating angina, hypertension, left ventricular hypertrophy and atherogenesis. 2. Minimal adverse side effect profile. 3. Enhanced quality of life.

A 67-year-old man with a history of hypertension, angina, and hypercholesterolemia presented to his physician with a drug regimen consisting of propranolol, hydrochlorothiazide, nitroglycerin, and potassium chloride (K-Lor®). A well-being and side-effect profile check was conducted during phase I and indicated general patient dissatisfaction with the current drug regimen. The patient was taking seven pills per day to treat angina and hypertension. The compliance profile with this drug regimen was estimated to be about 45%, with at least some patient dissatisfaction with having to take so many pills. Because the patient was taking four different prescription ingredients, the risk of incurring a drug-related adverse patient event was increased significantly. Nine potential adverse side effects or drug interactions were identified, including hypokalemia, sexual dysfunction, elevation of serum cholesterol levels, and a bad taste in the mouth following K-Lor administration.

The patient thought his quality of life was impaired, and aerobic exercise capacity was compromised by the inclusion of a beta blocker in the drug regimen. Two DRESC program cycles were required to convert this patient from seven pills a day to one pill per day, while achieving the stated clinical goals and improving quality-of-life parameters. On a once-daily 10 mg amlodipine regimen, the patient reported excellent control of his anginal symptoms, and repeated blood pressure measurements indicated satisfactory control. Moreover, there was no risk of drug interactions and the serum cholesterol level was reduced.

DRESC PROGRAM CASE STUDY NUMBER 2

Figure 6-8

ORIGINAL DRUG REGIMEN	→ ADRESC →	RECONSTRUCTED DRUG REGIMEN

■ FLURAZEPAM: 30 mg P.O. q.HS ■ DIPHENHYDRAMINE: 25 mg P.O. q.I.D. ■ AMITRYPTILINE: 10 mg P.O. q.HS ■ NAPROXEN: 375 mg P.O. T.I.D. ■ TYLENOL #3: T P.O. q.I.D.	■ TRAZODONE: 50 mg P.O. q.HS ■ NABUMETONE: 1000 mg q.HS ■ CETIRIZINE: 10 mg P.O. q.D.
1. Thirteen pills for insomnia, allergic rhinitis, depression and chronic osteoarthritis.	1. Three pills to treat depression, sleep disorder, allergic rhinitis, and osteoarthritis.
2. Compliance profile is about 30%.	2. No significant drug interactions.
3. Eight-fold increased risk of sustaining hip fracture.	3. Compliance rate is about 85%.
4. Compliance rate is about 35%.	4. Preserved CNS function.
5. Significant anticholinergic drug toxicity.	
6. Several drug interactions.	

A 73-year-old woman with a history of insomnia, allergic rhinitis, depression, and chronic osteoarthritis presented to her physician taking 13 pills and 6 different prescription ingredients. Her current drug regimen consisted of flurazepam, diphenhydramine, amitriptyline, naproxen, and acetaminophen with codeine (Tylenol #3®) as needed. The patient reported dissatisfaction with the drug regimen because of excessive daytime sleepiness, dry mouth, lack of energy, and general lethargy. The compliance profile survey conducted during phase I indicated a compliance profile of about 30%. It was estimated the patient had an eight-fold increased risk of falling and sustaining a hip fracture because of the use of a long-acting benzodiazepine, an antidepressant with potent anticholinergic properties (amitriptyline), and concurrent use of diphenhydramine. Several drug interactions were identified, and the patient indicated a strong willingness to have her drug regimen changed.

Because of the patient's age, drug alterations were conducted slowly and with careful clinical monitoring. The patient's clinical depression was treated with trazodone, which provided symptomatic relief of depressive symptoms, as well as slight sedation at night that was conducive to sleep. Diphenhydramine was replaced with astemizole. Failure to comply with the naproxen regimen was identified as an important problem, and the patient was given a once-daily NSAID to improve medication intake. The reconstructed drug regimen consisted of three pills to treat depression, sleep disorder, allergic rhinitis, and osteoarthritis. No significant drug interactions were identified, and the compliance rate improved to about 85%. Finally, the patient reported significant improvement in cognitive and behavioral function.

DRESC PROGRAM CASE STUDY NUMBER 3

Figure 6-9

ORIGINAL DRUG REGIMEN	RECONSTRUCTED DRUG REGIMEN

■ ASPIRIN: 160 mg P.O. q.D.	■ ASPIRIN: 30 mg P.O. q.D.
■ DIPYRIDAMOLE: 75 mg P.O. q.I.D.	■ AMLODIPINE 10 mg P.O. q.D.
■ ISOPROSTOL: 20 ug P.O. q.I.D.	■ NABUMETONE: 1000 mg q.HS
■ DICLOFENAC: 50 mg P.O. T.I.D.	■ SERTRALINE: 50 mg P.O. q.D.
■ ALPRAZOLAM: 25 mg P.O. T.I.D.	
■ VERAPAMIL: 80 mg P.O. T.I.D.	
■ PROPRANOLOL: 80 mg P.O. B.I.D.	
1. Twenty pills for hypertension, insomnia, arthritis, cardioprevention, prevention of NSAID-induced gastropathy.	1. Four pills for cardioprevention hypertension, angina.
2. Less than 20% compliance rate.	2. Compliance rate is about 82%.
3. Two unnecessary prescription medications.	3. Minimal drug-drug interactions.
4. One drug with high addiction potential.	
5. Several drug-drug interactions.	
6. Intolerable side-effect profile.	

This 65-year-old man was taking 20 pills for the treatment of hypertension, insomnia, arthritis, prevention of cardiac disease, and prophylaxis against NSAID-induced gastropathy. The patient had no previous documentation of peptic ulcer disease. The drug regimen consisted of aspirin, dipyridamole, misoprostol, diclofenac, alprazolam, verapamil, and propranolol. The patient presented to the emergency department with a heart rate of 36 and congestive heart failure. A well-being check and drug chronicle assessment had been conducted during phase I, just prior to the patient's acute hospitalization, which indicated profound dissatisfaction with the drug regimen. Specifically, the patient stated that the number of pills made it almost impossible for him to comply with the medications as prescribed. The patient reported shortness of breath, sexual dysfunction and constipation. The side effects of the drug regimen were characterized by the patient as intolerable, and he indicated that he would probably feel much better if he stopped taking all of his medications.

DRESC program strategies were applied to this drug regimen with the following results: the aspirin dose was reduced, thereby decreasing the risk of gastrointestinal side effects. The bradycardia and myocardial suppression caused by concurrent administration of verapamil and propranolol were eliminated by the introduction of amlodipine, a calcium channel blocker that does not suppress myocardial pump function and does not cause slowing of the sinoatrial node. Dipyridamole was eliminated from the drug regimen because there is no evidence that it is any better than aspirin at preventing transient ischemic attacks or recurrent myocardial infarction. The misoprostol also was discontinued, because the patient did not have a documented history of gastric or peptic ulceration. Depression and panic episodes that were treated with alprazolam were eventually managed with sertraline, a nonsedating, nonanticholinergic antidepressant. The alprazolam tapering required a 4-month period. Finally, the multiple dosing of diclofenac was replaced by an NSAID taken on an every-other-day basis. The net effect of the reconstructed drug regimen included an overall improvement in the patient's sense of well-being. The drug regimen was simplified by a reduction in the pill count from 20 to 4 pills per day. The compliance profile improved dramatically, and the risk of drug interactions was decreased.

[1]Stander PE, Yates GR. Modifying physician prescribing patterns of H2 receptor antagonists in an ambulatory setting. QRB 1988 July;14(7):206-9.

[2]Phillips SL, Carr-Lopez SM. Impact of a pharmacist on medication discontinuation in a hospital-based geriatric clinic. Am J Hosp Pharm 1990 May;47(5):1075-9.

[3]Schainen JS. Screening for polypharmacy in a nursing home care unit. Journal of Gerontol Nurs 1994 Mar;20(3):41,44.

[4]Sherman D. Reducing unnecessary psychoactive drugs. Contem Longterm Care 1992 Oct;15(10):76,78.

[5]Steiner JF, Fihn SD, Blair B, Inut TS. Appropriate reductions in compliance among well-controlled hypertensive patients. J Clin Epidemiol 1991;44(12):1361-71.

[6]Laucka PV, Hoffman NB. Decreasing medication use in a nursing-home patient-care unit. Am J Hosp Pharm 1992 Jan;49(1):96-9.

[7]Lipowski EE, Becker M. Presentation of drug prescribing guidelines and physician response. QRB 1992 Dec;18(12):461-70.

7

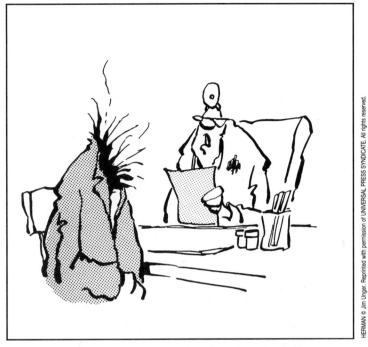

"I'm going to take you off the nitroglycerine pills."

Pharmatectural Strategies for Cardiovascular Drug Therapy and Disease Prevention in the Elderly

A rational, systematic approach to construction of drug regimens in the geriatric patient should be guided by several unique aspects of pharmacotherapy in this patient population. They include quality-of-life maintenance, the pitfalls of polypharmacy, prevention-oriented drug therapy, drug-drug interactions, and noncompliance-induced disease deterioration.[1-3] Even with meticulous attention to drug regimen design and vigilant monitoring of drug-related adverse patient events (DRAPEs), the older patient frequently requires pharmacologic maintenance with three or more medications, a therapeutic reality that places such individuals at high risk of incurring clinically important side effects and interactions.[4]

Oftentimes, side effects in the elderly are quietly festering, insidious, and ascribed by the patient or physician to nonpharmacologic factors, making drug regimen deconstruction and reconstruction especially difficult. In other cases, drug therapy may have been initiated without adequate indications. Consequently, pharmatectural strategies aimed at reducing the risk of drug-related problems in the geriatric patient must emphasize not only drug dose reduction but, when appropriate, drug elimination, simplification and consolidation. (See Chapters 5 and 6).

Put simply, the principal pharmatectural objective in treating the geriatric patient is to use as *few* pharmacologically active ingredients as possible to service as many of the patient's conditions as possible. Agents of low toxicity—aspirin, estrogen, antihypertensives, etc.—that have been shown to prevent coronary heart disease, stroke and renal deterioration, and which have significant potential for eliminating the need for more aggressive pharmacotherapy with more toxic drugs, offer special windows of opportunity.[2,5,6] By reducing pharmacologic burden, the risk of DRAPEs is minimized and quality-of-life maintenance is preserved.[7,8] The pharmatectural approach to constructing a therapeutically effective, prevention-oriented drug regimen in the older patient requires not only application of the principles emphasized in previous chapters, but a careful analysis of clinical trials that put specific pharmacotherapeutic options in the elderly into clearer focus.[9-11]

Background. As the United States enters the twenty-first century, a large fraction of its population will be elderly. Mean survival has increased more than 60% since the turn of the last century, and Americans 65 years and older will comprise 20% of the population by the year 2010.[12,13] Moreover, by the year 2000 there will be 15 million Americans over the age of 85, the fastest growing segment of the geriatric population.

With advancing age, individuals are susceptible to a number of clinical disorders. Current approaches to most geriatric disorders use drug therapy.[14] As a result, the elderly are burdened not only by diseases of old age, but with the consumption of an ever-increasing number of potent drugs, many of which can precipitate adverse side effects.[15-18]

No other risk factor compares with polypharmacy as a cause of adverse drug reactions and interactions in the geriatric population.[14,19] A number of British and American studies corroborate that persons over 65 years of age living independently take an average of 2.8 drugs per day. In skilled nursing facilities the number increases to an average of 3.4, while about 9 drugs per day are prescribed for the hospitalized elderly[20,21] (Table 7-1).

Table 7-1

Causes of Unintentional Drug Toxicity Among the Elderly	
• Duplications	• Omissions
• Self selection of drugs	• Pharmacy error
• Taking p.r.n. drugs too frequently	• Drug-induced confusion
• Automatic refills	• Recreational misuse
	• Multiple MDs

A study conducted by Larson at the University of Washington demonstrated that there is a ninefold increased risk of having an adverse drug reaction when four or more drugs are taken simultaneously.[22,23] Not surprisingly, 3% to 5% of all hospital admissions are related to adverse drug reactions, and of all hospital admissions for the elderly, 15% to 25% are complicated by an adverse drug reaction.[7,24,25] Some of these reactions are life threatening, and it is estimated that adverse drug reactions in the United States may account for up to 30,000 deaths each year.[19,26,27]

The potential toxicity of drugs in the elderly is exacerbated by a burgeoning and increasingly complex pharmaceutical landscape. At present, 13,000 prescription drugs are available in the United States, including at least 14 beta-blockers, 15 cephalosporins, 16 nonsteroidal anti-inflammatory drugs (NSAIDS), 8 oral sulfonylureas, 13 diuretic preparations, 8 ACE inhibitors, 15 penicillins, and 9 calcium channel blockers. A new entity is approved for human use every 2 to 3 weeks and two-thirds of all physician visits culminate in a prescription for a drug. In 1981, American physicians wrote 1.8 billion prescriptions, an average of 6.2 prescriptions for every person in the country. Over the past 8 years, it is estimated that the total number of prescriptions and "pills" have increased by 27% and 35%, respectively.[28]

Assessment of Drug Therapy. As the number of geriatric patients receiving pharmacologic treatment continues to rise, physicians are increasingly challenged with the diagnosis, identification, and management of adverse drug reactions among the elderly.[14,29] Inaccurate diagnoses of adverse drug reactions in elderly patients are common. Patients often experience multiple, nonspecific symptoms, a problem that is further complicated by the fact that many elderly patients suffer from dementia, depression, or other psychiatric disturbances. In addition, in this age group drug toxicity usually affects the central nervous system, and its symptoms are frequently attributed to other underlying causes, such as sepsis, neurologic disease, and metabolic derangements.[27,30,31]

Complicating assessment of drug-related toxicity is poor drug compliance,[32] which is frequent among the elderly (Table 7-2). In addition to not taking their medications, some elderly patients make unauthorized changes in their dosing intervals. Up to 70% of the geriatric population take OTC drugs that may interfere with, inhibit, or potentiate the effects of prescribed medications.[33,34]

Table 7-2

Risk Factors for Adverse Drug Reactions	
• Multiple drug regimens	• Changes in drug metabolism
• Incorrect diagnosis	• Changes in drug effect
• Lack of compliance	• Multiple physicians
• Poor OTC drug history	• Generic versus trade names

Complex drug regimens can confuse the geriatric patient, particularly if the patient has cognitive impairments. Physical limitations may also hinder drug compliance.

Pharmacologic therapy of the elderly, therefore, requires knowledge not only of appropriate drug dosages, potential side effects, and altered pharmacokinetics of drugs, but an increased awareness of potential drug interactions between chronic and acute medications.

Although it is generally assumed that the elderly are more susceptible to adverse drug reactions, some investigators argue that no good evidence exists in the medical literature to support this contention.[7] Rather, these experts suggest that drug treatment of the elderly is complicated by the presence of coexisting diseases, multiple medications, self-selection of drugs, inappropriate dosing, multiple doctors, difficulty with compliance, and other factors inherent to the geriatric age group.[16,19,35]

Based on numerous reports and clinical reviews, it is clear that to reduce the risks of drug therapy in the elderly, it is useful to categorize precipitating factors into physician-, patient-, and drug-related groups.[26,36-38]

Physician-Related Risk Factors for Adverse Drug Reactions

The majority of adverse drug reactions in the elderly are difficult to detect because symptoms are vague and nonspecific and, not infrequently, mimic symptoms of *illnesses* common to the geriatric age group. As a result, manifestations of many drug reactions and side effects are often overlooked or ignored by the physician. Difficulty in obtaining a history in this age group, the lack of specific physical findings, and the inability to alter the progression of disease can lull the clinician into unsafe prescribing habits and poor case detection patterns.

For example, physicians who prescribe drugs primarily in response to symptoms may fail to detect adverse drug reactions and interactions which, in many cases, obscure the underlying medical condition that prompted initial drug therapy.

Two common patterns that have emerged include prescribing an antidepressant to treat the depression caused by a lipophilic beta-blocker and the addition of a major tranquilizer to the drug regimen of patients with Alzheimer's disease to treat unrecognized benzodiazepine agitation. Another potential pitfall is the propensity of subspecialists to focus on a single organ system and prescribe drug therapy without regard for its effects on other organ systems, or drugs prescribed by other practitioners.

Prescribing new drugs that are thought to be effective in the elderly, but whose clinical safety and efficacy was proven primarily in only younger, otherwise well patients, is a particularly insidious problem. Until recently, the majority of clinical trials have tended to exclude the very old and extremely ill patient because of the difficulty in evaluating drug efficacy and side effects. Almost

Table 7-3

Causes of Adverse Drug Reactions in the Elderly
PHYSICIAN FACTORS
• Physician prescribes a high-risk drug to vulnerable host (i.e., ASA for patient with peptic ulcer disease) • Physician prescribes highly interactive drug to "pharmacologically vulnerable" patient (i.e., captopril to patient on potassium-sparing agent, diphenhydramine to patient on anticholinergics, etc.) • Physician prescribes inappropriate compensatory drug for unrecognized drug effect (i.e., tricyclic antidepressant to treat beta-blocker depression, major tranquilizer to treat benzodiazepine agitation, etc.) • Automatic drug prescribing (i.e., standard orders for ICU, CCU, or chronic care facilities) • Lack of follow-up on drug effects or poor longitudinal monitoring of drug interactions • Failure to adjust dosage

without exception, pharmaceutical trials are short-term, and, oftentimes, do not exceed 6 months in duration. Consequently, it is safest for the clinician to wait until careful trials with older patients are available.

It is estimated that 75% of all geriatric patient-physician contacts result in the addition of a prescription drug to the patient's therapeutic program (Table 7-4). Part of the problem is a discrepancy between physician and patient expectations regarding the necessity for drug administration. One large study has shown that 80% to 90% of physicians are under the impression that their patients expect a prescription drug as part of their outpatient therapy.[39] However, patients primarily indicate the need for a thorough examination, consultation, and reassurance and expect a prescription in only 30% to 50% of physician contacts. It appears that the unfounded expectations of both physicians and patients contribute to excessive prescribing of medications.

Table 7-4

Physician Prescribing Behavior: Patterns and Pitfalls
• Two thirds of all physician visits lead to prescription for drug. • American patients receive about four times more medication for a specific complaint than patients in Scotland. • In one study, 60% of physicians prescribed antibiotics for common cold. • Duke University study suggested 64% of antibiotic usage in hospitalized patients was either unnecessary or inappropriately dosed.

Until recently, physician prescribing knowledge in geriatric therapeutics was not examined in a systematic way. Early studies documented significant misuse of psychotropic drugs in nursing homes and suggested that the physician's knowledge base in geriatric clinical therapeutics may be inadequate. In one study, a questionnaire was devised to test the prescribing knowledge of primary care physicians in Pennsylvania. This investigation concluded that fewer than 30% of responding doctors "exhibited adequate knowledge of prescribing for the elderly." They also identified physician variables positively and negatively associated with an adequate knowledge of geriatric pharmacotherapy.[28] Positive associations included the importance of professional meetings, perception of the need for continuing medical education, board eligibility or certification, group (rather than solo) practice, and a practice which had at least 25% to 50% geriatric patients. Negative associations were the number of years since licensure and the belief that drug advertisements are an important source of drug information.[5,11,24]

Physician supervision of medications for the elderly, particularly in the nursing home environment, was judged inadequate by several authors in England who reviewed repeated prescriptions for psychotropic drugs without a physician visit.[41,42] These studies demonstrated a strong association between the number of times a prescription was refilled without seeing a physician and the age of the patient. In a large general practice in England, 70% of patients taking psychotropic or cardiovascular drugs had not contacted their physician in more than a month, and, of these, half had not been in contact with their physicians for a 6-month period.[43] Inasmuch as psychotropic drugs are capable of producing a variety of adverse reactions, their use demands constant vigilance. Ironically, those patients least able to monitor their own medications, (i.e., the oldest and most frail elderly) were most likely to be taking these drugs without supervision. Attitude surveys of these older patients found them very receptive to physician intervention aimed at withdrawing drugs judged detrimental or no longer useful.

Patient-Related Risk Factors for Adverse Drug Reactions

The two major patient-related risk factors associated with adverse drug reactions are compliance and age-associated changes in drug distribution and metabolism. Noncompliance with medications is an important therapeutic problem in patients taking multiple medications. Noncompliance with prescribed medications can lead to therapeutic failure and end-organ damage and, not infrequently, can induce the physician to prescribe additional—albeit unnecessary—medications to correct the clinical disorder.

Common noncompliance errors include: (1) deleting a prescribed drug; (2) continuing to take a dose of a drug that the physician has discontinued; (3) taking an incorrect dose; (4) taking the correct dose but at the wrong time interval. With respect to medication errors, polypharmacy drug regimens and daily dose frequency have been identified as important risk factors precipitating noncompliance.

If perfect compliance is defined as taking prescribed medications in a specified manner, then the elderly as a group are noncompliant at least 50% of the time in the community setting.[32] The complexity of a three-drug regimen, for example, is sufficiently great so that even patients under age 45 demonstrate noncompliance rates equal to those of the elderly. Patient noncompliance is a diverse category that includes errors of *omission* and *commission*. In a group of elderly diabetic patients with heart failure, analysis of noncompliance rates identified several factors that were associated with altered or inappropriate drug intake. These include age, number of associated diseases, functional impairment of the patient, and frequency of hospitalization. Only one factor clearly correlated with both errors of omission and commission: the *number* of drugs in the patient's regimen. Level of confusion and dementia were not assessed in this study, but other investigations suggest that compliance is threatened because of the forgetfulness so common in this age group.[7,21]

Compliance errors of commission include mixing of alcohol or over-the-counter drugs with prescribed drugs. It is estimated that alcoholism is present in up to 10% of the elderly population. Alcohol interacts adversely with all sedative drugs, and such OTC drugs as antihistamines may add to the anticholinergic effects of prescribed antipsychotics, antidepressants, and antiparkinsonian medications. Laxative abuse is thought to increase with age, and this may result in fluid and electrolyte disorders.

Environmental limitations are a major obstacle to compliance and play an important role in inappropriate drug intake in the elderly. For example, the elderly patient with arthritis may be unable to open childproof bottles or to split pills to obtain a fractional dose. A patient with limited mobility may have difficulty getting to the bathroom, and, therefore, discontinue regular use of diuretics. Retinopathy and peripheral neuropathy may preclude use of insulin for the older patient who lives alone.

Changes in drug effect and metabolism vary widely among individuals in old age. Biologic functions decline at varying rates. Consequently, the appropriate dose will usually follow the maxim, "Start low, go slow" to accommodate wide patient variability in the elderly. A number of recent studies and position statements published in the medical literature suggest that we are in the midst of an epidemic characterized by excessive, inappropriate, and suboptimal drug prescribing in middle-aged and older Americans. Less-than-satisfactory patient compliance with prescription medications ranks among the most problematic aspects of outpatient therapy, with some clinical experts claiming that poor drug compliance is a bona fide public health problem.

Poor medication compliance is a multifaceted problem that has the potential for: (1) preventing effective treatment of a clinical condition; (2) compromising the natural history of a disease; (3) coaxing out additional, unnecessary prescription medications to compensate for subtherapeutic drug levels and inadequate clinical effects; (4) inducing patients to self-medicate with OTC drugs or make alterations in their drug regimens; and (5) causing drug-induced side effects.

PATHOPHYSIOLOGY AND PHARMACOKINETICS

A number of age-related changes in pharmacokinetics can affect drugs commonly prescribed for the elderly. In this regard, alterations in absorption, distribution, metabolism, and elimination can precipitate adverse reactions or potentiate drug toxicity. Because drugs are absorbed passively and are not transported in active forms, absorption generally does not change with increasing age. However, distribution may be altered because the fat to muscle ratio increases with age. The fat portion of body weight increases from mid-life averages of about 18% for men and 33% for women, to 36% and 48% respectively for individuals aged 65 or over. As a result, the volume of distribution for water-soluble drugs decreases with age, whereas that for fat-soluble drugs increases.

Relatively water-soluble drugs include acetaminophen and alcohol. Diazepam and lidocaine are examples of fat-soluble drugs. In the elderly, acetaminophen and other water-soluble drugs will attain higher plasma levels. On the other hand, diazepam and lidocaine will be distributed across a greater volume of fat, causing markedly delayed metabolism and a prolonged half-life elimination.

Serum albumin also decreases with age.[4] This alteration is important for highly protein-bound drugs, such as sulfonylureas, for which effective concentrations depend on the amount of unbound drug. Accordingly, drug interactions that decrease protein binding for such drugs as chlorpropamide (Diabinese®) and tolbutamide (Orinase®) may lead to toxicity in the elderly patient.

Renal and hepatic clearance of drugs may also be affected by the aging process.[4,6] Liver blood flow is decreased 40% to 50% in the elderly. But hepatic drug metabolism varies widely with individuals, and there are no predictable age-related alterations.

The glomerular filtration rate (GFR), however, is reduced by approximately 35% in the geriatric age group.[46] Unlike hepatic clearance, the GFR reduction leads to predictable, directly proportional decreases in the clearance of drugs dependent on the kidney for excretion. Examples of such drugs include lithium, digoxin, cimetidine, procainamide, most commonly used antimicrobials, and chlorpropamide.[4] Age-related changes in pharmacodynamics affect the use of a number of drugs. For example, the number of beta-adrenergic receptors is markedly reduced on lymphocytes of elderly patients. Therefore, plasma levels of propranolol and metoprolol are higher and can cause marked hypotension, bradycardia, or central nervous system depression.

CATEGORIES OF ADVERSE DRUG REACTIONS

When evaluating and identifying potential drug reactions in the elderly, it is helpful to classify them into four groups (Tables 7-5 and 7-6):

1. Primary drug reactions
2. Secondary drug interactions
3. Drug withdrawal syndromes
4. Tertiary extrapharmacologic drug effects

Primary drug reactions. These occur when a single medication is responsible for the patient's symptoms. Examples include cimetidine psychosis, theophylline-induced seizures, propranolol depression, and digitalis toxicity. Other primary reactions are narcotic-induced respiratory depression, chronic salicylism, and lidocaine psychosis.

Secondary drug reactions. These reactions result from the interaction between two medications, with one causing an increased plasma level of the other drug. Examples include the interaction between first-generation sulfonylurea agents and sulfonamide antibiotics. The sulfonamides impair hepatic metabolism of sulfonylureas, causing elevated plasma levels, which may lead to increased insulin release and hypoglycemia. Salicylates and NSAIDs also can displace sulfonylurea from its serum protein binding sites, causing hyperinsulinemia and hypoglycemia.

Because it is a potent inhibitor of the p-450 cytochrome oxidase system in the liver, cimetidine has the potential for increasing the plasma concentration of several important drugs that undergo hepatic metabolism. These drugs include alcohol, lidocaine, phenytoin, aminophylline, benzodiazepines, propranolol, and warfarin. Thus, any elderly patient who is taking cimetidine in addition to one of these medications is at risk for developing a secondary drug interaction.

Alcohol, erythromycin, clarithromycin, and ciprofloxacin inhibit hepatic breakdown of theophylline compounds terfenadine, and carbamazepine and, therefore, can cause elevation in blood levels of these drugs into the toxic range. Other examples of secondary drug interactions include blunted beta-receptor site sensitivity to propranolol caused by indomethacin, and the mutual inhibition of cyclic antidepressants and centrally acting alpha-sympatholytic antihypertensive drugs such as alpha-methyldopa and clonidine.

Drug withdrawal syndromes. In the elderly, drug withdrawal syndromes caused by addicting medications such as phenobarbital and benzodiazepines usually do not differ in their clinical presentations from those seen in younger patients. However, older patients carry an additional risk of drug withdrawal syndromes from nonaddicting medications such as beta-blockers or other antihypertensives.

Sudden cessation of beta-blockers, for example, can produce angina and rebound hypertension in susceptible elderly patients. In fact, myocardial infarction is precipitated in 2% to 3% of patients when propranolol is abruptly withdrawn, especially in elderly patients at high cardiovascular risk. The proposed mechanism for rebound symptoms is an extended period of beta-receptor supersensitivity to endogenous catecholamine stimulation.

Extrapharmacologic effects. Finally, tertiary extrapharmacologic effects are a consideration for elderly patients taking many medications. One study reports that the elderly have a 50% to 150% increased risk of falling and sustaining a hip fracture when taking cyclic antidepressants, long-acting anxiolytics, or antipsychotic medications.[43]

Table 7-5

Evaluation of Drug Toxicity in the Elderly
TOXIC/THERAPEUTIC RATIO:
A time-honored concept that is valuable primarily when measuring dose-related adverse effects of a single drug in a patient with uncomplicated disease pattern.
INTERDRUG TOXICITY:
Much more applicable concept in the elderly, where there is a ninefold increase in adverse drug toxicity with consumption of four or more drugs.
EXTRAPHARMACOLOGIC TOXICITY:
Tertiary clinical pathology (falls, hip fractures) not included in classic categories of drug toxicity and measurable only through large-scale epidemiologic surveys; not included as "adverse" drug reaction in package insert (i.e., propensity to cause falling)

Table 7-6

Types of Adverse Drug Reactions in the Elderly
PRIMARY DRUG REACTIONS
(One drug—one side effect) • Cimetidine psychosis • Narcotic-induced respiratory depression • Lidocaine psychosis • Theophylline seizures • Insulin reaction • Chronic salicylism
SECONDARY DRUG INTERACTIONS
(Requires at least two drugs to cause interaction) • Sulfonylurea/sulfonamide • Cimetidine/lidocaine • Erythromycin/theophylline • Indomethacin/propranolol • Tricyclic antidepressant/alpha-sympatholytic
DRUG WITHDRAWAL SYNDROMES
(Addictive and nonaddictive withdrawal) • Beta-blocker withdrawal (angina) • Calcium channel-blocker withdrawal (angina, hypertension) • "Addictive drug" withdrawal syndromes (benzodiazepines, narcotics,etc.)
TERTIARY "EXTRAPHARMACOLOGIC" EFFECTS
(Measurable only by epidemiologic studies) • Falls caused by tricyclics, anxiolytics, and antipsychotics (short half-life versus long half-life agents) • Traumatic injuries caused by drug-induced orthostatic hypotension

GENERAL PRINCIPLES AND PATIENT EVALUATION

Clinical manifestations of drug toxicity may be particularly subtle in the elderly (Tables 7-7 and 7-8). In the case of digoxin or insulin toxicity, the nature of the drug reaction can frequently be diagnosed from the history, physical examination, and laboratory results alone. However, when a drug reaction produces a minimal alteration in mental status or mood, fatigue, focal neurologic lesion, coma, seizure disorder, cardiac arrest, myopathy, or nonspecific symptom complex, the diagnosis may be much more difficult. In such cases, if the clinician does not use a systematic approach to drug evaluation, the drug reaction may go undiagnosed and untreated.

A British study of nearly 2000 geriatric patients admitted to the hospital examined the drugs most often associated with adverse reactions.[44] Diuretics were responsible for the greatest absolute number of side effects, but they were also the most frequently used medications. Drug groups with the highest risk of adverse reactions were antihypertensives and antiparkinsonian drugs (13%), diuretics (11%), psychotropic drugs (12%), and digitalis (11.5%). Smaller studies in both the extended care and home settings have confirmed these findings.

Table 7-7

Some Presenting Symptoms of Drug Toxicity and Adverse Drug Reactions in the Elderly	
• Acute delirium	• Glaucoma
• Akathisia	• Hypokalemia
• Altered vision	• Orthostatic hypotension
• Bradycardia	• Paresthesias
• Cardiac arrhythmias	• Psychic disturbance
• Chorea	• Pulmonary edema
• Coma	• Severe bleeding
• Confusion	• Tardive dyskinesia
• Constipation	• Urinary hesitancy
• Fatigue	

To ensure rapid recognition of adverse drug reactions and the institution of appropriate therapy, familiarity with common medications and the ability to assess drug toxicity are essential. Aspirin-containing compounds can lead to chronic salicylism as well as gastritis. Moreover, antihistamines such as diphenhydramine can produce anticholinergic symptoms that may be potentiated by other commonly prescribed medications, such as cyclic antidepressants and antipsychotics. Finally, sympathomimetics such as pseudoephedrine and phenylpropanolamine-containing compounds can precipitate hypertension, angina, or even myocardial infarction.

Table 7-8

Indicators of Possible Toxicity	
Selected Drugs	**Reactions**
CHLORPROPAMIDE (DIABINESE)	
	Hepatic changes, signs of congestive heart failure, bone marrow depression, seizures, SIADH.
DIGITALIS	
	Anorexia, nausea, vomiting, arrhythmias, blurred vision, other visual disturbances (colored halos around objects)
FUROSEMIDE (LASIX)	
	Severe electrolyte imbalance, impaired hearing and/or balance (ototoxicity), hepatic changes, pancreatitis, leukopenia, thrombocytopenia
IBUPROFEN (ADVIL, MOTRIN, NUPRIN)	
	Nephrotic syndrome, fluid retention, ototoxicity, blood dyscrasias
LITHIUM	
	Diarrhea, drowsiness, anorexia, vomiting, slurred speech, tremors, blurred vision, unsteadiness, polyuria, seizures
METHYLDOPA (ALDOMET)	
	Hepatic changes, mental depression, nightmares, dyspnea, fever, tachycardia, tremors
PHENOTHIAZINE TRANQUILIZERS	
	Tachycardia, arrhythmias, dyspnea, hyperthermia, excessive anticholinergic effects
PROCAINAMIDE (PRONESTYL, PROCAN, OTHERS)	
	Arrhythmias, mental depression, leukopenia, agranulocytosis, thrombocytopenia, joint pain, fever, dyspnea, skin rash

Table 7-8

Indicators of Possible Toxicity — cont'd.	
Selected Drugs	**Reactions**
THEOPHYLLINE (BRONKODYL, ELIXOPHYLLIN, OTHERS)	
	Anorexia, nausea, vomiting, GI bleeding, tachycardia, arrhythmias, irritability, insomnia, muscle twitching, seizures
TRICYCLIC ANTIDEPRESSANTS	
	Arrhythmias, congestive heart failure, seizures, hallucinations, jaundice, hyperthermia, excessive anticholinergic effects

Alterations in body temperature such as hypothermia are associated with drug-induced hypoglycemia, whereas temperature elevations may be caused by anticholinergic drugs. Elevated blood pressure may reflect abrupt withdrawal from beta-blockers or clonidine. Increases in resting heart rate may indicate not only beta-blocker *withdrawal,* but occult toxicity due to cyclic antidepressants or aminophylline. Profound, symptomatic bradycardia may be the first manifestation of beta-blocker toxicity, which is potentiated by concomitant use of calcium channel blockers such as verapamil or diltiazem.

Hyperventilation, especially when associated with respiratory alkalosis, is a nonspecific finding but may be the first manifestation of chronic salicylism in the elderly patient. An irregular or rapid pulse may reflect digoxin, aminophylline, or cyclic antidepressant toxicity. Neurologic findings, such as nystagmus, may suggest sedative intoxication, while constricted pupils may reflect opiate intoxication. Wheezing may be the first sign of beta-blocker or salicylate toxicity.

The laboratory exam is invaluable and may reveal metabolic and electrolyte abnormalities associated with drug toxicity. Thiazide and loop diuretics may cause hyponatremia and hypokalemia, the former sometimes severe enough to induce coma and seizures. A decreased serum bicarbonate level may indicate chronic salicylism or anion gap acidosis. Azotemia may reflect not only excessive diuretic use, but also renal failure precipitated by NSAIDs of the propionic acid group.

CARDIOVASCULAR MEDICATIONS

Beta-Blockers

Toxicity from beta-blockers primarily affects the cardiovascular and central nervous systems. The most common cardiovascular side effects include hypotension, congestive heart failure, bradycardia, and heart block. The most common

respiratory manifestation is bronchoconstriction. Central nervous system alterations include depression, altered mental status, and decreased libido. Some of the
newer hydrophilic agents, such as atenolol, are associated with less CNS toxicity.

A number of medications, including cimetidine, oral contraceptives,
furosemide, and hydralazine, increase beta-blocker effects and may produce
clinical symptoms. Concomitant use of *intravenous* verapamil and propranolol is
contraindicated because the combination may produce profound hypotension and
profound bradycardia.

Beta-blockers may also block symptoms of hypoglycemia and should be
avoided in patients with diabetes mellitus. Diabetics who are taking insulin and a
beta-blocker should be treated with D-50-W intravenously if they present with
focal deficits or any mental status changes.

Timolol Maleate: Problematic Aspects In The Elderly

Primary open-angle glaucoma affects approximately 3% of all persons over
age 75. By damaging the optic nerve and retina, open-angle glaucoma is responsible for 15% to 20% of all blindness in this country. Because patients are generally
asymptomatic until neural damage is present, routine screening is warranted and
can be accomplished by use of the Schiotz tonometer. Patients with pressures
of > 20 mm Hg should be referred to an ophthalmologist, while pressures of
> 30 mm Hg represent an absolute indication for urgent treatment.

Treatment of open-angle glaucoma depends on miotics that facilitate the
outflow of aqueous humor, or beta-blocking agents, to reduce the amount of
production. Timolol maleate is a nonselective beta adrenergic receptor blocking
agent that reduces ocular pressure with minimal effect on pupil size, ciliary body
tone, or visual acuity. Because topically administered eyedrops forgo the significant first-pass metabolism of oral beta adrenergic antagonists, they tend to be
absorbed like an intravenous drug dose. It is estimated that 80% of ophthalmic
timolol is absorbed systemically. When used in the recommended dosage of one
drop of 0.25% solution in the affected eye twice daily, timolol is as effective and
better tolerated than the routinely used miotic preparations such as pilocarpine,
which may cause impaired night vision and visual blurring. Mild ocular irritation,
the most commonly reported side effect of ophthalmic timolol, is relatively
unusual. However, systemic side effects often encountered with orally administered beta-blocking agents have long been known.

An important study[46] reviewed the most serious adverse reactions reported to
the United States Food and Drug Administration (FDA) between 1978 and 1985,
during which time 40 million prescriptions for ophthalmic timolol were dispensed in the United States. Previously reported rates of systemic reactions
ranged between 15.9% and 50%. After excluding reports of hypertension, dizziness, headache, and hypotension not resulting in syncope, 450 case reports of
serious respiratory and cardiovascular events, and 32 deaths associated with the
use of ophthalmic timolol were documented. Consistent with the epidemiology of
open-angle glaucoma, the mean age of patients was 68 years (range 2 weeks to 95
years). Cardiac arrhythmias and bronchospasm-related events, including asthma,

were the most commonly reported adverse reactions (28.2% and 27.2% respectively).

The first week of therapy was critical for the elderly patients. All the deaths for which information was available (25/32) occurred within the first 2 days, 23% of the adverse effects occurred within the first 24 hours, and an additional 10% occurred within 2 to 7 days of initiation of therapy. Despite the apparent dangers associated with its use, ophthalmic timolol is one of the pharmacologic mainstays of glaucoma treatment. Rigid guidelines are suggested for its use, such as excluding patients with a history of bronchial asthma, chronic obstructive pulmonary disease, sinus bradycardia, second- or third-degree atrioventricular block, overt cardiac failure, or cardiogenic shock.

A recent article[47] reviewing four case reports of systemic symptoms associated with the use of ophthalmic timolol maleate indicates that inadvertent overdosage may be a major contributory factor. Four patients, aged 64 or older, reported such symptoms as weakness, unsteady gait, shortness of breath, nausea and confusion. Because almost all of the symptoms were temporally related to the morning instillation of timolol drops, home visits were made to assess the adequacy of its use and to establish a possible causative role. Self-administration of two to five drops of 0.25% timolol solution in each affected eye, rather than the prescribed one drop, was observed in each patient. Symptoms occurred 10 to 20 minutes after instillation and were associated with objective findings including hypotension, bradycardia, and expiratory wheezing. In all but one of the patients, the excessive doses were entirely inadvertent. After arrangements were made for correct administration of the medication, by enlisting the assistance of housemates or providing specially designed containers that would deliver only a single drop, all patients remained symptom-free.

Systemic side effects of beta-adrenergic blockade can be serious and even life threatening.[48] Because most patients receiving treatment for glaucoma are elderly, they are likely to have underlying medical conditions that increase their susceptibility to the adverse effects of beta-blockade, such as congestive heart failure and conduction disorders. The anticipated plasma levels of timolol resulting from a two- to nine-fold increase over the recommended dose could easily account for the side effects reported in many studies. This report indicates that elderly patients may have a difficult time with accurate instillation of ophthalmic drops, resulting in inadvertent overdosage. The authors suggest that a simple solution is to use droppers designed to withdraw and deliver only one drop at a time. Whether inadvertent overdosage is the only risk factor for adverse reactions to ophthalmic timolol is unclear. In the meantime, physicians and pharmacists should be aware of the potential for ophthalmic timolol to cause dizziness, unsteadiness, shortness of breath, and hypotension, as well as more serious respiratory and cardiovascular complications. Further studies are needed to establish the pharmacokinetics of ophthalmic timolol and to determine the definitive risk of potentially serious side effects after ophthalmic administration using the proper dosing regimen.

Withdrawal of Cardiac Medications

For a variety of reasons, patients with heart disease frequently require adjustments in their antianginal regimen. However, dramatic cardiac events, including unstable angina, rebound hypertension, and myocardial infarction, have been described following abrupt cessation of beta-blocking agents such as propranolol.[49] While such events are sufficient to argue persuasively against the abrupt withdrawal of antianginal agents in patients with chronic stable angina, the association and frequency of silent myocardial ischemia from withdrawal is less well studied. Furthermore, given the steadily increasing number of outpatients taking calcium antagonists alone and in combination with beta-blockers for treatment of chronic angina, two important questions surface: (1) does the presence of calcium blockers in individuals also taking beta-blockers protect against the beta-blockade withdrawal syndrome, and (2) what is the frequency of transient myocardial ischemia from abrupt cessation of calcium antagonist monotherapy?[50]

In an attempt to answer these questions, studies have investigated the occurrence of transient myocardial ischemia as detected by electrocardiographic monitoring. In 47 patients with chronic stable angina and proven coronary artery disease, abrupt withdrawal of beta-blockers, either as monotherapy or in combination with calcium antagonists (group 1, n = 25), was compared with abrupt cessation of calcium antagonism monotherapy (group 2, n = 22) for the occurrence of symptomatic cardiac events and ischemia. The first two monitorings were performed in the hospital (at entry into study and at 48 hours after withdrawal of drugs) and the third monitoring, 5 days after withdrawal, was performed out of the hospital and during daily activity (monitoring occasions 1, 2, and 3).[51,52]

The investigators found that in group 1, the frequency of total ischemia increased by 65% and 148% from monitoring occasions 1 to 2 and 1 to 3, respectively, and silent ischemia increased by 100% and 129%, respectively. However, no significant change in transient myocardial ischemia following cessation of drug was noted in group 2 (calcium monotherapy). The heart rate at onset of ischemia increased significantly in group 1 in contrast to group 2, which had significant increases only during out-of-hospital monitoring periods. Based on these results, the researchers concluded that a rebound in ischemia— predominantly silent ischemia—occurs after abrupt withdrawal of beta-blockers and that angina is not, in itself, a reliable parameter for assessing ischemia. Furthermore, it seems that combined therapy with calcium antagonists neither protects against the effects of beta-blocker withdrawal nor increases ischemic activity.

The results of this investigation make it clear that abrupt withdrawal from beta-blocker therapy may result in transient myocardial ischemia *whether or not* patients have angina. In fact, the finding of predominantly silent ischemia with beta-blocker cessation suggests that *all* patients should be considered at risk for potentially morbid cardiac events when such therapy is abruptly discontinued.

Unfortunately, this study did not address whether gradual withdrawal of beta-blocker therapy is preferable to sudden cessation.

The role of calcium antagonists has also been clarified. Based on this study, abrupt withdrawal of calcium antagonists is *not* associated with significant transient myocardial ischemia. Also, the presence of calcium antagonists does not protect against ischemic events produced by beta-blocker withdrawal.

Calcium Channel Blockers

Patients with calcium channel blocker toxicity usually present with an accentuation of the drug's desired clinical effects, such as high degree of atrio-ventricular (AV) block, hypotension, and CNS changes or congestive heart failure. Hypotension results from the drug's direct effect on ventricular and vascular smooth muscle and is reported in 3.4% to 6% of patients taking nifedipine, and in 5% to 10% of patients treated with verapamil for supraventricular tachycardia. Although most cases of hypotension are mild, some patients will require aggressive treatment.

Bradycardia and a high degree of AV block may also occur, and they are most often associated with verapamil or diltiazem, which can produce a negative chronotropic effect on the sinus and AV nodes. In such cases, temporary pacing may be required. Because of its potent, negative inotropic effects on the ventricle, verapamil or diltiazem can precipitate congestive heart failure in patients with depressed myocardial contractility. Headache is a common side effect and is most commonly seen in patients taking nifedipine GITS. Other CNS side effects include dizziness, sleep disturbance, and mood changes.

The variability of action among calcium antagonists is so pronounced that interchanging one calcium channel blocker for another can be difficult. In contrast to the case of beta-blockers or theophylline derivatives, in which differences among agents basically involve such minor factors as duration of action, appearance of CNS side effects, or receptor subselectivity, the various calcium channel blockers often cannot treat the same disease process.

However, such differences in clinical effect do offer distinct advances in terms of individualizing therapy. For instance, a patient with angina, AV node conduction disturbance, and mild congestive heart failure would benefit most from amlodipine. In this patient, amlodipine (1) relaxes coronary artery tone, which helps the angina; (2) does not affect SA or AV node conduction directly, which leaves the conduction disturbance unaffected; (3) dilates peripheral vessels (decreasing afterload and, thereby, myocardial oxygen demand); and (4) does not impair myocardial pump function. The use of either diltiazem or verapamil in the same patient would run the risk of increasing the conduction disturbance and exacerbating the congestive heart failure.

In contrast to verapamil and diltiazem, which should not be prescribed to patients with sinoatrial disease, atrioventricular block, congestive heart failure, or severe ventricular dysfunction (and only cautiously to those taking a beta-blocker), amlodipine does not affect electrical conduction in the heart and can be used safely in patients with the aforementioned conditions.[53]

Because amlodipine has a low risk of producing drug-drug or drug-disease interactions, it is suitable for combined therapy with a beta-blocker or digitalis. Its pharmacologic advantages make amlodipine the initial calcium channel blocker of choice in elderly patients with angina and/or hypertension who have marginal cardiac output, are prone to episodes of congestive heart failure, are taking beta-blockers or digitalis, or have a history of conduction disturbances. Amlodipine is also used as monotherapy in elderly patients and is very effective.[54]

Several studies conclude that combined treatment with beta-blockers and amlodipine increases antianginal efficacy compared with monotherapies, without increasing adverse effects. Moreover, amlodipine rarely precipitates congestive heart failure or profound bradycardia, two adverse consequences that can be observed with such agents as verapamil and diltiazem.

Antiarrhythmics

Appropriate therapy for ventricular arrhythmias remains a dilemma for the practicing clinician. While a host of potent antiarrhythmic agents are now available that can ameliorate or eradicate most serious rhythm disturbances, the long-term survival benefit of such therapy is unproven. Furthermore, these agents have numerous adverse effects well known to primary care practitioners, ranging from benign problems, such as rash or gastrointestinal intolerance, to serious hematologic or immunologic derangements.

In recent years, the paradoxical tendency for these drugs to induce rather than control arrhythmias has become more widely recognized and a cause for great concern. Drug-associated arrhythmias, or proarrhythmia, have ranged from an increase in premature ventricular contractions to life-threatening phenomena, such as refractory ventricular tachycardia, torsades de pointes, ventricular tachycardia associated with marked prolongation of the QT interval, and ventricular fibrillation.[55]

Primary care practitioners and pharmacists must recognize the significant potential hazards of antiarrhythmic drug therapy. In particular, the proarrhythmic potential of these agents can be life threatening. Left ventricular dysfunction and concomitant treatment with digitalis and diuretics predispose patients to the development of ventricular fibrillation during antiarrhythmic therapy. Drug-induced ventricular fibrillation is a very early event, frequently occurring within 3 days of initiating treatment and most often by 10 days.

It seems prudent to initiate antiarrhythmic therapy in a monitored inpatient setting whenever possible, especially in those at increased risk for ventricular fibrillation (e.g., those on digitalis therapy or in the presence of low left ventricular ejection fraction). Furthermore, until more data are available regarding the long-term survival benefit of antiarrhythmic therapy, these agents should be used very judiciously and reserved for those with malignant and symptomatic ventricular arrhythmias. Finally, physicians should maintain a high index of suspicion in those patients complaining of syncopal symptoms, palpitations, or other manifestations of cerebral hypoperfusion within a few days of initiation of antiarrhythmic therapy.

Given the number of patients who experience premature ventricular contractions (PVCs) following acute myocardial infarction (MI) and the documented adverse effects of potent antiarrhythmic agents, it is important to establish guidelines regarding the safety and efficacy of antiarrhythmic therapy in this patient population. Because sudden death following MI remains a significant public health concern, primary care practitioners sometimes feel compelled to initiate antiarrhythmic therapy in patients who have PVCs after their MI. The presence of PVCs is a risk factor for increased mortality and sudden death following MI, although whether such arrhythmias represent a primary myocardial derangement or underlying coronary artery disease is not yet established. Nevertheless, there have been several randomized clinical trials designed to test whether secondary prevention of sudden death following MI with Type I antiarrhythmic drugs is associated with improved survival. These investigations yielded mixed results.

Type I Antiarrhythmic Drugs. Harvard investigators conducted an English-language literature search of published studies that evaluated the use of prophylactic Type I antiarrhythmic drugs in patients with documented MI. Patients were enrolled within 60 days following MI, continued on therapy for at least 3 months, and only those trials about which a complete report was published in the medical literature were included. Ten such studies were examined. Not surprisingly, individual study designs differed with respect to follow-up (range, 3 to 24 months), Type I antiarrhythmic drug used, and underlying arrhythmia profile satisfying inclusion criteria, which ranged from the presence of simple PVCs to ventricular tachycardia. Investigators successfully isolated a total of 4122 patients randomized to either antiarrhythmic therapy or placebo. The ten studies tested nine antiarrhythmic agents including mexiletine hydrochloride, phenytoin sodium, tocainide hydrochloride, flecainide acetate, encainide hydrochloride, aprindine hydrochloride, imipramine hydrochloride, and moricizine.[56-59]

Precise risk profiles of enrolled patients were presented. Four studies specifically selected patients at relatively high risk for late mortality and sudden death following MI, such as those with mechanical complications or sustained ventricular tachycardia. Based on previously reported classifications of risk stratification following MI, two of the ten studies examined patients with low risk, such as no mechanical complications and infrequent PVCs. The remaining eight studies enrolled patients that would be considered at moderate to high risk following MI, such as patients with high-grade arrhythmias, complex PVCs, or mechanical complications.

The CAST report has done much to make physicians aware of the potential lethal consequences of treating unselected post-MI patients with such potent Type I antiarrhythmics as encainide and flecainide. In that study, which eventually prompted warnings about the use of these agents from their manufacturers, investigators reported 48 deaths in the treated group and 22 deaths in the placebo groups, resulting in a relative mortality rate of about 7.5% and 3.0% respectively.

These early mortality data ultimately precipitated discontinuation of the trial. The current meta-analysis study also is important, however, because it *extends the CAST-induced cautionary note to other Type I antiarrhthmics.* Given the inclusion criteria for enrolling patients in the 10 studies reviewed, it appears that even patients at moderate risk (e.g., those with complex PVCs mechanical complications, short runs of nonsustained ventricular tachycardia) for late mortality following MI *do not demonstrate any advantage over placebo when treated with Type I antiarrhythmic agents.* Given the potent and, sometimes adverse consequences associated with these drugs, primary care practitioners are best advised *not* to begin empiric prophylactic therapy with these agents, even when faced with post-MI patients whose ambulatory electrocardiograms demonstrate complete PVCs. It is conceivable that a small subset of patients who are at an usually high risk of sudden death following MI (e.g., those with mechanical complications, recurrent ventricular tachycardia, cardiac arrest) may, in fact, benefit from such therapy. At present, however, only invasive electrophysiologic studies can identify such patients, and, even in this subgroup, the benefits of therapy have not been conclusively proven. In any event, initiation of long-term, empiric antiarrhythmic therapy in these patients is probably better left to a cardiac specialist who has considerable experience in arrhythmia management.

Although six of the seven studies that specifically assessed arrhythmias found significantly reduced numbers of PVCs at some time during the trial period, the overall effects on mortality were discouraging. Overall, three studies showed small beneficial effects of treatment, two showed no difference, four showed small adverse effects of treatment, and one study showed a statistically significant deleterious effect on mortality. These investigators conclude that therapy of unselected patients with Type I antiarrhythmic agents is currently *unwarranted,* even in those individuals deemed to be at moderate risk for late mortality following MI.

Selected Agents. *Lidocaine.* Lidocaine toxicity alters conduction (high degree of atrioventricular block, asystole, and widened QRS complex) and impairs myocardial contractility. It most often affects the central nervous system and usually occurs during rapid intravenous infusion or with infusions greater than 24 hours in duration. CNS effects include lightheadedness, somnolence, coma, and seizures. Supportive care and discontinuation of lidocaine infusion are generally sufficient treatment in the emergency setting. Administration of fluid or pharmacologic cardiac acceleration may be necessary for hypotension caused by heart block or negative inotropic actions. Treat seizures with benzodiazepines rather than phenytoin.

Quinidine. Quinidine toxicity may be either acute or chronic. Many of the gastrointestinal, CNS, ECG and other findings (e.g., headache, flushed skin, blurred vision with mydriasis) are similar to findings seen in anticholinergic reactions. This suggests that quinidine and other anticholinergic drugs, such as cyclic antidepressants and antipsychotics, may produce an additive effect.

The ECG changes, which consist primarily of conduction delays including PR, QRS, and QT prolongation, correlate closely with the severity of the clinical course. Quinidine toxicity may also cause severe hypotension.

In addition to supportive treatment, studies suggest that alkalinization may be appropriate for quinidine toxicity, since alkaline serum decreases the free levels of this highly protein-bound drug.

The newer oral antiarrhythmic agents, (tocainide, mexiletine, and flecainide) produce a number of CNS and gastrointestinal side effects, some of which may necessitate discontinuing the drug in an elderly patient. Approximately 20% of all elderly patients taking tocainide stop the drug because of dizziness, confusion, nightmares, coma, or seizures. Gastrointestinal side effects that precipitate discontinuance include nausea, vomiting, and constipation. Mexiletine produces the same CNS and GI symptoms as tocainide, and discontinuance rates as high as 40% are reported.

Digitalis. Geriatric patients are at high risk for developing toxicity from digitalis glycosides. Several factors lead to increased risk, including concurrent administration of other drugs such as quinidine or disopyramide and metabolic abnormalities such as hypokalemia, hypomagnesemia, and renal failure. Toxicity should be suspected in any patient taking digoxin who develops new gastrointestinal, ocular, or central nervous system complaints, or in whom sinus bradycardia, AV conduction defects, junctional tachycardia, or PVCs develop without an underlying cause.

Anorexia, confusion, and depression are the most common symptoms of digoxin intoxication, while nausea, vomiting, and visual changes, so common in young patients, are frequently absent in the elderly. However, elderly patients may develop CNS symptoms of digoxin toxicity even with normal plasma digoxin levels. Serum digoxin levels should be obtained whenever progressive cardiac or renal failure occurs. Levels above 2 ng/ml are associated with increased risk of toxic effects.

Complaints in geriatric patients are nonspecific and include anorexia, abdominal pain, fatigue, malaise, headache, and visual disturbances (e.g., blurred vision, halos around objects or difficulty focusing). Cardiac toxicity may be present, with increased vagal tone or enhanced automaticity producing sinus bradycardia, variable degrees of AV conduct ion block, or ventricular ectopy. Ventricular arrhythmias are the most common dysrhythmic derangements, but atrial and junctional tachycardias with variable nodal conduction blocks also occur.

Management consists of stopping digoxin therapy, cardiac monitoring, maintaining normal to high-normal serum potassium levels, and when toxicity is life threatening, initiating appropriate antiarrhythmic therapy in combination with digoxin antibodies.

Antihypertensive Drug Toxicity

About 70% of elderly individuals treated with antihypertensive medications show symptoms of sadness, fatigue, apathy, agitation, or insomnia.[60] Reserpine, propranolol, and methyldopa cause these symptoms most often, but clonidine, guanethidine, and hydralazine are also capable of producing symptoms of mental depression. Other nonantihypertensive agents with similar effects include neuroleptics, tranquilizers, hypnotics, digoxin, antiparkinsonian drugs, anticancer agents, corticosteroids and NSAIDs. Drug interactions also are common (see Table 7-12).

Thiazide diuretics are associated with more adverse reactions than any other drug.[62] They are also among the most commonly prescribed drugs for the elderly. Hypovolemia and postural hypotension, electrolyte imbalances (hyponatremia, hypercalcemia, and hypokalemia), glucose intolerance, and hyperuricemia are the most common adverse reactions (Table 7-9).

Table 7-9

Side Effects of Commonly Used Diuretics			
Diuretic	**Thiazide**	**Loop Diuretic**	**Potassium-sparing**
Hypokalemia	+	+	−
Hyperkalemia	−	−	+
Acidosis	−	−	+
Alkalosis	+	+	−
Hyperuricema	+	+	−
Hypercalcemia	+	+	−
Hyperglycemia	+	+	−
Hypertriglyceridemia	+	+	−
Hyponatremia	+	+	−
Hypomagnesemia	+	+	+

Hypokalemia may induce or augment digoxin toxicity, while severe hyponatremia may produce stupor, seizures, and coma. Mild hyperuricemia is common but rarely induces an acute gout attack. Obtaining serum uric acid levels, however, can be helpful when the patient presents with a monarthric arthritis. Finally, loop diuretics can induce painful urinary retention and symptoms of prostatism in elderly men with gland enlargement. Spironolactone and triamterene may induce hyperkalemia in patients with reduced renal failure and in those taking ACE inhibitors.

Clonidine and methyldopa can cause postural hypotension, CNS depression, and sexual dysfunction (Table 7-10). The CNS depression associated with clonidine decreases mental acuity, causing patients to seem senile or demented in addition to feeling tired or drowsy. Moreover, sudden discontinuation of clonidine can cause a withdrawal syndrome of headache, sweating, and rebound hypertension. Consequently, if a patient on clonidine therapy presents with symptoms of rebound hypertension, insomnia, headache, or arrhythmia, inquire if the patient discontinued the drug abruptly.

Table 7-10

Adverse Side Effects of Antihypertensive Drugs				
	Impotence	Ejaculation difficulties	Decreased libido	Gyneco-mastia
Thiazides	?	−	+	−
Spironolactone	+	−	+	+
Methyldopa	+	+	+	+
Clonidine	+	+	−	+
Propranolol	+	−	+	−
Hydralazine	?	−	−	−
Prazosin	+	−	−	−
Doxazosin	−	−	−	−
ACE Inhibitors	−	−	−	−
Amlodipine	−	−	−	−

Elderly patients may experience sudden syncope after taking the first dose of prazosin or report some combination of dizziness, headache, or lethargy. Usually, these symptoms will subside after 2 or 3 days of therapy. The concomitant intake of beta-blockers or diuretics may enhance this first-dose side effect (Table 7-11). Hydralazine, which is contraindicated in coronary artery or valvular disease, can produce CNS manifestations, such as headache or depression. Reflex tachycardia, angina, lupus syndrome, and fluid retention are also reported.

Table 7-11

Drugs Causing Orthostatic Hypotension	
Benzothiadiazides	Methotrimeprazine
Bretylium	Methyldopa
Captopril	Methysergide
Clonidine	Minoxidil
Cyclic antidepressants	Nifedipine
Furosemide	Nitroglycerin
Guanethidine	Pentolinium
Guanidine	Phenothiazines
Hexamethonium	Phenoxybenzamine
Hydralazine	Prazosin
Iopanoic acid	Procarbazine
Levodopa	Reserpine
Lidocaine	Thiothixene

Table 7-12

Drug Interactions in Antihypertensive Therapy

Diuretics

- Diuretics can raise lithium blood levels by enhancing proximal tubular reabsorption of lithium
- NSAIDs, including aspirin, may antagonize antihypertensive and natriuretic effectiveness of diuretics
- ACE inhibitors magnify potassium-sparing effects of triamterene, amiloride, or spironolactone
- ACE inhibitors blunt hypokalemia induced by thiazide diuretics

Sympatholytic Agents

- Guanethidine monosulfate and guanadrel sulfate. Ephedrine and amphetamine displace guanethidine and guanadrel from storage vesicles. Tricyclic antidepressants inhibit uptake of guanethidine and guanadrel into these vesicles. Cocaine may inhibit neuronal pump that actively transports guanethidine and guanadrel into nerve endings. These actions may reduce antihypertensive effects of guanethidine and guanadrel
- Hypertension can occur with concomitant therapy with phenothiazines or sympathomimetic amines
- Monoamine oxidase inhibitors may prevent degradation and metabolism of released norepinephrine produced by tyramine-containing foods and may thereby cause hypertension
- Tricyclic antidepressant drugs may reduce effects of clonidine

Beta-blockers

- Cimetidine may reduce bioavailability of beta-blockers metabolized primarily by the liver by inducing hepatic oxidative enzymes. Hydralazine, by reducing hepatic blood flow, may increase plasma concentration of beta-blockers
- Cholesterol-binding resins, i.e., cholestyramine and colestipol, may reduce plasma levels of propranolol hydrochloride
- Beta-blockers may reduce plasma clearance of drugs metabolized by the liver (e.g., lidocaine, chlorpromazine, warfarin)
- Combinations of calcium channel blockers and beta-blockers may promote negative inotropic effects on the failing myocardium
- Combinations of beta-blockers and reserpine may cause marked bradycardia and syncope
- ACE inhibitors. Nonsteroidal anti-inflammatory drugs, including aspirin, may magnify potassium-retaining effects of ACE inhibitors

Calcium Antagonists

- Combinations of calcium antagonists with quinidine may induce hypotension, particularly in patients with idiopathic hypertrophic subaortic stenosis
- Calcium antagonists may induce increase in plasma digoxin levels
- Cimetidine may increase blood levels of nifedipine

Given the wide variety and proven efficacy of the many available agents, optimal antihypertensive therapy has become less a matter of selecting a drug that adequately controls diastolic and systolic blood pressure than of selecting an agent or regimen that is predictably associated with high patient compliance, a low incidence of adverse drug reactions, minimal interdrug toxicity, and preservation of quality of life, including cognitive and sexual function. As better-tolerated agents become available and long-term, large-scale studies on hypertension begin to yield statistically significant morbidity and mortality data, the focus has now shifted to the comparative ability of different antihypertensives to reduce total, cardiac, and stroke morbidity and mortality.

In general, the elderly respond to all available antihypertensive agents. Some trials suggest they may respond to a calcium channel blocker better than to a beta-blocker or an ACE inhibitor, although any one of these classes may be used as monotherapy in the elderly. Since concomitant diseases are prevalent in the elderly, tailoring therapy to these disorders and vigilant anticipation of side effects is the most important part of antihypertensive management. Hypertensives with angina may improve with a beta-blocker or a calcium channel blocker. Congestive heart failure is frequently accompanied by, and even caused by, hypertension. These patients benefit from diuretics and vasodilators of all types, especially ACE inhibitors.[61]

Studies show that physicians are notably poor at judging the effect of hypertensive therapy on quality of life. Interestingly, patients were found to be only marginally better at assessing their general well-being in a British study of the effects of antihypertensive therapy. The spouse or house mate was the most sensitive indicator of adverse effects on well-being and, thus, is the individual to best answer queries by the physician. Failure of an antihypertension regimen to lower blood pressure must not necessarily be assumed to be a failure of the drug. Compliance must be verified before additional drugs are added to prevent hypotension.

Nonpharmacologic therapy must be tried first, but the clinician must be realistic about expectations for a change of long-established behaviors. Salt restriction, weight reduction, and avoidance of alcohol are all admirable goals if the patient can be persuaded to modify their lifestyle.

Systolic Hypertension

In 1984, the Systolic Hypertension in the Elderly Program (SHEP) was instituted to investigate the potential benefits of the treatment of isolated systolic hypertension in the elderly.[63] The preliminary report from SHEP demonstrated the feasibility of safely and effectively lowering systolic blood pressure (SBP) in elderly individuals using a diuretic-based regimen with chlorthalidone.

SHEP consisted of a multicenter, randomized, double-blind, placebo-controlled trial conducted at tertiary centers involving 4,736 ambulatory patients (57% women, 14% black, mean age 72 years) older than 60 years of age. SBP on study entry ranged from 160 to 219 mm Hg, and diastolic blood pressure (DBP) was < 90 mm Hg. For subjects with SBP > 180 mm Hg, the goal of treatment was a reduction to < 160 mm Hg, whereas, for those with SBP of 169 to 179 mm Hg, the goal was reduction of at least 20 mm Hg. Patients randomized to active treatment or placebo were virtually identical in all important demographic and clinical parameters. Average follow-up for patients was 4.5 years.

Active treatment consisted of chlorthalidone, 12.5 mg/day initially with doubling of dosage if treatment goal was not attained. Up to 50 mg of atenolol or 0.1 mg reserpine could be added as a step 2 agent if the goal was not achieved with chlorthalidone alone. If blood pressure was markedly elevated on a single visit (SBP > 240 mm Hg, DBP > 115 mm Hg) or over a sustained period of time (SBP > 220 mm Hg, DBP > 90 mm Hg), patients in either group were released to obtain known active therapy. Study of the occurrence of stroke (both fatal and nonfatal) was the primary goal of therapy, while cardiovascular and coronary morbidity and mortality, all-cause mortality, and quality-of-life were secondary outcome measures.

Throughout the trial, the mean SBP of the active treatment group was about 26 mm Hg lower than at baseline, and DBP was lower by about 9 mm Hg, while in the placebo group SBP was lower by only about 15 mm Hg, and DBP was lower by about 5 mm Hg compared with baseline. Although the majority of patients in the placebo group received no active medication throughout the trial, the percentage released to active therapy increased progressively up to 44% at year 5. Stroke risk over 5 years in the active treatment group was 5.2/100 versus 8.2/100 in the placebo group, which represented a 36% reduction in risk (relative risk = 0.64; 95% confidence interval, 0.5 to 0.82; p = 0.003). This reduction was consistent across all age groups, including those older than 80 years.

The incidence of major cardiovascular diseases was reduced, including coronary heart disease (relative risk, 0.75; 95% confidence interval, 0.60 to 0.94) and left ventricular failure (relative risk, 0.46; 95% confidence interval, 0.33 to 0.65). Although there were trends toward reductions in overall mortality and total cardiovascular mortality (relative risk, 0.87 and 0.80, respectively), these were not significant. Reported rates of various side effects were somewhat higher in the active group than placebo, as were the number of patients with abnormal metabolic parameters (sodium, potassium, glucose, cholesterol, uric acid) at any time during the trial.

This was an extremely well-designed trial of large size that provides conclusive evidence, heretofore lacking, that treatment of isolated systolic hypertension can reduce the incidence of stroke in the elderly. The 36% reduction demonstrated in the trial may actually underestimate the true benefit because many subjects initially in the placebo group ultimately received active treatment. Treatment of systolic hypertension can also reduce other cardiovascular morbidity, although to a lesser degree. Some caution must be exercised in extrapolating these results to a less healthy population, since only 1% of all those initially screened for the trial were ultimately enrolled. Many were excluded because of co-existing cardiovascular disease or liver or renal dysfunction, which raises the possibility of significant selection bias.

This study further debunks numerous myths that are still somewhat prevalent regarding hypertension in the elderly: hypertension cannot be safely or effectively treated in the elderly, there are no benefits of therapy, and the elderly population does not tolerate treatment well. Based on this study, all persons older than 60 years of age (including those older than 75 years) with isolated systolic hypertension should be treated to reduce the risk of stroke and other cardiovascular diseases unless the presence of co-existent illness or poor overall functional status makes this unreasonable.[63]

Thromboembolic Prophylaxis

Overall, the stroke rate for patients with chronic atrial fibrillation is about 5% per year. However, this arrhythmia is a heterogeneous disorder, and in certain subgroups, (i.e., the elderly, those with recent myocardial infarction, and those with history of hypertension), the stroke rate is greater than 5% per year. At one time, rheumatic heart disease was the disorder most commonly associated with atrial fibrillation, but currently, nonvalvular heart disease accounts for more than 70% of the cases of atrial fibrillation. Despite the clear association between atrial fibrillation and stroke, the role of long-term anticoagulant therapy or long-term antiplatelet therapy for prevention of thromboembolic cerebral infarction remains unclear. However, four large prospective randomized trials have examined the risks and benefits of antithrombotic therapy for patients with nonvalvular atrial fibrillation.

The following studies examined the risks and benefits of antithrombotic therapy for patients with nonvalvular atrial fibrillation.

The Copenhagen Atrial Fibrillation, Aspirin, and Anticoagulant Study. The trial provided the first prospective, randomized evaluation of treatment options for patients with atrial fibrillation who were assigned to treatment with aspirin, 75 mg/day, warfarin (PT time ratio, 1.5 to 2.0) or a placebo. There was a 38% dropout rate in the warfarin group, 13% in the aspirin group and 15% in the placebo group.

The trial was stopped prematurely because a substantial reduction in thromboembolic complications was observed in the warfarin group. The intention-to-treat analysis showed a significant reduction in total thromboembolic events (risk reduction, 56%) in the warfarin group but no such reduction in thromboembolic events among those receiving 75 mg/day of aspirin.

The Stroke Prevention in Atrial Fibrillation Study. The study was a multicenter trial comparing warfarin and aspirin therapy with a placebo in patients with nonrheumatic atrial fibrillation. The design called for the enrollment of 1,644 patients during a 3-year period, with an additional year of follow-up observation before termination. The study was terminated because significant benefit was found with active aspirin or warfarin therapy.

Analysis of the data demonstrated an acceptably low bleeding risk and a thromboembolic event rate of 2.3% per year in the warfarin group, 3.6% in the aspirin group, and 7.4% in the placebo group, for an overall warfarin-associated risk reduction of 67%.

Boston Area Anticoagulant Trial for Atrial Fibrillation. This unblinded, randomized, controlled study was performed to test the safety and efficacy of low-dose warfarin therapy for preventing stroke in patients with nonrheumatic atrial fibrillation. Overall, 212 patients received anticoagulant therapy for an average of 2.3 patient years, and the control group consisted of 208 patients. The average PT ratio of those with active warfarin therapy was 1.33. Thirteen strokes occurred in the control group and two occurred in the warfarin group, yielding a stroke rate of 0.4% per patient year and 3.0% in the control group. The Boston study demonstrated that low-intensity anticoagulation in patients with nonrheumatic atrial fibrillation was safe and effective and could yield a stroke reduction as high as 86% per patient year.

The Canadian Atrial Fibrillation Anticoagulation Study. The study was a randomized, double-blind, multicentered, placebo-controlled trial of warfarin in patients with nonrheumatic atrial fibrillation. Consisting of 187 patients in the warfarin group and 191 in the placebo group, the study yielded an annual combined event rate for nonlacunar stroke and noncentral nervous system embolism of 2.5% in the warfarin group and 5.2% in the placebo group.

Although the study lacked statistical power, it emphasized that the trend in warfarin is consistent with and supportive of the positive results with warfarin found in the other three aforementioned studies.

Not surprisingly, these studies focused on elderly patients, and the average age in most trials was about 70 years. All studies showed a substantially reduced incidence of stroke and a low incidence of significant bleeding in patients taking warfarin. Overall, the benefits in stroke reduction appear to outweigh the risks for serious bleeding in patients with atrial fibrillation. Further studies will be required to identify the precise role of aspirin in such patients and the relative risks and benefits of using warfarin for prevention of stroke in patients with lone atrial fibrillation.

Prescribing Implications. With its propensity for causing thromboembolic cerebrovascular infarction, atrial fibrillation is a common disease that has the potential for killing and disabling thousands of elderly Americans each year. It should be emphasized that atrial fibrillation has a prevalence of about 2% in the general population and is more common in the elderly, affecting about 5% of persons older than 60 years of age. Clinicians now recognize that chronic atrial fibrillation in older patients with coronary artery disease is a quietly festering but deadly condition. Previously, many physicians chose not to treat it because of the perception that the hemorrhagic risks of anticoagulant therapy would outweigh the benefits.

It now appears that most patients with nonvalvular atrial fibrillation, especially those at high risk for stroke and who are candidates for anticoagulation therapy, will benefit from chronic warfarin therapy. The elderly patient with chronic nonvalvular atrial fibrillation and underlying coronary heart disease is perhaps the most likely to benefit from chronic low-intensity warfarin therapy. If attempts at restoration of normal sinus rhythm have failed or are contraindicated, patients should be started on long-term warfarin therapy, although it should be stressed that the precise benefits and risks of long-term anticoagulation are simply not known.

Monitoring Anticoagulation Therapy. An important empirical observation is that a significant minority of patients who sustained a thromboembolus while taking warfarin had a subtherapeutic PT ratio at the time of their morbid event. This observation stresses the importance of vigilant monitoring of warfarin therapy to prevent morbidity.

Warfarin and Myocardial Infarction. Following a myocardial infarction (MI), reinfarction and stroke are major causes of subsequent morbidity and mortality. Arterial thrombosis (or embolism in the case of stroke) is the primary pathogenic event in each of these, implying that anticoagulant therapy after a MI might be a beneficial prophylactic measure. In the past, high dose warfarin was often used during the postinfarction period, but hemorrhagic complications were common, and studies evaluating this therapy reached conflicting conclusions regarding the risk to benefit ratio. Therefore, routine administration of anticoagulants in the post-infarction period fell out of favor.

At present, routine warfarin therapy cannot be recommended for patients: (1) who have had thrombolytic therapy, a revascularization procedure, or are taking aspirin for secondary prevention of MI; and 2) who have had an inferior, uncomplicated MI, inasmuch as the morbidity and mortality is already so favorable in these groups that the benefits of warfarin therapy may outweigh the risks.

Who then should receive warfarin therapy following MI? Patients who have had a large anterior MI, as well as those at high risk for subsequent complications and increased mortality but who have not been thrombolyzed, revascularized, and are not *already* on aspirin for secondary prevention, can be expected to benefit from warfarin therapy, if this therapy is started within 1 month following acute MI.

Finally, it should be emphasized that some kind of therapy directed at thrombus prevention is essential following MI. Whether aspirin or warfarin is preferable is still a matter of debate, inasmuch as at least one study has shown that 650 mg aspirin is just as effective as warfarin in preventing thrombus formation in high-risk patients.

Thromboembolism and Mechanical Heart Valves

There is general agreement that patients with mechanical heart valves require lifelong anticoagulation therapy with warfarin to reduce the risk of systemic embolization associated with the use of these prostheses. Controversy remains, however, regarding the optimal dosage. The major controversy concerns weighing the potential risk of increased thromboembolic events seen with inadequate anticoagulation against the increased bleeding complications seen with more intensive warfarin therapy. Recent randomized studies of anticoagulation for other medical conditions, such as venous thromboembolism, have shown that less intense anticoagulation therapy was just as effective as, but safer than, the usual recommended dose of warfarin therapy. It is important to determine the efficacy and safety of different anticoagulation regimens in patients with mechanical heart valves.

Long-term anticoagulation therapy is effective in limiting thromboembolic events in many clinical situations, including patients with mechanical heart valves. Such therapy is not benign, however, and can be complicated by potentially serious bleeding episodes. Several studies have demonstrated equal efficacy but greater safety with lower-intensity anticoagulation regimens than previously recommended. It appears prudent for clinicians to strive for an INR of 1.5 when treating patients with mechanical heart valves with oral warfarin. Lower prothrombin ratios (i.e., < 1.5) are likely to be associated with a greater risk of thromboembolic events, while higher ratios are known to cause more bleeding complications.

Aspirin and Transient Ischemic Attacks

Aspirin reduces the risks of vascular death, stroke, and nonfatal MI in patients with a prior stroke or (TIA). Dosages ranging from 300 to 1500 mg/day have been used. Such doses diminish platelet adhesiveness by inhibiting thromboxane A2 production. Theoretically, a lower dose of aspirin sufficient to inhibit thromboxane, but not prostacyclin, may be even more effective in preventing vascular complications in high-risk patients. In patients with a history of TIA or ischemic stroke, the annual risk for a serious vascular event is almost 10%. Even a very small dose of aspirin (30 mg/day) effectively reduces the chances of a thrombotic event in high-risk patients, with fewer minor bleeding complications. However, the degree of thrombotic risk reduction equals, but does not exceed, that of a higher-dose regimen. Even at low doses, aspirin retains a potent antiplatelet effect that should be respected. The decision to implement low-dose antiplatelet therapy must still be made with the risk of a hemorrhagic complication in mind. In the future, a low-dose aspirin regimen will probably be the preferred program for prevention of a thrombotic event in high-risk patients because it is equally effective, better tolerated, and associated with a reduction in risk of minor bleeding episodes. On a practical note, there remains some question as to the bioavailability of low doses of aspirin in the plain aspirin formulation.

Aspirin Therapy and Myocardial Infarction

Aspirin inhibits platelet aggregation. It serves as an effective agent for secondary prevention of MI and nonhemorrhagic stroke in patients with unstable angina, myocardial infarction, stroke, or TIA. However, its usefulness for primary prevention remains to be determined. In healthy men older than 50 years of age, aspirin prophylaxis was shown to reduce the risk of MI by almost 50%, but there is the question of a slight increase in the risk of hemorrhagic stroke. A patient at low risk of underlying heart disease might be reluctant to take aspirin for primary prevention, but one with a higher risk of infarction, such as those with stable angina, might be more willing if the potential benefits were compelling.

Primary prevention of MI is certainly a worthwhile goal, given the 25% to 30% mortality rate for the periinfarction period. Patients with stable angina are at greatly increased risk of cardiovascular events, with mortality rates of 2% to 10% per year. Thus, the potential benefit of low-dose aspirin therapy in primary prevention of MI seems great. The unanswered question is the risk of stroke, which remains to be quantified. Until this risk is better defined, we suggest limiting prophylactic aspirin therapy to patients with chronic stable angina who are judged to be at no additional risk of hemorrhagic stroke (e.g., no history of hypertension, diabetes, bleeding diathesis, previous hemorrhagic stroke). Also undefined is the safety of very prolonged aspirin prophylaxis (greater than 60 months). There is some evidence that aspirin exposure, especially in high doses, may be injurious to vessel walls, making it important to further define the risks of very long-term, low-dose aspirin use. For now, adding a single dose of aspirin every other day to the regimen of carefully selected patients with chronic stable angina deserves serious consideration. More widespread implementation of aspirin therapy must await larger scale studies to address the issues of stroke risk and reduction in cardiovascular mortality.

SALICYLATES

More than 200 OTC preparations contain aspirin, which can adversely affect the elderly. Presenting symptoms can include gastritis with gastrointestinal blood loss leading to iron deficiency anemia and peptic ulcer with or without serious hemorrhagic manifestations. The elderly are particularly prone to chronic salicylate intoxication, which presents as tinnitus, confusion, respiratory alkalosis, and noncardiogenic pulmonary edema. Even patients taking therapeutic analgesic doses of salicylates are prone to chronic salicylism. Consequently, any elderly patient who presents with confusion, respiratory alkalosis, and pulmonary edema of unknown etiology should have a salicylate blood level determined. The diagnosis depends on a thorough drug history and elevated blood salicylate level.

Treatment for primary prevention of stroke in high-risk patients has been rather disappointing. Endarterectomies, bypass procedures, and dipyridamole therapy are without proven efficacy. There is no evidence that anticoagulant therapy prevents strokes due to atheromatous cerebrovascular disease, although it is useful for prevention of systemic embolization. Aspirin lowers the risk of stroke in men, but the effect has not been demonstrated convincingly in women.

Ticlopidine is a new antiplatelet agent. Its mode of action is the irreversible inhibition of ADP-dependent platelet aggregation pathways. Unlike aspirin and NSAIDs, it does not impair prostaglandin synthesis and thromboxane production. Ticlopidine is capable of lowering the risk of fatal and nonfatal stroke in high-risk patients and is more effective than aspirin, the only other agent previously shown to have such an effect. However, the risk of severe neutropenia, although infrequent and fully reversible, means that ticlopidine should be used cautiously, with blood counts monitored frequently. Most episodes of neutropenia occurred within 1 to 3 months of onset of therapy. Moreover, diarrhea can be a troublesome side effect. Nonetheless, if prescribed carefully, this agent is a useful and important addition to the limited choices available for stroke prevention in patients unable to take aspirin.

MANAGEMENT OF HYPERCHOLESTEROLEMIA IN THE ELDERLY

Patients over 60 years of age have a higher prevalence of elevated serum cholesterol and coronary heart disease than any other segment of the population, yet no prospective trial has been performed solely to examine the benefits of treating hypercholesterolemia in the elderly. Consequently, the decision to initiate therapy in these patients is often difficult. Furthermore, concern has been raised over the value of the total serum cholesterol level for predicting coronary artery disease in the geriatric population.

Total cholesterol levels generally increase with age. In men, cholesterol rises continuously between the ages of 18 and 55, while in women a large increase in cholesterol occurs at menopause. By the age of 60, these levels reach a plateau, but by this time one third of men and one half of women have total cholesterol levels > 240 mg/dl, and low-density lipoprotein levels > 160 mg/dl. By consensus of the National Cholesterol Education Program, these individuals fall into the high-risk group. The number of elderly candidates for lipid-lowering therapy is, therefore, immense, and policy regarding management has an enormous impact on society.

Several studies have demonstrated diminution in the predictive value of total cholesterol levels with increasing age. In the Framingham Heart Study, the relative risk of developing coronary artery disease for patients younger than 50 years of age with severe hypercholesterolemia was 3.58%; but in similar patients older than 50 years, the risk ratio fell to 2.18%. This is due in part to the increased impact of competing risk factors such as diabetes and hypertension in the elderly, which tend to obscure the relationship between hypercholesterolemia and coronary artery disease. However, in the Multiple Risk Factor Intervention Trial (MRFIT), although the risk ratio declined with age, the attributable risk of coronary artery disease related to hypercholesterolemia actually increased between the ages of 35 and 60 years.

Although definitive, prospective data specific to the elderly are as yet unavailable, the potential benefits of lowering cholesterol may be greater in the elderly than in any other age group. Other studies also have suggested that lipid-lowering therapy in the elderly is effective.[64] For instance, the Lipid Research Clinics Primary Prevention Trial (LRC-PPT) enrolled male patients up to 59 years old and followed them for up to 10 years. It documented substantial reductions of LDL levels with combined dietary and pharmacologic intervention in elderly subjects; there were significant reductions in myocardial infarction, cerebrovascular accidents, and cardiovascular mortality. It is important to note that in this and most other trials, 2 to 3 years of follow-up were necessary before significant benefits became apparent. LDL and HDL levels retain strong relative risk values with advancing age. The inverse correlation between HDL and coronary disease is the most powerful of these relationships. HDL and LDL levels should, therefore, be determined in elderly patients with total cholesterol levels > 200 mg/dl, even in the absence of other risk factors.

Three main questions emerge that should be answered before embarking on lipid lowering therapy in the elderly. First, does the patient have a reasonable remaining life expectancy? Advanced age alone should not exclude a patient from therapy, but an octogenarian should probably be treated only if the patient is physiologically young and able to enjoy an active lifestyle. Second, does the patient have an acceptable quality of life that would be lost if cardiovascular disease became apparent? The authors suggest that patients with end stage diseases such as crippling rheumatoid arthritis or dementia are unlikely to benefit from aggressive treatment of hypercholesterolemia. Third, can the patient be reasonably expected to comply with therapy? It is often difficult for elderly patients to make major changes in dietary habits, to pay for expensive medications, or to tolerate side effects. The decision to treat hypercholesterolemia in the elderly must be viewed in perspective. Furthermore, since hypertension and diabetes increase morbidity and mortality in the elderly, treatment of these disorders should always take precedence.

When the decision to institute treatment for hypercholesterolemia is made, dietary modification is the first step and should be carried out for at least 6 months before drug therapy is instituted. The authors suggest that, in general, drug therapy should be started only when the LDL remains above 160 mg/dl and that lovastatin-like drugs be the first-line therapy. The authors consider gemfibrozil, which primarily lowers triglycerides while raising HDL, as a second-line agent. Niacin and probucol are not recommended.[65]

Until definitive, prospective data exist regarding the treatment of hypercholesterolemia in the elderly, decisions about such therapy will be difficult to make and steeped in some controversy. It seems reasonable at this point to base decisions about therapy primarily on the levels of LDL and HDL rather than on total serum cholesterol. Overly aggressive interventions to lower cholesterol should be avoided in most elderly patients because of cost, practicality, and the lack of definitive proof of uniform efficacy. However, age alone should not be an exclusion for any particular treatment regimen in an otherwise healthy elderly individual. As with virtually all disorders in the geriatric population, the physiologic age and functional status of the patient are far more important determinants of the value of therapy than chronologic age.

Nitrate Therapy

The sublingual (nitroglycerin) and oral (isosorbide dinitrate) nitrate preparations are antianginal agents that promote vasodilation of both venous and, to a lesser extent, arterial vascular beds. In the coronary beds, nitrates redistribute blood flow along collateral routes to the underperfused myocardium.

Orthostatic hypotension occurs commonly in the elderly. Tolerance and cross-tolerance between nitrates develops with prolonged usage. Headache occurs early after consumption and with excessive doses. Angina may develop or worsen with sudden withdrawal of nitrates.

Orthostatic hypotension occurs with the antihypertensives, especially the calcium channel blockers, phenothiazines, and alcohol.

Patients inexperienced with nitrates should lie down for the first few doses in case of hypotension, which is usually due to dehydration or excessive preload reduction. The onset of action of nitroglycerin topical ointment takes 20 to 60 minutes, and the transdermal patch takes 40 to 60 minutes. These preparations are adequate for prophylaxis, but their onset of action is too slow for acute angina. Only sublingual nitroglycerin or sublingual-chewable isosorbide, with an onset of action of 1 to 3 minutes, should be used for acute anginal attacks.

ESTROGEN AND CARDIOVASCULAR DISEASE IN POSTMENOPAUSAL WOMEN

All postmenopausal women should be considered candidates for ERT. The final decision as to whether estrogen is appropriate should be made by the patient and her physician after weighing all relevant factors. A history of breast cancer or other estrogen-sensitive malignancy is the only true absolute contraindication to estrogen use. A history of thromboembolic disease is a common relative contraindication but does not generally preclude therapy. In women who were treated with a hysterectomy, the benefits of ERT generally greatly outweigh the risks because there is obviously no risk of endometrial cancer or the annoying recurrence of menstrual bleeding.

In women who still have a uterus, progestins should be added to the regimen to minimize the risk of endometrial cancer. There is no evidence that this combination blunts the beneficial lipid-lowering effects of estrogen. The standard cyclical estrogen/progestin regimen frequently results in withdrawal bleeding, which usually affects long-term compliance. The use of continuous low-dose progesterone along with daily estrogen use can greatly reduce the frequency of bleeding and thereby improve the tolerability of ERT. Unusually heavy or irregular bleeding should be investigated by endometrial biopsy or curettage. Doses greater than 1.25 mg of conjugated estrogen (or its equivalent) per day should be avoided.

Estrogen Replacement Therapy and Risk of Venous Thrombosis

Of special concern is the possible risk of venous or arterial thrombosis in patients receiving ERT. Although epidemiologic data fail to demonstrate an association between ERT and thrombosis, the well-known and documented association between contraceptive estrogens and thrombosis has deterred some practitioners from long-term ERT in women suspected to be at high risk for thrombotic complications.[67]

Characterizing the precise relationship between estrogen use and thrombosis in middle-aged and older women is problematic because idiopathic thrombosis and conditions that predispose to thrombosis are more commonly seen with increasing age, making it difficult to implicate estrogens as independent risk factors for thrombosis. Clearly, this issue must be clarified, and the safety of postmenopausal estrogen use should be well-established before women are encouraged to consider long-term ERT for cardioprotection. In addition, there is some debate as to the best oral estrogen replacement drug. Although the use of synthetic oral estrogens is discouraged by most experts, these preparations are the most widely used. Additional data regarding their safety would be useful.

A study at the University of California,[67] was conducted to test the association of estrogen with thrombophlebitis in postmenopausal women. The investigators reviewed consecutive hospital admissions of women aged 45 years or older from 1980 through 1987. Cases were defined as all women with a diagnosis of thrombophlebitis, deep venous thromboembolism, or pulmonary embolism. Women were considered current hormone users if they were taking hormones at the time of admission. Two controls per case were identified through a computer search of women aged 45 years or older whose diagnoses did not include one of the thrombotic diagnoses listed above. There were 121 cases and 236 controls identified, with a mean age of 65.4 years (range, 48 to 87). Overall, the three most common nonthrombotic diagnoses were hypertension, diabetes, and coronary artery disease.

Current use of exogenous estrogens was reported by 5.1% of cases and 6.3% of controls. Hormone regimens varied considerably, so that determining an average dose for controls and cases was not possible. Although not statistically significant, several purported risk factors for thrombosis were more prevalent in estrogen users than nonusers. The presence of these factors would tend to increase the incidence of thrombosis, thus strengthening the probability that there was no association demonstrated between estrogen use and thrombosis.

The investigators conclude that although an estrogen-mediated shift toward hypercoagulability would be expected to increase the incidence of thrombosis, this study found no evidence that long-term estrogen therapy was a risk factor for clinically significant venous thrombosis. This study should be reassuring to physicians and patients who are considering the use of ERT but are concerned about the potential for venous or arterial thrombosis.[67]

Although the study finds no increased risk of thrombosis with estrogen use, unfortunately, the investigators were not able to determine the precise dose of estrogen, a central issue in risk-factor analysis. At present, ERT can be prescribed for women at low risk for endometrial carcinoma and for those without a prior risk of thrombotic episodes. In women with a history of thrombotic episodes, lower doses of non-oral estrogen are preferred. Generally, on the basis of current information, postmenopausal estrogen therapy is of proven value and should be prescribed routinely unless contraindicated.[68]

VITAMIN D AND OSTEOPOROTIC FRACTURES IN POSTMENOPAUSAL WOMEN

Osteoporosis is now widely recognized as a major public health problem in the United States that results in significant morbidity and mortality, particularly among postmenopausal women. Estrogen, calcium supplementation, weight-bearing exercise, calcitonin, and diphosphonates are all effective to varying degrees in preventing or treating osteoporosis. Calcitriol, the physiologically active form of vitamin D, is also considered potentially useful therapy for osteoporosis because of its ability to enhance calcium absorption in the gastrointestinal tract and, at least in vitro, to stimulate bone mineralization.

Three previous studies of calcitriol for osteoporosis produced conflicting results. Two studies showed bone-mass stabilization in patients who received calcitriol, while the third showed no difference from placebo in slowing bone loss. No study showed that calcitriol improved bone formation, and all the trials were too small to evaluate fracture rates. The criteria for efficacy and the numbers of patients in these studies were all different, making it difficult to draw definite conclusions about the benefits of calcitriol.

Investigators at the University of Otago in New Zealand performed a prospective, randomized trial of the effects of calcitriol on the development of new vertebral fractures in 622 ambulatory postmenopausal women.[72] All subjects had osteoporosis but no other severe medical problems. None of the women was taking estrogen before or during the study. Subjects were randomized to receive either 0.25 pg calcitriol twice daily or 1 g calcium daily. The subjects and the physicians were aware of the treatment assignment after randomization.

Subjects were observed for 3 years and were assessed periodically regarding routine biochemical and renal function, calcium absorption, and urinary calcium excretion. The major outcome studied was the development of new vertebral fractures. Roentgenograms of the thoracic and lumbar spine were obtained each year. A fracture was defined as the decrease of 15% or more in any 1 year in the anterior or posterior height of the body of any vertebra from T4 through L4.

Treatment with calcitriol for 3 years resulted in a three-fold reduction in the rate of new vertebral fractures as compared with treatment with calcium alone. The effect of calcitriol was evident only during the second and third years of therapy (second-year fracture rate 9.3, versus 25 fractures per 100 patient years; third year, 9.9, versus 31.5 fractures per 100 patient years; $p < 0.001$). The benefit from calcitriol was clear *only* in women with *mild to moderate* osteoporosis, defined as those with five or fewer vertebral fractures at baseline entry into the study. Calcitriol treatment was effective in women with normal calcium absorption as well as those with calcium malabsorption and was not associated with hypercalcemia or other side effects.

Therapy for osteoporosis should be directed toward those at highest risk by taking steps to prevent falls, eliminate smoking and excessive alcohol intake, and to avoid medications known to increase bone loss, such as corticosteroids and high doses of thyroid hormone. Moderate degrees of weight-bearing exercise and calcium supplementation are prudent and helpful for most individuals. ERT is effective in reducing bone loss and fractures even in older women and exerts benefits on the cardiovascular system as well. Calcitonin is effective in preserving bone mass, but it must be given by injection and is expensive. Etidronate improves spinal bone mass and prevents spinal fractures.

Based on this trial, calcitriol should potentially be considered for treating patients with osteoporosis. Further studies are required to define its exact role. Until then, its use is most appropriate in high-risk individuals, without severe osteoporosis and multiple fractures. For instance, those with inadequate calcium intake, evidence of calcium malabsorption, or limited sun exposure may be particularly appropriate candidates for vitamin D supplementation. Close monitoring of serum and urine calcium levels and renal function is essential during therapy with calcitriol. Therapy should be prolonged because it appears that no benefit accrues until after at least several years of treatment.

PROSTATIC HYPERTROPHY

Benign prostatic hypertrophy (BPH) is an extremely common condition among elderly men. Accordingly, transurethral resection of the prostate (TURP), the mainstay of therapy for symptomatic BPH, is one of the most frequently performed surgeries in the elderly population. For years, medical alternatives for the treatment of BPH were sought but remained limited. Because of the rich alpha-adrenergic innervation of the smooth muscles in the prostate and the bladder neck, medical therapy directed at blockade of these receptors, resulting in smooth muscle relaxation, relieves symptoms of prostatism. This was the basis of the treatment of BPH with phenoxybenzamine, a pure alpha blocker, which although somewhat effective, had unacceptable side effects making clinical use impractical. Terazosin and doxazosin are approved as useful and safe options for medical therapy of BPH. Although there are numerous reports of efficacy for these agents in improving symptoms of prostatism, there are relatively little data that assess the safety, compliance, and effectiveness of these agents during longer periods in patients with BPH. Although transurethral resection remains the definitive treatment for this disorder, patients with mild to moderate prostatism and those who are poor surgical candidates or wish to avoid surgery should be considered for medical therapy to relieve symptoms.

Doxazosin and terazosin (and probably other alpha$_1$ blockers) provide symptomatic relief without significant side effects in approximately one half of these individuals. If improvement is to occur, it is generally present by 2 months after starting therapy; if no benefit is noted by then, the medication should be stopped.

Caution is urged in the use of alpha$_1$ blockers in frail, elderly patients. This subgroup of patients is particularly susceptible to postural hypotension with the use of these agents. This can be avoided by prescribing a low dose to be taken at bedtime. Elderly patients who are prescribed alpha blockers should be instructed about the risk of first-dose syncope and how to prevent it.

[1]Ahronheim J. Practical pharmacology for older patients: avoiding adverse drug effects. *Mt Sinai J Med* 1993 Nov;60(6):497-501.

[2]Canadian Medical Association. Medication use and the elderly. *Can Med Assoc J* 1993 Oct 15; 149(8):1152A-D.

[3]Hallas J, Worm J, Beck-Nielsen J, Gram LF, Grodum E, Damsbo N, Brosen K. Drug related events and drug utilization in patients admitted to a geriatric hospital department. *Dan Med Bull* 1991 Oct;38(5):417-20.

[4]Lamy PP. Comparative pharmacokinetic changes and drug therapy in an older population. *J Am Geriatr Soc* 1982;30:S11-9.

[5]Delafuente JC. Perspectives on geriatric pharmacotherapy. *Pharmacotherapy* 1991;11(3):222-4.

[6]Greenblatt DJ, Sellers EM, Shader RI. Drug therapy: drug disposition in old age. *N Eng J Med* 1982;306(18):1081.

[7]Hutchinson TA, et al. Frequency, severity, and risk factors for adverse drug reactions in adult outpatients: prospective study. *J Chronic Diseases* 1986;39(7):533.

[8]Kernan WN, Castellsague J, Perlman GD, Ostfeld A. Incidence of hospitalization for digitalis toxicity among elderly Americans. *Am J Med* 1994 May;96(5):426.

[9]Lamy PP. Drug therapy in the elderly. *Pharmacy International* 1986;7:46.

[10]Lamy PP. Geriatric pharmacology. *Geriatrics* 1986;36(12):41-49.

[11]Lamy PP. Medication management. *Clin Geriatr Med* 1984;4:623-638.

[12]U.S. Department of Health and Human Services *Guidelines for the study of drugs likely to be used in the elderly.* Rockville, Md: FDA, Center for Drug Evaluation and Research, 1989.

[13]World Health Organizations. Health care in the elderly: report of the technical group on the use of medications in the elderly. *Drugs* 22:279.

[14]Michocki RJ, Lamy PP, Hooper FJ, Richardson JP. Drug prescribing for the elderly [see comments] [Review]. *Arch Fam Med* 1993 Apr;2(4):441-4.

[15]Lamy PP. *Prescribing for the Elderly.* Littleton, Mass: PSG Publishing, Inc., 1980.

[16]Leach S, Roy SS. Adverse drug reactions: an investigation on an acute geriatric ward. *Age Ageing* 1986;15:241.

[17]Fletcher A, Bulpitt C. Quality of life and antihypertensive drugs in the elderly [Review]. *Aging (Milano)* 1992 Jun;4(2):115-23.

[18]Hall RCW, et al. Anticholinergic delirium: etiology, presentation, diagnosis, and management. *J Psychedelic Drugs* 1978;10:237.

[19]Pollow RL, Stoller EP, Forster LE, Duniho TS. Drug combinations and potential for risk of adverse drug reaction among community-dwelling elderly. *Nurs Res* 1994 Jan-Feb;43(1):44-9.

[20]Christopher CD. The role of the pharmacist in a geriatric nursing home: a literature review. *Drug Intell Clin Pharm* 1984;18:428-33.

[21]Darnell JC, et al. Medication used by ambulatory elderly: an inhome survey. *J Am Geriatr Soc* 1986;34:1.

[22]Larson EB, Kukull WA, Buchner D, et al. Adverse drug reactions associated with global cognitive impairment in elderly persons. *Ann Intern Med* 1987;107:169-73.

[23]Craft JC, Siepman N. Overview of the safety profile of clarithromycin suspension in pediatric patients. *Pediatr Infect Dis J* (12 Suppl 3):S142-7.

[24]Knapp DA, et al. Drug prescribing for ambulatory patients 85 years of age and older. *J Am Geriatr Soc* 1984;32(2):138.

[25]Wilcox SM, Himmelstein DU, Woolhander S. Inappropriate drug prescribing for the community-dwelling elderly. *JAMA* 1994 July 27;272(4):292-6.

[26]Shrimp LA, et al. Potential medication-related problems in noninstitionalized elderly. *Drug Intell Clin Pharm* 1985;19:766.

[27]Williamson J, Chopin JM. Adverse reactions to prescribed drugs in the elderly: a multicenter investigation. *Age Ageing* 1980;9:73.

[28]American College of Physicians. Improving medical education in therapeutics. *Ann Intern Med* 1988;108:145-147.

[29]Newton PF, Levinson W, Maslen D. The geriatric medication algorithm: a pilot study. *J Gen Intern Med* 1994 Mar;9(3):164-7.

[30]Symposium: managing medication in an aging population: physician, pharmacist, and patient perspectives. *J Am Geriatr Soc* 1985;Supp 30:11.

[31]Vestal R.E. Drug use in the elderly: a review of problems and special considerations. *Drugs* 1978; 16:358.

[32]Gryfe CI, Gryfe BM. Drug therapy for the aged: the problems of compliance and the roles of physicians and pharmacists. *J Am Geriatr Soc* 1984;32(4):301.

[33]Hale WE, May FE, Marks RG, Stewart RM. Drug use in an ambulatory elderly population: a five-year update. *Drug Intell Clin Pharm* 1987;21:530-5.

[34]Helling DK, Lemke LH, Semia TP, et al. Medication use characteristics in the elderly: the Iowa 65+ Rural Health Study. *J Am Geriatr Soc* 1987;35:4-12.

[35]Report of the Royal College of General Physicians: Medication for the elderly. *J R Coll Physicians Lond* 1984;18:7.

[36]Sloan RW. Principles of drug therapy in geriatric patients [Review]. *Am Fam Phys* 1992 June; 45(6):2709-18.

[37]Thomas DR. The brown bag and other approaches to decreasing polypharmacy in the elderly. *N C Med J* 1991 Nov;52(11):565-6.

[38]Thompson JF, et al. Clinical pharmacists prescribing drug therapy in a geriatric setting: outcome of a trial. *J Am Geriatr Soc* 1984;32(2):154.

[39]Furguson RP, Wetle T, Dubitzky D, Winsemius D. Relative importance to elderly patients of effectiveness, adverse effects, convenience and cost of antihypertensive medications. A pilot study. *Drugs Aging* 1994 Jan;4(1):56-62.

[40]Nathan A, Sutters CA. A comparison of community pharmacists' and general practitioners' opinions on rational prescribing, formularies and other prescribing-related issues. *J R Soc Health* 1993 Dec;113(6):302-7.

[41]Gosney M, Tallis RL. Prescription of contraindicated and interacting drugs in elderly patients admitted to hospital. *Lancet* 1984;2:564-567.

[42]Jue SG, Vestal RE. Adverse drug reactions in the elderly: a critical review. O'Malley K. Ed. *Medicine in Old Age-Clinical Pharmacology and Drug Therapy* London, 1985.

[43]Ray WA, Griffin MR, Schaffner W, et al. Psychotropic drug use and the risk of hip fracture. *N Engl J Med* 1987;316:363.

[44]Montamat SC, Cusak B. Overcoming problems with polypharmacy and drug misuse in the elderly. *Clin Geriatr Med* 1992 Feb:8(1):143-58.

[45]Hallas J, Worm J, Beck-Nielsen, Gram LF, Grodum E, Damsbo N, Brosen K. Drug related events and drug utilization in patients admitted to a geriatric hospital department. *Dan Med Bull* 1991 Oct; 38(5):417-20.

[46]Haves LP, Stewart CJ, et al. Timolol side effects and inadvertent overdosing. *J Am Geriatr Soc* 1989;37:261-2.

[47]Nelson WL, Fraunfelder FT, et al. Adverse respiratory and cardiovascular events attributed to timolol ophthalmic solution, 1978-1985. *Am J Ophthalmol* 1986;102:606-11.

[48]Diggory P, Heyworth P, Chau G, McKenzie S, Sharma A. Unsuspected bronchospasm in association with topical timolol—a common problem in elderly people: can we easily identify those affected and do cardioselective agents lead to improvement? *Age Ageing* 1994 Jan;23(1):17-21.

[49]Psaty BM, Koepsell TD, et al. The relative risk of incident coronary heart disease associated with recently stopping the use of B-blockers. *JAMA* 1990; 263.

[50]Vidt DG, Borazanian RA. Calcium channel blockers in geriatric hypertension [Review]. *Geriatrics* 1991 Jan;46(1):28-30, 33-4, 36-8.

[51]Schwartz JS, Abernethy DR. Cardiac drugs: adjusting their use in aging patients. *Geriatrics* 1987; 42(8):31.

[52]Held PH, Yusuf S, Furberg CD. Calcium channel blockers in acute myocardial infarction and unstable angina: an overiew. *BMJ* 1989;299:1187-1192.

[53]Tonkin A, Wing L. Aging and susceptibility to drug-induced orthostatic hypotension. *Clin Pharmacol Ther* 1992 Sept;52(3):277-85.

[54]O'Malley K, Cox JP, O'Brien E. Choice of drug treament for elderly hypertensive patients [Review]. *Am J Med* 1991 Mar;90(3A):27S-33S.

[55]Nestico PF, Morganroth J. Cardiac arrhythmias in the elderly: antiarrhythmic drug treatment. *Cardiol Clin; 4(2):285-303. 1998*66

[56]Hine LK, Laird NM, et al. Meta-analysis of empirical long-term antiarrhythmic therapy after myocardial infarction. *JAMA* 1989;262:3037-40.

[57]Morganroth J. Bigger JT Jr, Anderson JL. Treatment of ventricular arrhythmias by United States cardiologists: a survey before the Cardiac Arrhythmia Suppression Trial results were available. *Am J Cardiolog* 1994 Feb;23(2):283-9.

[58]Peters RW, Mitchell LB, Brooks MM, Echt DS, Barker AH, Capone R, Liebson PR, Greene HL. Circadian pattern of arrhythmic death in patients receiving encainide, flecainide or moricizine in the Cardiac Arrhythmia Suppression Trial (CAST). *J Am Coll Cardiol* 1994 Feb;23(2):283-9.

[59]Willund I, Gorkin L, Pawitan Y, Schron E, Schoenberger J, Jared LL, Shumaker S. Methods for assessing quality of life in the cardiac arrhythmia suppression trial (CAST). *Qual Life Res* 1992 Jun;1(3):187-201.

[60]Burris JF. Hypertension management in the elderly [Review]. *Heart Disease Stroke* 1994 Mar-Apr; 3(2):77-83.

[61]Flack JM, Wolley A, Esunge P, Grimm RH. A rational approach to hypertension treatment in the older patient [Review]. *Geriatrics* 1992 Nov;47(11):24-8,33-8.

[62]Warram JH, Laffel LMB, et al. Excess mortality associated with diuretic therapy in diabetes mellitus. *Arch Intern Med* 1991;151:1350-6.

[63]SHEP Cooperative Research Group. Prevention of stroke by antihypertensive drug treatment in older persons with isolated systolic hypertension. *JAMA* 1991;265:3255-65.

[64]Lewis B, et al. On lowering lipids in the post-infarction patients. *J Intern Med* 1991;229:483-8.

[65]Denke MA, Grundy SM. Hypercholesterolemia in the elderly: resolving the treatment dilemma. *Ann Intern Med* 1990;112:780-92.

[66]Stampfer MJ, et al. Postmenopausal estrogen therapy and cardiovascular disease. *N Engl J Med* 1991;325:11.

[67]Devor M, Barrett-Connor E, et al. Estrogen replacement therapy and risk of venous thrombosis. *Am J Med* 1992;92:271-82.

[68]Falkeborn M, et al. Hormone replacement therapy and the risk of stroke. *Arch Intern Med* 1993;153:1201-9.

[69]Tilyard MW, et al. Treatment of postmenopausal osteoporosis with calcitriol or calcium. *N Engl J Med* 1992;326(6):33357-362.

[70]Prince RL, Smith M, Dick IM, et al. Prevention of postmenopausal osteoporosis: A comparative study of exercise, calcium supplementation, and hormone replacement therapy. *N Engl J Med* 1991;325:1189-95.

[71]Dawson-Hughes B, Dallal GE, Krall EA, et al. Effect of vitamin D supplementation on wintertime and overall bone loss in healthy postmenopausal women. *Ann Intern Med* 1991;115:505-12.

[72]Aloia JF, Vaswani A, Yeh JK, et al. Calcium supplementation with and without hormone replacement therapy to prevent postmenopausal bone loss. *Ann Intern Med* 1994;120:97.

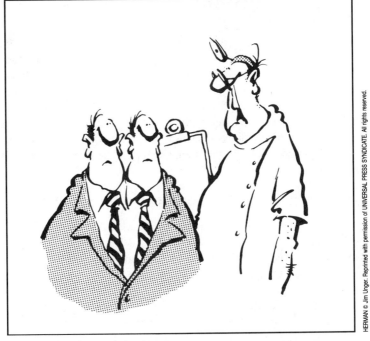

"Take four aspirin and call me in the morning."

Pharmatectural Strategies for Psychiatric, Arthritic, Pulmonary, and Gastrointestinal Drug Therapy in the Elderly

Nonsteroidal anti-inflammatory drugs (NSAIDs) (See Table 8-1) including aspirin, are an important cause of drug-related morbidity and mortality in the elderly. Important forms of toxicity include gastritis, peptic ulceration, and renal insufficiency.[2,3] All NSAIDs can cause these adverse drug reactions, although some studies identify piroxicam (Feldene®) and sulindac (Clinoril®) as clinically safer with respect to renal toxicity.[4,5] All NSAIDs, except aspirin, cause reversible inhibition of platelet function. Aspirin has an *irreversible* effect on platelet function that lasts for the life of the platelet (4 to 7 days). NSAIDs can cause allergic reactions, ranging from rash to anaphylaxis in patients allergic to aspirin.[6] Chronic consumption of aspirin, even in recommended amounts, may lead to chronic salicylism, which is characterized by deafness, marked fatigue, confused and withdrawn behavior, metabolic acidosis, and noncardiogenic pulmonary edema.[7] CNS effects include dizziness, anxiety, tinnitus, and confusion, which may occur in up to 10% to 20% of the elderly on chronic salicylate therapy. Hepatic reactions are usually mild when they occur, but severe hepatitis has been reported. Aplastic anemia is also reported with NSAIDs.

Women older than 65 are at greatest risk of gastrointestinal bleeding and gastric perforation associated with NSAIDs.[8] A history of gastrointestinal bleeding and concomitant diuretic therapy are the two risk factors identified in this group of patients that predict poor outcome. These patients are also frequently dehydrated.

Renal Impairment Associated with NSAIDs

A review of elderly patients on Medicaid with diagnoses of nephritis, nephropathy, and hyperkalemia showed a strong correlation with NSAID use. Three distinct renal syndromes are now associated with NSAIDs.[9]

1. Patients with dehydration, congestive heart failure, nephrosis, or preexisting renal insufficiency who develop acute renal failure within days of starting NSAID therapy. The urine sediment is normal.
2. Acute interstitial nephritis may occur at any time but usually presents after months of NSAID exposure. There is no eosinophilia, eosinophiluria, or rash. Patients present with the nephrotic syndrome (usually edematous).
3. Chronic interstitial nephritis is associated with high-dose NSAID therapy and other analgesics. Papillary necrosis is frequently present.

Table 8-1

Current NSAIDs
Aspirin
Diclofenac
Diflunisal (Dolobid)
Etodolac
Fenoprofen (Nalfon)
Flurbiprofen
Ibuprofen
Indomethacin (Indocin)
Ketoprofen (Orudis)
Ketorolac
Meclofenamic acid (Ponstel)
Mefenamic Acid
Nabumetone
Naproxen (Naproxyn)
Oxaprozin
Piroxicam (Feldene)
Sulindac (Clinoril)
Tolmetin (Tolectin)

Numerous clinical studies have raised questions regarding the overall safety of ibuprofen and other NSAIDs with respect to renal toxicity.[9] Based on acute interventional studies, patients at unusually high risk for NSAID-associated renal impairment are those with clinical disorders and underlying conditions that depend on renal prostaglandin synthesis, such as renal disease, heart failure, cirrhosis, old age, volume depletion, ACE inhibitor therapy, and diuretic use. Despite the lack of well-designed, large-scale investigations, smaller trials have caused some experts to recommend that all elderly patients taking NSAIDs have their renal function closely monitored.

Some authorities, it should be pointed out, are less certain about the evidence linking ibuprofen to renal damage. They emphasize that, in contrast to experimental and interventional studies, previous epidemiologic investigations did not show a major degree of ibuprofen-associated renal impairment. Critics of these findings, however, note that such studies may have lacked the sensitivity to detect ibuprofen-associated renal impairment, since investigators used a diagnosis of renal disease as opposed to a deterioration in serum creatine or creatinine clearance as the primary criteria for renal impairment from NSAIDs. They also emphasize that other epidemiologic studies of ibuprofen-associated renal impairment may have excluded patients at high risk for adverse toxicity from these agents.

Not surprisingly, the seemingly contradictory findings between acute interventional studies and epidemiologic data have left many clinicians in a quandary as to precisely what the actual risks of adverse renal effects of NSAIDs are and, as a corollary, what the parameters for appropriate patient monitoring should be. Given the widespread use of ibuprofen and other NSAIDs, it is critical to clarify these issues for the primary care practitioner so that subgroups of patients who might be at increased risk can be identified.

To address the aforementioned issues, investigators from the Indiana University School of Medicine performed a controlled, retrospective cohort study using a computerized medical record system that contained complete patient laboratory and clinical data, diagnoses, and drug prescriptions for patients in a large internal medicine practice.[9] In particular, they studied the medical records of 1908 patients taking ibuprofen for about 15 months, and compared them to 3933 patients from the same practice who were taking acetaminophen for a similar duration of time. They attempted to: (1) determine the incidence of renal impairment in patients taking ibuprofen; (2) identify predictors for the development of renal impairment; (3) determine which univariate predictors are independently predictive of renal impairment and which ones are merely confounders of this event; and (4) determine whether the risk of renal impairment among patients taking ibuprofen differs from that of a control group of patients taking acetaminophen.

Only those patients who had at least one determination of serum creatinine (SCR) and blood urea nitrogen (BUN) within the year preceding the first ibuprofen or acetaminophen prescription date, and at least one SCR and BUN determination within the year following this date were included in the study. Renal impairment was defined according to either SCR or BUN criteria as follows: (1) In patients with a normal initial creatinine level, ibuprofen-associated renal impairment was defined by a post-prescription date determination documenting an increase in SCR >1.2 mg/dl. Serious impairment was defined as a two-fold increase in SCR, or any final SCR value >2.5 mg/dl; (2) patients with an elevated initial SCR (>1.2 mg/dl) were defined as having ibuprofen-associated renal impairment if the post-prescription SCR determination revealed a 10% increase over baseline, while serious impairment was defined as any two-fold increase in SCR; (3) in patients with a normal initial, pre-prescription BUN level, ibuprofen-associated renal impairment was defined as an increase >40 mg/dl; (4) in patients with elevated BUN levels, a 10% increase in BUN was considered indicative of ibuprofen-induced renal impairment, whereas any two-fold increase was defined as serious renal impairment.

Risk Factors. Of the 1,908 patients in the study group, investigators found that renal impairment occurred in 343 patients (18%). Of the 1,658 ibuprofen-treated patients with normal baseline SCR and BUN, 8.6% developed renal impairment, whereas, of the 250 patients with elevated initial renal function parameters, 25.2% developed renal impairment, 0.7% of which could be characterized as serious. Multivariate analyses indicated five independent predictors of renal impairment: age, prior renal insufficiency, coronary artery disease, elevated systolic blood pressure, and diuretic use. Interestingly, when these investigators tested the degree to which ibuprofen contributed to renal impairment by evaluating the control group of 3,933 acetaminophen recipients, they found that neither ibuprofen nor acetaminophen was among the independent predictors of risk when all the patients were considered. Rather, as these researchers carefully note, these risk factors reflect the likelihood of developing renal impairment by general internal medicine patients and are not specific to ibuprofen therapy.

However, multivariate analyses of patients in both study and control groups at high-risk for renal impairment revealed that compared to the acetaminophen recipients, ibuprofen was indeed a risk factor for renal impairment in patients more than 65 years of age (odds ratio, 1.34) and those with a diagnosis of coronary artery disease.

These investigators conclude that within the year following the receipt of a prescription for ibuprofen, patients over the age of 65 years and those with clinically documented coronary artery disease are at greater risk of renal impairment than patients receiving acetaminophen. Because ibuprofen does not appear to contribute to renal impairment in healthier, younger patients, the authors suggest that such individuals do not require special monitoring of renal function. In contrast, however, they note that in the elderly and in patients with known or suspected coronary heart disease, renal monitoring is warranted with long-term ibuprofen therapy.[5]

NSAIDS and Gastrointestinal Hemorrhage

Although NSAIDs are effective in the management of acute and chronic pain syndromes associated with osteoarthritis and other inflammatory musculoskeletal disorders, the propensity of these drugs to cause gastrointestinal side effects remains a significant deterrent to their use, especially in the elderly.[1,4] Fortunately, the incidence of consequential gastrointestinal hemorrhage, defined as the need for hospitalization, or death resulting from ulcer-induced bleeding, is reported to be 1.6% to 1.8% among long-term users of NSAIDs.[10] These data provide some comfort for practitioners who rely on NSAIDs to improve functional status in patients with chronic, debilitating disease. However, the risk of ulceration in the elderly may be higher, with many recent studies reporting a threefold risk or greater for peptic ulcer disease and upper gastrointestinal tract bleeding associated with NSAID use. The problem with most of these studies, however, is that they fail to generate conclusions and guidelines regarding the effect of NSAID drug dose, duration of use, and specific drug therapy on the development of gastrointestinal hemorrhage, ulceration, or both. Clearly, a need exists for a large-scale investigation that would help clinicians identify factors that increase or, conversely, decrease the risk of NSAID-induced toxicity.[2,3]

To address these issues, a group of investigators from Vanderbilt University School of Medicine conducted a case-control study of Tennessee Medicaid enrollees who were 65 years of age or older.[11] The study included 1,415 patients who were hospitalized for confirmed peptic ulcer disease or upper gastrointestinal tract hemorrhage sometime between 1984 and 1986. The 7,063 control persons represented a stratified random sample of other Medicaid enrollees. Subjects with confirmed peptic ulcer disease or hemorrhage were then categorized according to recency of NSAID use, filled prescriptions, dose, and duration of use. The investigators then defined four categories of exposure according to recency of use.

Current users were defined as patients who had filled a prescription before the index date with a supply of the drug that ended on or after the index date. Indeterminate users were defined as those persons whose prescribed supply of NSAIDs ended 1 to 60 days before the index date. Former users were defined as persons who had received a prescription for NSAIDs 365 days before the index date, but whose supply ended more than 60 days before the index date. Nonusers were classified as subjects with no prescription for NSAIDs for 365 days before the index date.

Overall, of those patients hospitalized with peptic ulcer disease, 34% were *current* users of NSAIDs, compared with 13% of control persons, for an estimated relative risk of 4.1 for development of peptic ulcer disease or upper gastrointestinal tract hemorrhage among NSAID users. Current NSAID use was associated with an elevated risk of development of peptic ulcer in each of three diagnostic categories. The risks were 5.5 for gastric ulcer, 4.3 for duodenal ulcer, and 2.4 for upper gastrointestinal tract hemorrhage. Moreover, the risk of developing peptic ulcer disease increased with increasing dose. It appears as if subjects with a short duration of exposure to the NSAID were at increased risk for developing peptic ulcer disease (i.e., that risk for NSAID-induced complications was greater during the first month of therapy).

Relative Risks. Although the design of this study did not permit investigators to monitor compliance associated with specific NSAIDs, they attempted to compare risks for peptic ulcer disease among current users of specific agents. The relative risks of current users of naproxen, piroxicam, tolmetin, and meclofena-mate were significantly greater than those of current users of ibuprofen.

These investigators conclude that current elderly users of prescription nonas-pirin NSAIDs are about four times more likely to be hospitalized for confirmed peptic ulcer disease or upper gastrointestinal tract hemorrhage than a control group not on NSAID therapy.

The authors note that the finding of reduced risk among ibuprofen users must be interpreted cautiously because: (1) the lower risk associated with this drug might have resulted from poorer compliance associated with agents given on a three or four times daily basis, as opposed to other NSAIDs (piroxicam, sulindac, etc.), which are given once or twice daily; (2) the 1200 mg standard daily dose of ibuprofen used in this study is, in fact, much lower than the dosage rate customarily used by most practitioners to achieve anti-inflammatory effects and substantial improvements in functional capacity (i.e., 1600 to 2400 mg of ibuprofen daily); and (3) the 1200 mg standard daily dose of ibuprofen used as a benchmark in this study probably does not have the same anti-inflammatory activity or therapeutic efficacy as do the other agents evaluated at their recom-mended daily dose. As a result of these clinically important dose- and compli-ance-dependent limitations and variations, interdrug comparisons, especially as they relate to the propensity of therapeutically equivalent doses of NSAIDs to cause peptic ulcer pathology, cannot be fully substantiated from the results reported in this study.

Prescribing Guidelines. This study provides further confirmatory evi-dence that non-aspirin prescription NSAID use is associated with an increased risk of developing peptic ulcer disease, upper gastrointestinal tract disease, or both, in patients 65 years of age or older. This is not new information. What this study reports, however, that *is* new and clinically useful is: (1) the significant association between increasing dose of NSAIDs and the risk of developing peptic ulcer disease and complications requiring hospitalization; and (2) the finding that the greatest risk for developing NSAID-induced complications is observed during the first 30 days of drug therapy. Based on these findings, prescribers are advised to use the lowest dose of NSAID possible to achieve acceptable functional status and pain control in patients with osteoarthritic disorders. It should be emphasized, however, that achieving an adequate clinical response at the standardized recom-mended dose of ibuprofen (1200 mg) cited in this study will not be possible in a significant percentage of cases, and that higher and, therefore, potentially more toxic doses of ibuprofen may be required. Moreover, given the increased risk observed early in the course of NSAID therapy, patients should be followed very carefully, especially during the first month of NSAID therapy. The presence of gastrointestinal complaints, weakness, melena, or other symptoms referable to the gastrointestinal or cardiovascular system necessitate immediate follow-up. Stool guaiac monitoring is strongly recommended in older patients using NSAIDs.

Elderly patients at risk of renal failure or GI bleeding need to be advised of these risks when taking ibuprofen. If at all possible, NSAID use should be reserved for acute inflammation associated with rheumatoid arthritis or osteoarthritis. GI blood loss is usually minimal even in predisposed patients during the first 7 to 10 days unless an active ulcer is present. After the acute flare, NSAIDs should be withdrawn in favor of acetaminophen for chronic pain control. Hypertensive patients should be advised that OTC ibuprofen and all NSAIDs may elevate blood pressure. Patients should be warned to stop NSAID use if they become weak or dizzy or develop diarrhea, vomiting, or loss of appetite.

Misoprostol for Preventing NSAID Gastropathy

Nonsteroidal anti-inflammatory drugs (NSAIDs) continue to be among the most widely prescribed medications in ambulatory populations for a variety of rheumatologic and pain disorders. The chronic use of NSAIDs is also associated with an increased frequency of peptic ulcers and ulcer complications, including bleeding and perforation. Although endoscopically confirmed upper gastointestinal ulcers have been estimated to occur in between 15-31% of chronic NSAID users, the incidence of clinically significant ulcers is certainly less than this although not exactly defined. The morbidity, mortality and overall costs of NSAID induced gastrointestinal problems are quite substantial and have led to efforts to use other agents to help prevent or lessen their severity. H_2 receptor antagonists such as ranitidine (Zantac®) have been shown to inhibit the development of duodenal ulcers in NSAID users but neither these agents nor sucralfate (Carafate®) are useful in reducing the incidence of NSAID induced gastric ulcers. Misoprostol (Cytotec®), a synthetic prostaglandin analog, affords significant protection against NSAID-induced gastropathy. This has been documented in terms of both reduced endoscopic lesions as well as fewer clinically significant ulcers and upper gastrointestinal bleeding episodes in *high risk individuals.* The usual dose of 200 µg of misoprostol four times per day is associated with frequent gastrointestinal side effects (primarily nausea, dyspepsia, diarrhea), which, although usually mild, often seriously diminishes patient compliance. Lower doses of misoprostol are likely to have fewer associated adverse events but have not previously been demonstrated to be as efficacious. Such a regimen, however, could enhance patient compliance and reduce the cost of misoprostol therapy.

Prophylactic Effects. In one study[62-64] patients with chronic rheumatologic disorders who were expected to require at least three months of therapy with either ibuprofen, piroxicam, naproxen, sulindac, tolmetin, diclofenac, or indomethacin were evaluated. Subjects were randomized to receive misoprostol 200 µg four times daily or placebo in a double-blind fashion and to continue their NSAIDs in the same dosage as before the study. Endoscopy was performed at 4, 8 and 12 weeks. In the intent-to-treat cohort, 0.6% of patients randomized to receive misoprostol developed a duodenal ulcer compared with 4.6% of those who received the placebo. Misoprostol also prevented gastric ulcers: 1.9% developed a gastric ulcer in the misoprostol group versus 7.7% on placebo. In the misoprostol patients 32.3% developed diarrhea versus 17.9% of placebo subjects.

In another trial, investigators at several academic centers conducted a six month randomized, double-blind, placebo-controlled trial involving patients with rheumatoid arthritis (RA) in 664 clinical practices of internal medicine, family medicine and rheumatology throughout the United States and Canada who were receiving NSAIDs. A total of 8,843 subjects age 52 or greater (71% women, mean age 68) who were receiving any of ten different NSAIDs were enrolled. Patients were randomly assigned to concurrent misoprostol, 200 μg, or placebo four times daily. The overall incidence of these clinically significant UGI events was low (less than 1%), but there was a 40% reduction in serious UGI complications in the misoprostol group. A substantial number of subjects withdrew from the study prematurely—42% in the misoprostol group and 36% in the placebo group. This difference was attributed to the diarrheal symptoms in the misoprostol group.

In a third trial, investigators at 135 centers across the United States conducted a twelve week, randomized, double-blind, placebo-controlled, parallel, four-limbed study of different dosing regimens of misoprostol. The study involved 1,623 pstients (59% women, median age 58) with a variety of rheumatologic disorders who were receiving standard doses of any of nine different NSAIDs. Subjects were randomly assigned to one of four regimens: placebo four times daily, misoprostol 200 μg twice daily and placebo twice daily, misoprostol 200 μg three times daily and placebo once daily or misoprostol 200 μg four times daily. Misoprostol significantly reduced the incidence of both forms of endoscopically documented ulcer compared to the placebo. The incidence of gastric ulcers was 15.7% in patients taking the placebo but in patients taking misoprostol two times daily was only 8.1%, in those taking it three times daily 3.9% and for four times daily 4.0%. There was a statistically significant dose-response effect of misoprostol in preventing gastric ulcer. For duodenal ulcers the incidence was 7.5% in the placebo group but in the group receiving misoprostol twice daily was 2.6%, three times daily 3.3% and four times daily 1.4%. No difference or dose-response effect was noted between the two or three times daily doses of misoprostol in preventing duodenal ulcers. Fewer subjects withdrew due to adverse effects in the twice (12%) or three times (12%) daily misoprostol groups compared to the four times per day group (20%).

Prescribing Guidelines. There is now ample evidence that misoprostol can reduce the risk of both endoscopically-documented and clinically serious UGI complications in patients taking NSAIDs. Unfortunately, because of its expense, inconvenient dosing regimen and frequent side effects of misoprostol, many questions remain about the cost-effectiveness and practicality of misoprostol therapy. Most estimates of misoprostol therapy indicate that routine preventive therapy with traditional doses of 200 μg four times daily is as much as six or seven times as expensive as that of no treatment (in view of the expense of the medication and the relatively low incidence of serious clinical events it is designed to prevent). Therefore, routine use of misoprostol in all patients taking NSAIDs can not be recommended.

A more practical cost-effective approach for misoprostol use, therefore, consists of the following: (1) stop NSAIDs in high risk individuals whenever possible; (2) when NSAIDs can't be discontinued, target misoprostol mainly for individuals at *high risk* for serious UGI complications (e.g., previous UGI bleeding, previous peptic ulcer, age over 75, history of cardiac disease). The presence of *all four* of these factors confers a risk of serious UGI event of 9% within 6 months compared to 0.4% in individuals with none of these; (3) when using misoprostol start with lower doses (400-600 mg daily in divided doses) to improve convenience and tolerability. Doses of 600 μg per day appear optimal for preventing gastric ulcer while doses of 400 μg daily appear to afford sufficient protection against the development of duodenal ulcer. Exact doses need to be individualized based on risk status and incidence of adverse events in specific patients.

In summary, misoprostol reduces the risk of clinically serious UGI complications in patients taking NSAIDs. *Routine use* of misoprostol in all patients taking NSAIDs cannot be recommended, however, because of its expense, inconvenient dosing regimen and frequent side effects. A more practical approach for misoprostol use, therefore, is to stop NSAIDs in high risk individuals whenever possible, target misoprostol mainly for individuals at high risk for serious UGI complications, and when using misoprostol start with lower doses (400-600 mg daily in divided doses) to improve convenience and tolerability. Exact doses need to be individualized based on risk status and incidence of adverse events in specific patients.

HYPOGLYCEMIC AGENTS

Management of non-insulin-dependent, type II diabetes mellitus usually includes diet, weight control, exercise, and use of oral sulfonylurea agents (See Table 8-2, page 336).[12] Although newer oral sulfonylureas, such as glipizide (Glucotrol®), offer significant advantages in reducing adverse side effects, one should be aware of unusual manifestations of hypoglycemic syndromes in the geriatric population. Hypoglycemia, which can be precipitated by oral agents, is a frequently encountered metabolic derangement, especially in the frail elderly, and can present a broad range of neuropsychiatric syndromes and dysfunctions. Typically, CNS findings in the acutely hypoglycemic geriatric patient consist of confusion, mental impairment, delirium, focal deficits, or frank coma.

Risk Factors. Physicians should look for hypoglycemic reactions in elderly patients with mild or progressive renal impairment (reflected in a decreased glomerular filtration rate) who are concomitantly taking an oral hypoglycemic agent. Because approximately two thirds of circulating insulin is metabolized in the renal parenchyma, patients with reduced renal mass who are taking insulin-releasing agents are especially prone to elevated insulin levels and secondary hypoglycemia. Consequently, in this clinical situation, oral sulfonylurea agents may precipitate hypoglycemia, even though the drug is being taken *as prescribed* and with adequate food intake. Initial treatment consists of intravenous glucose administration with D-50-W followed by patient education and readjustment of the sulfonylurea dose.

Large studies usually point to the first-generation sulfonylureas such as chlorpropamide (Diabinese®) and tolbutamide (Orinase®) as the agents most likely to cause hypoglycemia in the elderly population. Chlorpropamide has a long duration of effect (24 to 60 hours) and elimination half-life (35 hours) and should be used with caution in the elderly. Moreover, secondary drug interactions with phenylbutazone, sulfonamides, salicylates and NSAIDs can precipitate an increased hypoglycemic effect among the first-generation oral agents.

A newer, more potent second-generation oral sulfonylurea agent, glipizide (Glucotrol XL®), has a shorter half-life and more rapid onset of action, making it the current oral sulfonylurea of choice in the elderly population.[13] Glyburide (Micronase®, Diabeta®) is another second-generation agent, but one study of its effects reported 57 cases of severe hypoglycemia, including 24 protracted cases and 10 fatalities.[14] In contrast, glipizide caused neither long-lasting cases of hypoglycemia, nor hypoglycemia-induced fatalities in a seven-year study conducted by the Swedish Board of Health and Welfare's Adverse Drug Reaction Advisory Committee.

Glipizide has the unique capacity to induce a selective glucose (nutrient)-mediated insulin release that closely mimics *in vivo* insulin release patterns in response to postprandial nutrient loading. This selective release, which is maintained as long as 48 months after glipizide therapy, offers special advantages and reduces adverse side effects in the elderly patient with type II diabetes. Finally, because glipizide, unlike the first-generation agents, is bound nonionically to serum proteins, it is less prone to producing hypoglycemia due to secondary drug interactions. Glipizide has a potency equivalence with glyburide and has been shown to reduce insulin requirements when used in type I diabetics.

Insulin Versus Oral Agents For Adult-Onset Diabetes. A major unresolved issue in management of non-insulin-dependent diabetes mellitus (NIDDM) is whether insulin or an oral agent is the treatment of choice. An intense debate has raged ever since the University Group Diabetes Program (UGDP) study cast some doubt on the safety of oral agent therapy. Proponents of oral agent therapy criticized the UGDP study design and argued that oral agents are ideally suited for NIDDM, since they act to lessen peripheral resistance to endogenous insulin, a major cause of NIDDM.

The issue of cardiovascular morbidity remains unresolved, although new data may be forthcoming. In the meantime, the advent of a more potent generation of oral agents raises the issue of how well these new preparations compare with insulin regarding control of hyperglycemia, risk of hypoglycemia, correction of hyperlipidemia, and other important parameters. A randomized, double-blind, placebo-controlled study of glyburide versus insulin for long-term metabolic control of NIDDM has been reported, providing a prospective, controlled comparison of these two modes of therapy.

Both agents produced similar improvements in fasting blood sugar and hemoglobin A_1C levels, similar degrees of weight gain, similar frequencies of mild symptomatic hypoglycemia, and significant reductions in serum lipid levels. Nearly normal degrees of blood glucose control were achieved. Patients in both treatment groups showed significant improvements in HDL levels and HDL cholesterol, but those treated with insulin had a significantly greater improvement in these parameters than did those treated with glyburide.

The authors concluded that glyburide and once-per-day insulin therapy provide similar and very adequate degrees of glucose control in NIDDM patients.

Insulin has the advantage of producing a more favorable lipid profile, although the long-term benefits of this effect are not known.

CHOLESTEROL-REDUCING AGENTS

According to the Framingham Heart Study, the prevalence of coronary artery disease in the diabetic patient is about twice that in the general Population. Although the increased susceptibility to heart disease is almost certainly related in part to impaired glucose homeostasis, the patient with NIDDM is also susceptible to abnormalities in the lipoprotein metabolism that include increases in plasma VLDL triglycerides and VLDL and LDL cholesterol, and decreases in HDL cholesterol. Based on epidemiologic studies in the general population, there is evidence to suggest that pharmacologic and dietary interventions that achieve beneficial effects on plasma lipid levels (i.e., reduction in serum LDL and VLDL cholesterol and elevation of HDL cholesterol) may decrease the risk of coronary heart disease in patients with NIDDM.

According to available data, an average reduction in total cholesterol levels of 26%, as observed with lovastatin therapy, should reduce the risk of coronary heart disease by about 50%. This reduction in risk should put patients with NIDDM at about the same baseline risk for heart disease as the general population.

The relative importance of multiple factors that place patients with NIDDM at increased risk for heart disease is not precisely known. Nevertheless, reduction of elevated plasma cholesterol and triglyceride levels with dietary or pharmacologic intervention is advisable in diabetic patients with risk factors for coronary artery disease.

Guidelines for Screening and Treatment of Hypercholesterolemia

Hypercholesterolemia remains one of the leading risk factors for coronary heart disease (CHD), affecting over 20% of the population. Effective means for its detection and treatment are available, but many unresolved issues remain, including whom to screen, what to screen for, whom to treat, and what is the best approach to treatment. Several years ago the National Institutes of Health established the Expert Panel on the Detection, Evaluation, and Treatment of High Blood Cholesterol in Adults. This consensus panel established the National Cholesterol Education Program and has just issued its Second Report, which addresses many of the basic questions related to screening and treatment of hypercholesterolemia.

Table 8-2

Pharmacologic and Pharmacokinetic Activity of Sulfonylurea Agents

Generic name	Brand	Daily dose range (mg)	Duration of effect (hr)	Elimination of half-life (hr)
Tolbutamide	Orinase	500-3,000	6-12	4-5
Tolazamide	Tolinase	100-750	10-16	7
Acetohexamide	Dymelor	500-1,500	12-24	5
Chlorpropamide	Diabinese	100-500	24-60	35
Glyburide	Micronase	2.5-20	24	10
Glipizide	Glucotrol	2.4-50	24	2-4

Table 8-3

Sedative-Hypnotic and Anxiolytic Drugs in the Elderly

Drug	FDA approved	Half-life (hr)	Usual initial dose for the elderly	Brand
Flurazepam	Hypnotic	50-100 (major metabolite)	15 mg at bedtime	Dalmane
Temazepam	Hypnotic	5-15	15 mg at bedtime	Restoril
Oxazepam	Anxiolytic	5-20	10 mg three times a day	Serax
Diazepam	Anxiolytic	20-100 (major metabolite)	2 mg per day or twice a day	Valium
Lorazepam	Anxiolytic	10-20	0.5-2 mg/day	Ativan
Triazolam	Hypnotic	2,3	0.125 mg or 0.0612 mg	Halcion
Alprazolam	Anxiolytic	12-15	0.25 mg-1.0 mg three times a day	Xanax

In formulating its Second Report,[60] the panel considered the expanding body of new data that has become available since its First Report in 1988. The basic approach to screening is reasserted, namely that a non-fasting cholesterol be obtained every 5 years in adults 20 years of age and older. Added to this position is the recommendation that an HDL cholesterol be obtained at the same time, provided the means are available for its accurate detection. This addition of an HDL cholesterol determination is based on recognition of the emerging importance of a low HDL cholesterol (<35 mg/dl) as an independent risk factor for coronary disease. The use of total CHD risk as the basis for management decision continues to be recommended and reemphasized. A gradient of risk is identified and based in part on CHD risk factors in addition to degree of LDL cholesterol elevation, which continues to be the predominant determinant of CHD risk due to hypercholesterolemia. Hypercholesterolemic patients with established CHD or another form of atherosclerotic disease (peripheral arterial insufficiency, symptomatic carotid artery disease) are assigned to the highest category of risk. Those with 2 major CHD risk factors (smoking, hypertension, diabetes, family history of premature CHD, male sex, age >45 in men and >55 in women, low HDL cholesterol) but no established CHD are in the next highest risk category. Those with hypercholesterolemia and less than 2 major risk factors are in the last of the increased risk categories.

Management decisions are based predominantly on this risk assessment and can be summarized in the following table adopted from the Second Report:

Patient Category	Initial LDL Level (mg/dl)	LDL Goal (mg/dl)
DIETARY THERAPY		
No CHD, <2 risk factors	>160	<160
No CHD, >2 risk factors	>130	<130
With CHD	>100	<100
ADD DRUG TREATMENT		
No CHD, <2 risk factors	>190	<160
No CHD, >2 risk factors	>160	<130
With CHD	>130	<100

Also addressed was the finding of an increase in non-cardiac deaths among those treated with lipid-lowering medication but not among those treated with diet alone. The reasons for this finding are unknown at present. The increase nullifies the reductions achieved in cardiac deaths and caused the panel to recommend delaying use of drug therapy in most young persons and pre-menopausal women who are at otherwise low CHD risk.

The panel recommended more attention be given to recognition and treatment of low HDL cholesterol because of its role as a major CHD risk factor. Finally, the benefits of exercise and weight reduction are emphasized and urged as important complements to a dietary program.

The Second Report goes a long way toward correcting some of the deficiencies of the first, particularly the inattention to the potential importance of HDL cholesterol, exercise, and weight reduction. The panel's special contribution of basing management recommendations on total CHD risk and not just degree of lipid abnormality is strengthened and made even more clinically useful. Finally, the recognition of a potential risk associated with use of pharmacologic therapy is an important caution—one that should encourage more emphasis on non-pharmacologic efforts, especially in young, lower risk persons. However, pharmacologic therapy remains very important in very-high-risk persons, such as those with established CHD. Their reduction in CHD risk with use of drug therapy far exceeds the observed increase in risk of noncardiac deaths.

ANXIOLYTIC AND SEDATIVE-HYPNOTIC DRUGS

Although morbidity precipitated by psychoactive drug use in the elderly is well recognized, recent epidemiologic data suggest that the geriatric population,[15] especially the institutionalized elderly, are at continued risk for experiencing toxicity and functional impairment associated with polypharmacy. Given the potential morbidity associated with suboptimal drug administration in this vulnerable subgroup, a Harvard-based study[16] attempted to characterize patterns of psychoactive medication use for 850 residents of intermediate-care facilities (ICF) in Massachusetts. The investigators reported all prescriptions and patterns of actual drug use for patients during a 1-month period to arrive at a comprehensive profile of how such medications are being prescribed and consumed in these facilities.

On average, ICF residents were prescribed 8.1 medications during the study month and actually received 4.7 medications during this period. Nearly two-thirds (65%) of the residents were prescribed psychoactive medications. Of ICF inhabitants, 53% actually received psychoactive drugs on 5 or more days during the month, with 26% receiving antipsychotic medication; haloperidol (Haldol®) was given to 43% of those receiving antipsychotics and to 10% of the total sample. Twenty-eight percent of patients were receiving sedative/hypnotic drugs, primarily on a scheduled (82%) rather than on an as-needed basis. Of all patients receiving a sedative/hypnotic, about one-fourth (26%) were taking diphenhydramine hydrochloride (Benadryl®), a strongly anticholinergic agent used frequently for nighttime sedation. Of those residents receiving one or more of the benzodiazepines as a sedative/hypnotic, 30% were receiving such long-acting drugs as flurazepam (Dalmane®), diazepam (Valium®), and chlordiazepoxide (Librium®); 87% of benzodiazepine orders were prescribed as a standing order.

Of special note is the fact that 41% of patients with a diagnosis of Alzheimer's disease were receiving sedative/hypnotic drugs, although most experts agree that these agents have little therapeutic value in these patients and, in some studies, have been shown to induce agitation and increase the frequency of cognitive dysfunction. Amitriptyline hydrochloride, the most sedating and anticholinergic antidepressant presently available, was the most commonly prescribed agent in this therapeutic class. Overall, 14% of all patients studied were prescribed an antidepressant, although only 31% of this group had a *diagnosis* of depression noted in the record. Based on their findings, the investigators conclude that ICF patients were exposed to high levels of sedative/hypnotic and antipsychotic drug use. Suboptimal choice of medications within a drug class was common, and use of standing versus as-needed orders was often not in keeping with current concepts in geriatric psychopharmacology.

Prescribing Guidelines. Despite a barrage of carefully wrought admonitions regarding excessive prescribing and misuse in the geriatric age group,[17-18] practitioners frequently encounter geriatric patients for whom a sedative/ hypnotic, antidepressant, or antipsychotic, either alone or in some combination, is indicated.[19-22] Although this study concentrated on psychoactive drug use in ICF residents, the conceptual points and suboptimal prescribing patterns flagged by this important investigation can easily be applied to the outpatient sphere, where psychoactive drugs are so often prescribed in geriatric patients.[23]

Anticholinergic toxicity in the elderly must be avoided.[24-26] Amitriptyline, for example, is a highly sedating drug with potent anticholinergic activity, two properties that make it especially undesirable for elderly patients.[27-29] Such newer agents as fluoxetine (Prozac®), sertraline (Zoloft®), and trazodone (Desyrel®), which possess no or significantly less anticholinergic toxicity, are now available and preferable for the treatment of depression.[30] The use of diphenhydramine,[31-33] a strongly sedating agent whose use is also characterized by undesirable anticholinergic side effects, can be especially problematic when combined with other strongly anticholinergic agents in the antipsychotic and antidepressant class.[34,35] Practitioners, therefore, should recognize that diphenhydramine is not the sedative of choice for the elderly,[36,37] nor are such long-acting benzodiazepines as flurazepam hydrochloride, diazepam, or chlordiazepoxide, which also present an increased risk of toxicity for this vulnerable population. When benzodiazepines are required, low doses of shorter-acting agents are generally preferable.

Ultimately, mastering the fine art of drug prescribing in the elderly requires the recognition that subtle, incremental forms of drug-induced functional or cognitive impairment can produce profound and sometimes devastating consequences.

Benzodiazepines. These agents are frequently used to relieve short-term anxiety in geriatric patients.[38] In general, agents with long half-lives should be avoided in the elderly population (See Table 8-3, page 336). Somnolence, confusion, and depression are the most common presenting symptoms of anxiolytic toxicity associated with long-acting benzodiazepines. Drugs with shorter half-lives, such as triazolam (Halcion®), oxazepam (Serax®), alprazolam (Xanax®), and lorazepam (Ativan®) are preferable anxiolytics for the elderly. Benzodiazepines are also effective sedative hypnotics. Flurazepam is the most common but has a long half-life. Thirty-nine percent of elderly patients receiving the usual 30 mg dose of flurazepam have significant CNS depression due to accumulation of the drug. A shorter-acting benzodiazepine, such as temazepam (Restoril®) or alprazolam, may be better choices.[38]

Triazolam is the most widely prescribed hypnotic in the United States. Its relatively short serum half-life (approximately 6 hours) reduces the risks of daytime sedation and cumulative sedation compared with longer-acting hypnotics such as flurazepam. However, behavioral disturbances and impairment of memory have been reported,[39] with particular concern for the elderly who seem to be more sensitive to the medication. The mechanism(s) and severity of the adverse effects of triazolam remain incompletely defined and the subject of considerable research.[39]

The approximately 50% reduction in drug clearance and the absence of evidence for a specific drug sensitivity suggests that reduced single doses of triazolam can be used in the elderly for sleep. Dosage should be cut by 50% from that which would be appropriate for a young patient. A reasonable single dose might be 0.125 mg. One might even consider prescribing just half of a 0.125 mg tablet, as this is likely to have the same sedative effect 0.125 mg would have in a young person. It is important to note that the etiology of insomnia must be determined before it can be deemed safe to use any sedative. Nocturnal heart failure, sleep apnea, and depression are among the very important conditions that might cause insomnia but not be appropriate for sedative use. Even when it is deemed appropriate to use triazolam, only a small number of pills should be dispensed at any one time, and the patient and family should be carefully instructed against the routine or daily use of the medication.[40] The issue of an idiosyncratic behavioral disturbance triggered by triazolam remains a concern and the literature should be followed carefully for more details about its occurrence and identifying patients at risk.[41]

MANAGEMENT OF PAIN IN PATIENTS WITH CANCER

The prevalence of cancer in the United States continues to increase. Cancer is newly diagnosed in approximately one million individuals per year and one out of every five deaths in the US (about 1400 per day) is caused by cancer. One of the most debilitating and recalcitrant symptoms in patients with metastatic or recurrent cancer is severe pain, which often develops well before the terminal stages of disease. Even when pain is treated, relief is often inadequate and patients have persistent functional impairment in their activities of daily living. Despite guidelines for pain management in cancer patients, there remains significant variability in treatment regimens. This is unfortunate since in the majority of patients, pain can be controlled through a comprehensive, multidisciplinary approach that incorporates both pharmacologic and non-pharmacologic modalities. Many factors contribute to the inadequacy of pain management in cancer patients incuding inadequate knowledge amongst clinicians, negative attitudes of patients and clinicians toward medications and a variety of reimbursement problems.

In order to address the scope of pain management regimens employed and characteristics of cancer patients whose pain is well controlled versus those in whom it is not, investigators at multiple academic cancer centers around the United States evaluated 1,308 patients with metastatic or recurrent cancer.[61] Sixty-seven percent of the subjects admitted having pain beyond common everyday types (headache, sprains, etc.), reported that they took analgesic medications on an everyday basis, or were identified by their physicians as having pain. Of those with pain, 62% were considered to have substantial pain, defined as a score of at least 5 on a scale of zero to ten, that was sufficient to interfere with activities of daily living. At subsequent office visits, all patients completed a pain severity scale as well as rating how much the pain interfered with their enjoyment of life and their activities of daily living and the degree of pain relief (pain management index) they were receiving from treatment (a negative score represented inadequate treatment). Physicians caring for the subjects were asked to assess the same features in order to determine the degree of discrepancy between the two.

In 42% of those with pain, there were negative pain management scores indicating inadequate analgesia. Factors associated with increased likelihood of inadequate analgesia included discrepancy between patients and physician in judging the severity of pain, pain not attributed to cancer by the physician, better functional status, age greater than 70, female sex and being seen at a center that predominantly cared for minority groups. Patients with less adequate analgesia also reported greater pain-related impairment of function.

Prescribing Guidelines. Pain management is frequently inadequate for many patients with cancer. In order to minimize this, clinicians need to take a collaborative, interdisciplinary approach to pain management, develop an individualized plan for pain management with patients and their families, perform thorough ongoing assessments of the patient's pain and effects of treatment, and use both pharmacologic and non-pharmacologic interventions for pain relief. In assessing pain, patients should be the primary source of information, but they need to be questioned frequently since some may be reluctant to volunteer information. In addition to obvious sources of pain (e.g., bone fractures), clinicians must be able to recognize other common conditions that can cause pain in cancer patients (e.g., bone metastases, epidural metastases with spinal cord compression, peripheral neuropathies, mucositis).

Medications are the cornerstone of pain management in the cancer patient because they are relatively inexpensive, usually work fairly quickly and generally entail acceptable risks. Although the specific regimen needs to be tailored to the individual patient, a workable protocol has been developed by the World Health Organization. Initially, aspirin, acetaminophen or a non-steroidal anti-inflammatory drug is instituted followed by the addition of an opioid such as codeine or hydrocodone (often as a fixed combination pill because of synergistic effects). These more potent agents should be started initially for patients who present with moderate to severe pain. More potent opioids such as morphine, methadone and fentanyl should be instituted for patients with persistent severe pain and should be given on an around-the-clock basis with additional doses available on an as-needed basis.

Tolerance and dependence are predictable consequences of use of potent high dose opioid analgesics, but this should not preclude the use of adequate doses to achieve acceptable pain relief while balancing side effects (constipation, sedation, nausea, etc.). The sequential trial of more than one opioid is usually preferable before switching to another method of administration of medication or more invasive procedures. Patient-controlled analgesia involving programmable pumps to deliver drugs intravenously, subcutaneously or epidurally are most useful to treat breakthrough pain. Physical modalities such as cold, heat, electrical stimulation, and acupuncture may reduce the need for medication but should not be used as a substitute for drugs. Furthermore, psychosocial support and antidepressant and other medications (e.g., carbamazepine, phenytoin) may be useful adjuncts to opioid medications. For severe, refractory pain syndromes, radiation therapy, nerve blocks or invasive surgical procedures should be considered.

Aspirin, acetaminophen or non-steroidal anti-inflammatory drugs are the initial agents of choice followed by the addition of an opioid such as codeine or hydrocodone (often as a fixed combination pill because of synergistic effects). Morphine, methadone and fentanyl are appropriate for patients with persistent severe pain and should be given on an around-the-clock basis with additional doses available on an as-needed basis. Tolerance and dependence are predictable consequences of use of potent high dose opioid analgesics, but this should not preclude the use of adequate doses to achieve acceptable pain relief. Antidepressant and other medications (e.g., carbamazepine, phenytoin) may be useful adjuncts to opioid medications.

ANTIDEPRESSANTS

The elderly are particularly sensitive to the adverse effects of tricyclic antidepressants (See Table 8-4).[42] As discussed previously, these agents are *not* recommended as drugs of choice for treatment of depression in the elderly. The most common presenting symptoms of toxicity include sedation, anticholinergic effects, adrenergic hyperactivity (tremulousness, sweating), and cardiovascular toxicity. Anticholinergic effects include dry mouth, constipation, blurred vision, urinary retention, decreased sweating, and hyperthermic reactions.

Researchers at the National Institutes of Health conducted a series of randomized, double-blind, crossover studies of patients with painful diabetic peripheral neuropathy, comparing amitriptyline, desipramine and fluoxetine. The study objectives were to assess relative efficacy and to better understand the mechanism(s) of action on diabetic neuropathic pain.

Two separate studies were conducted: one compared desipramine with amitriptyline; the other compared fluoxetine with a placebo. The outcome measures examined were daily pain score and end-of study global pain rating. Each treatment phase lasted 7 weeks, followed by a washout period and crossover for another 7 weeks of treatment. Recruitment was done by advertisement: 57 patients qualified and entered one or both studies.

Mean daily dose was 105 mg for amitriptyline, 111 mg for desipramine and 40 mg for fluoxetine. Seventy-four percent of patients reported moderate or greater pain relief during the blinded use of amitriptyline; 61% during the use of desipramine; and 41% during the use of the placebo. The differences between amitriptyline and desipramine were not significant, nor were those between fluoxetine and the placebo. Amitriptyline and desipramine were effective even in

Table 8-4

		Adverse Effects and Toxicity of Tricyclic and Tetracyclic Antidepressants			
Structural class	**Trade name**	**Young adult daily dose**	**Elderly daily dose**	**Sedative properties**	**Anticholinergic properties**
Tricyclic					
Tertiary amine					
Amitriptyline	Elavil	100-300 mg	25-150 mg	+++	++++
Imipramine	Tofranil	100-300 mg	25-150 mg	++	+++
Doxepin	Sinequan	100-300 mg	25-150 mg	+++	++++
Trimipramine	Surmontil	100-300 mg	25-150 mg	+++	+++
Secondary amine					
Nortriptyline	Pamelor	50-100 mg	10-60 mg	+	+++
Desipramine	Norpramin	100-300 mg	25-150 mg	0	++
Protriptyline	Vivactil	20-60 mg	5-30 mg	0	+++
Dibenzoxazepine (amoxapine)	Asendin	150-300 mg	25-150 mg	++	+++
Triazolopyridine (trazodone)	Desyrel	150-400 mg	50-300 mg	+++	+
Tetracyclic maprotiline	Ludiomil	100-300 mg	25-150 mg	++	+++
Selective serotonin reuptake inhibitor (SSRI)					
Sertraline	Zoloft	50-200 mg	50-100 mg	0	0
Fluoxetine	Prozac	20-40 mg	10-20 mg	0	0
Paroxetine	Paxil	20-50 mg	10-40 mg	0	0
Venlafaxine	Effelor	75-150 mg	75-150 mg	0	0

patients who were not depressed, whereas fluoxetine worked only when there was an underlying depression. Some of the study's findings include:

Amitriptyline and desipramine are equally effective for treatment of pain caused by diabetic peripheral neuropathy, regardless of the presence of depression. Fluoxetine appears to work *only in the context of depression,* suggesting it has no direct effect on the mechanism of pain in diabetic peripheral neuropathy. Desipramine and other tricyclics with lesser anticholinergic activity (e.g., nortriptyline), might be reasonable alternatives to amitriptyline, which many patients find difficult to tolerate.

The reason for the beneficial effects of these agents is related to their blockade of norepinephrine reuptake, distinguishing them from fluoxetine, which does not block norepinephrine reuptake and which did not provide significant pain relief.

Anticholinergic effects—which may cause delirium, agitation, visual hallucinations, and decreased thirst—precipitated by tricyclic antidepressants are frequently underdiagnosed. Lack of sweating and decreased thirst can produce dehydration and electrolyte imbalances that can be fatal in the elderly population. Orthostatic hypotension due to anticholinergic toxicity can cause falls, myocardial infarction, and cerebrovascular events.[43] Cardiovascular effects due to antidepressant toxicity in the elderly include an anticholinergic effect that can increase the heart rate and a quinidine-like effect that may increase PR, QRS, and QTC intervals.

Tricyclic antidepressant overdose has serious cardiotoxic effects that are not usually present at the therapeutic doses. Because of the cardiovascular effects associated with overdose, researchers anticipated an increased incidence of sudden death and arrhythmia among elderly patients using these antidepressants. The Boston Collaborative Drug Surveillance Program, however, has demonstrated that neither occurs, even in the presence of organic heart disease, which is so common in the elderly.[39]

Although pharmacologic treatment of depression is effective in the elderly, monoamine oxidase inhibitors should be avoided because of the risks of serious drug interactions and the frequency of orthostatic hypotension. Common practice dictates that agitated or anxious depressions should be treated with sedating drugs (amitriptyline or doxepin), and retarded depressions should be treated with less sedating agents (nortriptyline or desipramine). Orthostatic hypotension, which can cause falls, is probably the most dangerous side effect. Doxepin and nortriptyline cause fewer incidents of postural hypotension. Their major cardiac toxicity is interference with cardiac conduction. At high risk are patients with preexisting bundle branch block or sinus node dysfunction.

Doxepin has the fewest adverse effects on the heart. However, anticholinergic effects are common. The most serious anticholinergic effect is confusion or delirium, for which the underlying cause frequently goes unrecognized. Amitriptyline and doxepin are the most potent anticholinergics, and desipramine is the least. Other miscellaneous side effects include increased appetite and weight gain, decreased seizure threshold, and increased anxiety.[44,45]

ANTIPSYCHOTIC DRUGS

Several major psychiatric disorders in the elderly are treated with antipsychotic and neurologic drugs (See Table 8-5). Complications of this treatment include tardive dyskinesia (five times more common in the elderly), akathisias, dystonias, pseudoparkinsonism, and anticholinergic side effects.[46,47] A major adverse reaction to neuroleptics is neuroleptic malignant syndrome (NMS), which is frequently unrecognized in the elderly. NMS consists of fever, rigidity, autonomic instability, and mental status changes.

With the widespread use of both tricyclic antidepressants and antipsychotics, 12% of all elderly ambulatory patients and 25% of those hospitalized in nursing homes now receive two or more drugs with anticholinergic effects.[48] In general, studies show that clinicians do not choose drugs within a given class to minimize anticholinergic effects. Consequently, suspect an anticholinergic reaction in elderly patients with symptoms of urinary retention, acute glaucoma, delirium, hallucinations, seizures, dysarthria, hyperthermia, tachycardia, and even heart block—especially if the patient has taken drugs in one or more of the anticholinergic classes.[49,50]

MANAGEMENT OF DEPRESSION FOLLOWING MYOCARDIAL INFARCTION

Depression is not uncommon following acute, life-threatening illnesses, but the majority of patients have resolution of depressive symptoms and return to normal function. It is estimated, however, that 15-20% of patients who suffer an acute myocardial infarction (MI) have a major depressive episode in the post-infarction period, and a substantial number of these individuals have persistent emotional difficulties which have been correlated with increased mortality. Surprisingly, the severity of the cardiac illness and the degree of emotional problems are unrelated in these patients. Although persistent depression has been linked to increased mortality following myocardial infarction, less is known about outcomes in *survivors* of MI who have persistent depression.

In one analysis,[65] 552 male myocardial infarction patients between the ages of 29 and 65 years were evaluated beginning 17 to 21 days following an acute myocardial infarction with follow-up six months later. Subjects underwent a comprehensive phychodiagnostic evaluation and were allocated into one of three groups: low, moderate or severe depression. At baseline, 15% patients were identified with severe depression, 22% with moderate depression, and 63% with a low degree of depression. Follow-up information on fatal and nonfatal cardiac events (reinfarction, syncope, severe angina, coronary bypass surgery, coronary angioplasty) and functional and emotional status after discharge were obtained for all 552 subjects for the six month study. Taking all of these assessments into account, the relative risks were significantly increased for those patients with high degrees of post-MI depression at baseline in terms of ongoing angina, emotional instability, and continued smoking, and the likelihood of return to work was significantly less in the high depression group.

Table 8-5

Adverse Effects of Antipsychotic Medications in the Elderly						
Drug and dose for elderly	Relative potency	Sedation	Extra-pyramidal	Anticholinergic	Orthostatic hypotension
Chlorpromazine					
(Thorazine) 10-25 mg b.i.d. t.i.d.	100	+++	++	+++	++
Thioridazine					
(Mellaril) 10-25 mg b.i.d. t.i.d.	95-100	+++	+	+++	++
Thiothixene					
(Navane) 2-3 mg	5	+	+++	+	+
Haloperidol					
(Haldol) 0.5-2 mg	2	+	+++	+	+
Fluphenazine					
(Prolixin) 0.5-2 mg	2	+	+++	+	+

Cardiac patients who develop significant post-MI depression fail to convalesce as well as those who are without significant symptoms of depression. Depressed individuals are in a psychological state of reduced vigor, with a lack of initiative and detachment from activities of daily living. They have a reduced ability to comply with risk factor modification efforts and may develop feelings of hopelessness. Ultimately, individuals with significant depression can lapse into a prolonged invalid state with a tendency to remain in the sick role for possible secondary benefits. Patients with depression have increased episodes of angina, an increased risk for recurrent infarction and a reduced quality of life. The exact reasons for this are not entirely clear. While the degree of myocardial damage and consequent left ventricular function are critical factors in determining post-MI morbidity and mortality, the degree of depression and emotional difficulties following MI, surprisingly, is not well correlated to the severity of the cardiac problem itself.

Clinicians need to be vigilant in identifying patients with depression following an MI and stratify the individual into a higher risk status. As with other cases of depression, it may be misdiagnosed or under-recognized in cardiac patients who may deny or downplay depressive symptoms. The exact role of anti-depressant medication in this situation is not entirely defined but certainly should be considered for those individuals with persistent significant symptoms. Avoidance of agents with high anti-cholinergic potential that carry some added risk in the cardiac patient is advisable.

Post-MI depression is an independent and significant source of morbidity and reduced quality of life at least for the first six months (the highest risk period) following myocardial infarction. Depression appears to have the greatest impact on pain perception and illness behavior. The diagnosis of depression can be difficult in cardiac patients who may deny or downplay depressive symptoms. Patients with depression following an MI should be considered at high risk status. Antidepressants are generally indicated for those individuals with persistant significant symptoms. Tricyclic agents with low anticholinergic potential (e.g. nortryptiline, desipramine) or serotonin reuptake inhibitors (sertraline, fluoxetine) are preferred agents.

Predicting Major Bleeding Complications in Patients on Long-Term Anticoagulants

It is estimated that two million Americans are treated with warfarin as outpatients each year. Although long-term anticoagulant therapy has been demonstrated to be effective in preventing thromboembolism, the key issue for these patients is whether the benefit of such therapy outweighs the risk of hemorrhagic complications in an individual patient. Predictors of major bleeding complications at the start of outpatient therapy in those treated with warfarin would be of great benefit to clinicians faced with the challenge of initiating and monitoring the effects of anticoagulation. In addition to knowing just how frequently bleeding complications occur and what subgroups are at greatest risk, practitioners would also benefit from knowing: (1) the relationship of bleeding to prothrombin time during outpatient therapy with warfarin; (2) the yield of diagnostic evaluation of bleeding in terms of previously unknown, remediable lesions; and (3) whether the yield of discovering a remediable lesion varies according to the prothrombin time at the time of hemorrhagic episode.

Two back-to-back, retrospective studies shed important new light on these critical issues in outpatient drug therapy. The records of 565 patients starting outpatient therapy with warfarin upon discharge from a university hospital were reviewed. Bleeding was classified as *major* if it was fatal, life-threatening, led to severe blood loss, to surgical intervention, or to moderate blood loss that was acute or subacute and could not be explained by trauma or surgery. *Minor* bleeding included other internal bleeding (including overt or occult gastrointestinal bleeding, hemoptysis, and gross hematuria), symptomatic anemia ascribed to acute but occult blood loss, or chronic bleeding with moderate blood loss.

Based on these criteria, investigators found that major bleeding occurred in 65 patients (12%) and was fatal in 10 patients (2%). Minor bleeding also occurred in 65 patients (12%). The cumulative incidences of major bleeding at 1, 12, and 48 months were 3%, 11%, and 22% respectively. Five independent risk factors for major bleeding—age 65 years or greater, history of stroke, history of gastrointestinal bleeding, a serious comorbid condition (recent myocardial infarction, renal insufficiency, or severe anemia), atrial fibrillation—predicted bleeding in the test group. The cumulative incidence of major bleeding was 2% in 57 low-risk patients and 63% in 20 high-risk patients. As expected, the gastrointestinal tract was the most frequent location of bleeding but was fatal in only one case. Intracranial bleeding was the most common cause of fatal hemorrhage. It is important to note that the researchers observed a significant association between a history of hypertension and intracranial bleeding. This association was significant even if blood pressure was adequately controlled at the time of warfarin therapy. Interestingly, patients with a history of stroke had increased rates of gastrointestinal bleeding as well as intracranial hemorrhage.

Those 130 patients (24%) with either major or minor bleeding were then studied to determine the relation of bleeding to prothrombin times and important *remediable* lesions. Important remediable lesions were classified as those lesions or injuries for which specific therapy is routinely indicated (i.e., esophageal, gastric, or duodenal ulcers; colonic diverticula, colon cancer; bladder cancer, etc.). Using these criteria, it was found that for each 1.0 increase in the prothrombin time-to-control ratio, the odds ratio for major bleeding during the week after a prothrombin time measurement increased 80%; the odds ratio for minor bleeding increased 50%. Bleeding complications are related to important remediable lesions in 49 of 130 cases (38%), although these lesions were unknown before bleeding in only 22 cases (17%). New, previously unknown lesions were discovered in 20 of 59 case subjects of (34%) with gastrointestinal bleeding or hematuria, but in only 2 of 71 case subjects (3%) with bleeding from other sites. Finally, of special clinical importance is the observation that prothrombin times rose precipitously at the time of bleeding in patients *without* important remediable lesions, whereas prothrombin times tended to be in the therapeutic range in those *with* significant remediable lesions.

The overall rates of major and fatal bleeding (12% and 2%, respectively) as well as for the rates of major and fatal bleeding *per year of outpatient anticoagulant therapy* (7% and 1%, respectively) are striking. Put simply, these investigations dramatize the potential risks of long-term warfarin therapy and convincingly demonstrate that this form of pharmacologic intervention is associated with significantly higher morbidity in individuals 65 years of age or older, in those with recent myocardial infarction or a comorbid condition, and in patients with atrial fibrillation. Clinicians should also note that a previous history of stroke or hypertension (even if blood pressure is normal at the time anticoagulant therapy is initiated) is associated with a significantly increased risk of intracranial hemorrhage.

With respect to the prothrombin time, it appears as if increases in the ratio of measured to controlled values are related to predictable increases in major and minor bleeding during the weeks following such measurements. Moreover, it appears that remediable lesions most often surface at a time when prothrombin times or INR are in the therapeutic range, whereas nonremediable lesions declare themselves following precipitous rises in prothrombin time. Given these observations, clinicians should aggressively pursue diagnostic evaluation in all patients who present with bleeding, especially when their prothrombin times or INR are in the therapeutic range and have been stable for quite some time prior to the hemorrhagic complication. For now, the decision to proceed with long-term anticoagulation continues to present a formidable dilemma in which the predictable risks must be weighted against not-so-predictable benefits in a vulnerable patient population. See Tables 8-6 through 8-8 for possible drug interactions that can effect bleeding times.

Table 8-6

Possible Drug Interactions with Anticoagulants			
Decrease vitamin K	**Displace anticoagulant**	**Inhibit metabolism**	**Other**
Antibiotics Cholestyramine Mineral oil	Salicylates Sulfonamides Sulfonylureas Ethacrynic acid Mefenamic acid Naldixic acid Diazoxide	Chloramphenicol Allopurinol Nortriptyline Disulfiram Metronidazole Alcohol (acute ingestion) Cimetidine Fluconazole	Thyroid drugs Anabolic steroids Quinidine Glucagon

Table 8-7

Drugs That Diminish Anticoagulant Drug Activity	
Induction of Enzymes	**Increased Procoagulant factors**
Barbiturates	Estrogens
Glutethimide	Oral contraceptives
Ethchlorvynol	Vitamin K
Griseofulvin	
Phenytoin	
Carbamazepine	
Rifampin	
Chlorinated insecticides	

Table 8-8

Drugs Potentiating Anticoagulant Drug Effects		
Inhibition of platelet aggregation	**Inhibition of procoagulant factors**	**Ulcerogenic drugs**
Salicylates	Quinidine	Sulfinpyrazone
Sulfinpyrazone	Antimetabolites	Salicylates
Dipyridamole	Alkylating agents	Adrenal corticosteroids
NSAIDs	Salicylates	

H₂ ANTAGONISTS

A commonly prescribed drug among the elderly population, cimetidine (Tagamet®) can cause sedation and confusion, especially in doses above 1000 mg/day. Aside from this direct adverse reaction, side effects are very usually tolerable. However, because cimetidine is a potent inhibitor of the p-450 hepatic microsomal oxidation enzymes, it blocks metabolism of many other drugs that may be taken concurrently, increasing their effect on plasma levels. This leads to a number of potentially dangerous drug interactions. In patients taking warfarin, the prothrombin time can rise 20% to 200%. Both diazepam and chlordiazepoxide can cause increased sedation. Theophylline levels can increase from the therapeutic to the toxic range in patients who are on cimetidine therapy. Toxic effects, such as bradycardia, hypotension, and arrhythmias, may appear with beta-blockers. Elevated levels of anticonvulsants, especially in the elderly, can be seen within a period of several days in patients taking carbamazepine (Tegretol®) and phenytoin (Dilantin®). With lidocaine, an increase in serum levels of 60% to 90% can occur with maintenance infusions in patients on cimetidine therapy.

Table 8-9

Adverse Drug Interactions in Combination with Cimetidine (Tagamet)
• With warfarin, prothrombin time rises 20 to 200%.
• With benzodiazepines, increases sedation.
• With theophylline, increases in theophylline from therapeutic to toxic range (narrow therapeutic range).
• With beta-blockers, toxic effects may appear, such as bradycardia, hypotension, arrhythmias.
• With carbamazepine (Tegretol) and phenytoin (Dilantin), elevated levels of anticonvulsants, especially in the elderly, over several days.
• With lidocaine, 60 to 90% increase in serum levels occurred with maintenance infusion; study conducted in the elderly. Cimetidine therapy was new in these patients.

The newer, selective H_2 antagonists, ranitidine (Zantac®) and famotidine (Pepcid®), produce very mild CNS depression and have the distinct advantage of producing less inhibition than hepatic microsomal oxidation system.

BRONCHODILATORS

Aminophylline and theophylline once represented the cornerstone of oral bronchodilator therapy for the elderly asthmatic, bronchitic. These drugs are metabolized by the liver, and clearance is remarkably sensitive to hepatic dysfunction. Complications of aminophylline include seizures, which may even occur at therapeutic levels, increased angina, palpitations, and arrhythmias. Nervousness and lack of sleep are also encountered in the geriatric population. Theophylline toxicity in the elderly may also mimic chronic organic brain syndrome, multiinfarct dementia, and psychosis. Draw blood levels on patients who have this constellation of symptoms and are taking a theophylline preparation.

Certain drug interactions may precipitate aminophylline toxicity. Cimetidine and other liver-metabolized antibiotics (erythromycin) decrease excretion of aminophylline. Ephedrine and other sympathomimetic agents in combination with aminophylline may cause excessive CNS stimulation, precipitating bizarre behavior and sleeplessness.

Salmeterol Use in Asthma Patients

Most trials on asthma medications have focused on clinical outcomes such as airway caliber and responsiveness, patient symptoms, and protection against stimuli such as allergens. Although these are important, they do not necessarily indicate whether patients truly feel better and can function better physically, emotionally and socially in their day-to-day lives. Salmeterol (Serevant®) is a long-acting beta-2 agonist for which there is a large amount of data to support its clinical efficacy; one trial also reported a better quality of life (QOL) with salmeterol than with a placebo. Another important question is how salmeterol compares with a more commonly prescribed beta-2 agonist, albuterol (Ventolin®, Proventil®), in improving asthma-specific QOL.

Investigators in one trial enrolled 140 adult patients (age 18 to 70) with mild to moderate asthma into a 12 week, double-blind, crossover comparison of salmeterol 50 μg twice daily versus albuterol 200 μg four times daily versus placebo, with each medication taken for 4 weeks.[61] Patients were randomly assigned to one of six treatment orders (i.e., all possible treatment orders). Outcomes were assessed primarily with the Asthma Quality of Life Questionnaire, a 32-item instrument using four domains identified as important by asthma patients: symptoms, emotions, exposure to environmental stimuli and activity limitations. Conventional clinical efficacy was also checked during the last part of each treatment cycle via patient-report of symptoms (chest tightness, wheezing, cough, dyspnea and phlegm production), use of "rescue" albuterol inhalations, and measurement of Peak Expiratory Flow Rate (PERF).

Of the 140 subjects initially enrolled, 17 (10 placebo, 3 albuterol, 4 salmeterol) withdrew because of exacerbation of symptoms and three (one placebo, one albuterol, one salmeterol) because of side effects. Salmeterol was superior to both placebo and albuterol as measured by the overall Quality of Life Questionnaire. In the symptom and emotional function domains, the differences between salmeterol and albuterol were also statistically and clinically significant. In the areas of activity limitations and exposure to allergens the differences between salmeterol and albuterol were statistically significant but not clinically important. In measurement of conventional clinical outcomes, the results were similar to other trials in that salmeterol showed greatest benefit over albuterol in measurement of morning PEFR, morning asthma symptoms, bedtime PEFR and nights with no sleep disturbances.

There is no doubt that a major advantage of salmeterol over albuterol is its long duration of action. The largest differences between the two agents in conventional clinical outcomes occur at night and on waking in the morning. Asthma patients with significant nocturnal symptoms and poor sleep patterns are particularly appropriate for this medication. In addition to improvements in purely physiologic parameters, salmeterol may also improve asthma-specific QOL. This benefit is unlikely to be due solely to differences at night and awakening. Although cost may limit use of salmeterol in some circumstances, it is an excellent long-acting agent for chronic management of asthmatics, particularly those with nocturnal problems. Albuterol may be most appropriate for use on an as needed, "rescue" basis without regular administration in patients with milder or less frequent symptoms.

The long-acting agent salmeterol has clinically important effects on improving asthma-specific QOL compared to albuterol and placebo. A dose of 50 μg twice daily is effective in asthma patients. Those individuals with worsened symptoms at night and upon awakening in the morning are most appropriate for this long-acting agent. Albuterol and other shorter duration beta-2 agonists may be better used on an as-needed basis or for those with less serious or infrequent episodes of bronchospasm.

ANTIHISTAMINES

The early stages of diphenhydramine intoxication are characterized by acute psychosis, hallucinations, autism, loosened associations, affective blunting, and inappropriate behavior.[54] As time passes, the symptom complex may become more similar to an acute brain syndrome with confusion, disorientation, inability to concentrate, and loss of short-term memory.[34] These symptoms present an interesting differential diagnosis. However, based on the physical exam, drug overdose should always be suspected. Initial lab analysis should include serum electrolytes, prothrombin time, calcium, BUN, glucose, arterial gases, blood alcohol, and urine toxicologic screening. In addition, an ECG, chest and skull x-rays, and lumbar puncture may be necessary, depending on the clinical presentation.

A history of drug ingestion is frequently unreliable or unobtainable from the patient. Friends or relatives may be questioned concerning the drug intake. Autonomic signs or symptoms may be the key to diagnosis. Anticholinergic poisoning is associated with tachycardia, mydriasis, flushing, hyperpyrexia, urinary retention, decreased intestinal motility, hypertension, dry skin and decreased salivation.

Table 8-10

Anticholinergic Agents
Antihistamines
Antiparkinsonian drugs
Antipsychotics (phenothiazines and butyrophenones)
Antispasmodics
Belladonna alkaloids
Ophthalmic products (myriatics)
Plants (jimsonweed)
Thioxanthenes
Tricyclic antidepressants

A vast array of antihistamines, hypnotics, antidepressants, and tranquilizing agents pose significant anticholinergic activity (Table 8-10). An increasing number of these drugs are now available in OTC preparations and may, in acute poisoning, produce a picture typical of central anticholinergic toxicity. This syndrome refers to an acute psychosis of delirium resulting from a primary blockade of cerebral cholinergic inhibitory pathways accompanied by signs of peripheral muscarinic blockage.[55]The presentation may vary from confusion, hallucinations, and convulsions to deepening coma and respiratory arrest (Table 8-11). Toxic psychosis is a recognized complication of antihistamine poisoning.

Table 8-11

Central Effects of Anticholinergic Toxicity	
Anxiety	Hyperactivity
Ataxia	Lethargy
Choreoathetoid movements	Loss of short-term memory
Coma	Myoclonus
Delirium	Paranoid ideation
Disorientation	Respiratory failure
Dizziness	Seizures
Dysarthria	Tinnitus
Expressive aphasia	Tremor
Frank psychosis	
Hallucinations (visual/auditory)	

The treatment of a diphenhydramine overdose is generally supportive, particularly in regard to airway management and the maintenance of vital signs.[31] The patient in a psychotic episode may require constant supervision for up to several days to guard against potentially serious complications such as aspiration, accidental injury, hyperthermia, and seizures. Diphenhydramine is well absorbed following ingestion and is widely distributed throughout the body, including the CNS. The drug appears in plasma within 15 minutes and may reach peak concentrations within 1 hour. Gastric lavage or emesis should be initiated immediately on the patient's arrival at the emergency department. After emesis, administration of activated charcoal and a cathartic may help to minimize absorption. Forced diuresis, hemodialysis, and hemoperfusion are generally ineffective since little free drug remains in the plasma.

For a mild case of intoxication, or in elderly, confused patients with uncertain cardiac status, one can manage the patient with conservative treatment and reassurance. Central nervous system depressants, which themselves have anticholinergic properties, should be avoided. Convulsions may be treated with phenytoin at 10 to 15 mg/kg intravenously. Patients with severe intoxication should be admitted to intensive care and monitored closely for cardiac arrhythmias, hypotension, and cardiovascular collapse.

Any patient with an acute onset of bizarre mental and neurologic symptoms should be suspected of poisoning by an anticholinergic drug, including antihistamines. A careful history, with specific attention to OTC drugs, is vital for confirming the diagnosis.

VACCINES

Pneumococcal infection represents a substantial threat to the health of the elderly, the immunocompromised, and those with serious underlying illness. Polyvalent pneumococcal polysaccharide vaccine was developed to address this threat. There are two formulations of the vaccine: the original one contained the polysaccharides of 14 species, whereas the currently available vaccine contains the polysaccharides of 23 species of Streptococcus pneumoniae. Although the vaccine has been available for more than a decade, evidence of its efficacy is limited. One study demonstrated the vaccine to be effective, but the protection decreases with time (especially after 5 years), advancing age, and immuno-incompetence.

Despite being effective and safe, pneumococcal vaccine is underused. It should be administered to all patients with moderately high risk of serious pneumococcal infection, including the elderly.

Investigators designed a case-control study comparing pneumococcal vaccine status in 1,054 patients with documented pneumococcal infection and in 1,054 carefully matched controls (similar age, gender, underlying illnesses) who had not had pneumoccal infection. Thirteen percent of those with pneumococcal infection had received the vaccine versus 20% of the controls (P<0.001).

Aggregate protective efficacy of the 14-and 23-valent vaccines was 56% against serotypes represented by the vaccines. Efficacy was 65% in immunocompetent patients but fell to 21% in immuncompromised persons. In addition, efficacy declined with age and time from immunization, five-year protective efficacy was 85% in patients less than age 55, but declined to 32% in those aged 75 to 84. Efficacy declined by about 30% after five years from the time of vaccination. There was no difference among the vaccinated and the nonvaccinated in terms of mortality from pneumococcal infection.

SUMMARY

Although the elderly constitute only 12% of the U.S. population, they consume approximately 20% to 30% of all drugs.[56,57] Moreover, many of the elderly are simultaneously taking prescription drugs for more than one chronic condition over variable periods of time, and they may supplement their prescription drugs with OTC medications and alcohol. For these reasons, this age group is at high risk for sustaining drug toxicity and adverse drug interactions.[58]

One large study of hospitalized elderly patients with a mean age of 71 years found that each patient consumed an average of 3.1 prescription drugs and one OTC preparation. Initially, one sixth of the persons surveyed denied using OTC medications, but further questioning revealed that these patients did, in fact, take OTC drugs. Moreover, 50% of these elderly patients needed prompting to remember to take their medications, so noncompliance was a serious problem.[59]

Among the implications of that study for the diagnosis and identification of adverse drug reactions in the emergency setting is the importance of focused assessment and interview techniques to examine drug-taking behavior and compliance in the elderly, particularly for OTC drugs.

Finally, any elderly patient with nonspecific CNS, cardiac, or gastrointestinal signs and symptoms must provide a careful drug history, including OTC medications, antiulcer agents, cardiac medications, and antihypertensive drugs. Always consider adverse drug reactions, especially the anticholinergic syndrome, and secondary drug interactions, as a cause of illness.

[1]Albrich JM. Geriatric pharmacology. In: Schwartz GR, Bosker G, Grigsby JW, eds. Geriatric Emergencies. Bowie, Md.: Robert J. Brady Co., 1984.

[2]Walt RP. Misoprostol for the treatment of peptic ulcer and antiinflammatory-drug-induced gastroduodenal ulceration. *N Engl J Med* 1992;327:1575.

[3]Graham DY, White RH, Moreland LW, et al. Duodenal and gastric ulcer prevention with misoprostol in arthritis patients taking NSAIDs. *Ann Intern Med* 1993;119:257.

[4]Lamy PP. A consideration of NSAID use in the elderly. *Geriatric Medicine Today* 1988;7(4):30.

[5]Lamy PP. Renal effects of nonsteroidal anti-inflammatory drugs. Heightened risk to the elderly? *J Am Geriatr Soc* 1986;34:361-7.

[6]Hogan DB, Campbell NR, Crutcher R, Jennett P, MacLeod N. Prescription of nonsteroidal anti-inflammatory drug for elderly people in Alberta. *Can Med Assoc J* 1994 Aug 1;151(3):315-22.

[7]Durnas C, Cusak BJ. Salicylate intoxication in the elderly. Recognition and recommendations on how to prevent it [Review]. *Drugs Aging* 1992 Jan-Feb;2(1):20-34.

[8]Sager DS, Bennett RM. Individualizing the risk/benefit ration of NSAIDs in older patients [Review]. *Geriatrics* 1992 Aug;47(8):24-31.

[9]Whelton A, et al. Renal effects of ibuprofen, piroxican, and sulindac in patients with asymptomatic renal failure. *Ann Intern Med* 1990;112:568-76.

[10]Shorr RI, Ray WA, Daugherty JR, Griffin MR. Concurrent use of nonsteroidal antiinflammatory drugs and oral anticoagulants places elderly persons at high risk for hemorrhagic peptic ulcer disease. *Arch Intern Med* 1993 July 26;153(14):1665-70.

[11]Griffin MR, et al. NSAID use and death from peptic ulceration in the elderly. *Ann Intern Med* 1988;109:359-63.

[12]Melander A. Clinical pharmacology of sulfonylureas. *Metabolism* 1987;36(2)(supp 1).

[13]Leichter S. A prospective double-blind clinical trial of glipizide and glyburide in type II diabetes mellitus. *Communication* 1986.

[14]Asplund K, Wilholm BE, Lithner F. Glibenclamide-associated hypoglycemia: a report on 57 cases. *Diabetologia* 1984;26:412.

[15]Cadieux RJ. Geriatric psychopharmacology. A primary care challenge [Review]. *Postgrad Med* 1993 Mar;93(4):281-2, 285-8, 294-30.

[16]Mayer-Oakes SA, Kelman G, Beers MH, DeJong F, Matthias R, Atchison KA, Lubben JE, Schweitzer SO. Benzodiazepine use in older, community-dwelling southern Californians: prevalence and clinical correlates. *Ann Pharmacother* 1993 Apr;27(4):416-21.

[17]Stewart RM, Marks RG, Padgett PD, Hale WE. Benzodiazepine use in an ambulatory elderly population: a 14-year overview. *Clin Ther* 1994 Jan-Feb;16(1):118-24.

[18]Takami N, Okada A. Triazolam and nitrazepam use in elderly outpatients. *Ann Pharmacother* 1993 Apr;27(4):506-9.

[19]Cancellaro LA. Appropriate use of neuroleptics and antidepressants in the geriatric patient. *South Med J* 1991 May;84(5 Suppl):S53-6.

[20]Freeman C. Drug treatment of insomnia in the elderly. *Conn Med* 1992 Jan;56(1):35-7.

[21]Garrard J, Makris L, Dunham T, Heston LL, Cooper S, Ratner ER, Zelterman D, Kane RL. Evaluation of neuroleptic drug use by nursing home elderly under proposed Medicare and Medicaid regulations [see comments]. *JAMA* 1991 Jan 23-30;265(4):463-7.

[22]Katz IR. Drug treatment of depression in the frail elderly: discussion of the NIH Consensus Development Conference on the Diagnosis and Treatment of Depression in Late Life [Review]. *Psychopharmacol Bull* 1993;29(1):101-8.

[23]Monroe R, Jacobson G, Ervin F. Activation of psychosis by combination of scopolamine and alpha-chloralose. *Arch Neurol* 1957;76-536.

[24]Blazer DG, et al. The risk of anticholinergic toxicity in the elderly: a study of prescribing practices in two populations. *J Gerontol* 1983;38(1):31.

[25]Granacher RP, Baldessarini RJ. Physostigmine: its use in acute anticholinergic syndrome with antidepressant and antiparkinson drugs. *Arch Gen Psychiatry* 1975;32:375.

[26]Kulig K, Rumack BH. Anticholinergic poisoning. In Haddad LM, Winchester JF, eds. Clinical management of poisoning and drug overdose. Philadelphia: W.B. Saunders Co., 1983

[27]Bressler R, Katz MD. Drug therapy for geriatric depression [Review]. *Drugs Aging* 1993 May-Jun;3(3):195-219.

[28]Cassel CK, Walsh JR, eds. Medical, psychiatric, and pharmacological topics. *Geriat Med* 1984;1:554.

[29]Glassman AH, Roose SP. Risks of antidepressants in the elderly: tricyclic antidepressants and arrhythmia-revising risks [Review]. *Gerontology* 1994;40(Supp):15-20.

[30]Dunner DL. An overview of paroxetine in the elderly [Review]. *Gerontology* 1994;40(Supp):21-7.

[31]Sachs BA. The toxicity of benadryl: report of a case and review of the literature. *Ann Intern Med* 1948;29:135.

[32]Tune L, Carr S, Hoag E, Cooper T. Anticholinergic effects of drugs commonly prescribed for the elderly: potential means for assessing risk of delirium [see comments]. *Am J Psychiatry* 1992 Oct;149(10):1393-4.

[33]Wyngaarden JB, Severs MH. The toxic effects of antihistamine drugs. *JAMA* 1951;145:277.

[34]Hestand HE, Teske DW. Diphenhydramine hydrochloride intoxication. *J Pediatr* 1977; 90(6):1017.

[35]Iserson KV, Hackney KU. Antihistamines. In Haddad LM and Winchester JF. Clinical management of poisoning and drug overdose. Philadelphia: WB Saunders Co., 1983

[36]National Poison Center Network. Annual statistical report. Pittsburgh 1979.

[37]Nigro SA. Toxic psychosis due to diphenhydramine hydrochloride. *JAMA* 1968;203(4):139.

[38]Shorr RI, Robin DW. Rational use of benzodiazepines in the elderly [Review]. *Drugs Aging* 1994 Jan;4(1):9-20.

[39]Greenblatt DJ, Harmatz JS, et al. Sensitivity to triazolam in the elderly. *N Engl J Med* 1991;324:1691-8.

[40]Michocki RJ, Lamy PP, Hooper FJ, Richardson JP. Drug prescribing for the elderly [see comments] [Review]. *Arch Fam Med* 1993 Apr;2(4):441-4.

[41]Longe RL. Triazolam dose in older patients [letter]. *J Am Geriatr Soc* 1992 Jan;40(1):103-4.

[42]McCue RE. Using tricyclic antidepressants in the elderly [Review]. *Clin Geriatric Med* 1992 May; 8(2):323-34.

[43]Smith M, Buckwalter KC. Medication management, antidepressant drugs, and the elderly: an overview [Review]. *J Psychosoc Nurs Ment Health Serv* 1992 Oct;30(10):30-6.

[44]Thapa PB, Meador KG, Gideon P, Fought RL, Ray WA. Effects of antipsychotic withdrawal in elderly nursing home residents. *J Am Geriatr Soc* 1994 Mar;42(3):280-6.

[45]Todd B. Drugs and the elderly: identifying drug toxicity. *Geriatr Nurs* 1985;12:213.

[46]Lindley CM, Tully MP, Paramsothy V, Tallis RC. Inappropriate medication is a major cause of adverse drug reactions in elderly patients. *Age Ageing* 1992 July;21(4):294-30.

[47]Livingston J, Reeves RD. Undocumented potential drug interactions found in medical records of elderly patients in a long-term care facility. *J Am Diet Assoc* 1993 Oct;93(10):1168-70.

[48]Raskind MA. Geriatric psychopharmacology. Management of late-life depression and the noncognitive behavioral disturbances of Alzheimer's disease [Review]. *Psychiatr Clin N Am* 1993 Dec;16(4):815-27.

[49]Stewart RB. Advances in pharmacotherapy: depression in the elderly—issues and advances in treatment [Review]. *J Clin Pharm Ther* 1993 Aug;18(4):243-53.

[50]Swift CG. Prescribing in old age. *BMJ* 1988;296:913-15.

[51]Gurwitz JH, Avorn J, Ross-Degnan D, Choodnovskiy I, Ansell J. Aging and the anticoagulant response to warfarin therapy [see comments]. *Ann Intern Med* 1992 June 1;116(11):901-4.

[52]Stroke Prevention in Atrial Fibrillation Study Group. Preliminary report of the stroke prevention in atrial fibrillation study. *N Engl J Med* 1990;322:863-8.

[53]Becker RC, Ansell J. Antithrombotic therapy. An abbreviated reference for clinicians. *Arch Intern Med* 1995;155:149.

[54]Gibian T. Rational drug therapy in the elderly or how not to poison your elderly patients [Review]. *Aust Fam Physician* 1992 Dec;21(12):1755-60.

[55]Sternberg L. Unusual side reactions of hysteria from Benadryl. *J Allergy* 1947;18:417.

[56]Benson JW. Drug utilization patterns in geriatric drugs in the US-1986. *J Geriatric Drug Ther* In press.

[57]Bloom JA, Frank JW, Shafir MS, Martiquet P. Potentially undesirable prescribing and drug use among the elderly. Measurable and remediable [see comments]. *Can Fam Physician* 1993 Nov;39:2337-45.

[58]Eng HJ, Lee ES. The role of prescription drugs in health care for the elderly. *Journal of Health and Human Resources Administration* 1987;9:306-18.

[59]May FE, Stewart RM, Hale WE, et al. Prescribed and nonprescribe drug use in an ambulatory elderly population. *South Med J* 1982;75:522-8.

[60]Expert Panel on Detection, Evaluation, and Treatment of High Blood Cholesterol in Adults. Summary of the Second Report of the National Cholesterol Education Program. *JAMA* 1993;269:3015.

[61]Cleeland CS, et al. Pain and its treatment in outpatients with metastatic cancer. *NEJM* 1994 March 3;330:592-6.

[62]Graham DY, et al. Duodenal and gastric ulcer prevention with misoprostol in arthritis patients taking NSAIDs. *Ann Int Med* Aug 15, 1993;119:257-62.

[63]Silverstein FE, et al. Misoprostol reduces serious gastrointestinal complications in patients with rheumatoid arthritis receiving nonsteroidal anti-inflammatory drugs. *Ann Int Med* Aug 15, 1995;123:241-49.

[64]Raskin JB, et al. Misoprostol dosage in the prevention of nonsteroidal anti-inflammatory drug-induced gastric and duodenal ulcers: a comparison of three regimens. *Ann Int Med* Sept 1, 1995;123:344-50.

[65]Ladwig KH, et al. Post-infarction depression and incomplete recovery six months after acute myocardial infarction. *Lancet* 1994 Jan 1;343:20-3.

[66]Juniper EF, et al. Quality of life in asthma clinical trials: comparison of salmeterol and salbutamol. *Am J Respir Crit Care Med* 1995;151:66-70.

Pharmatecture Index

About The Author

Dr. Gideon Bosker is a widely published clinical scholar, educator, and author whose work in clinical pharmacology, primary care medicine, geriatrics, and emergency medicine has been recognized in national and international circles. An Associate Clinical Professor at Oregon Health Sciences University, Dr. Bosker has co-authored or edited numerous journal articles and seven medical textbooks including, **Principles and Practice of Geriatric Emergency Medicine, The Manual of Emergency Medicine Therapeutics, Prehospital Pharmacology,** and **The Quick Consult Manual for Primary Care Medicine.** Dr. Bosker's lectures on Pharmatecture™ have been presented at more than 1,000 hospitals across the country. He is currently the Editor-in-Chief of **The Primary Care Medicine Bulletin, Emergency Medicine Reports®,** and **The Emergency Medicine Desk Reference®.** His current book, **Pharmatecture™: Minimizing Medications to Maximize Results,** represents more than 10 years of clinical experience and research in the areas of geriatric pharmacology, drug selection systems, drug-related adverse events, medication compliance, pharmacoeconomics, and formulary management.